MIDDLE EAR MECHANICS IN RESEARCH AND OTOLOGY

MIDDLE EAR MECHANICS IN RESEARCH AND OTOLOGY

Proceedings of the 4th International Symposium
Zurich, Switzerland 27 – 30 July 2006

Editors

Alexander Huber

University Hospital Zurich, Switzerland

Albrecht Eiber

University of Stuttgart, Germany

World Scientific

NEW JERSEY • LONDON • SINGAPORE • BEIJING • SHANGHAI • HONG KONG • TAIPEI • CHENNAI

Published by

World Scientific Publishing Co. Pte. Ltd.
5 Toh Tuck Link, Singapore 596224
USA office: 27 Warren Street, Suite 401-402, Hackensack, NJ 07601
UK office: 57 Shelton Street, Covent Garden, London WC2H 9HE

British Library Cataloguing-in-Publication Data
A catalogue record for this book is available from the British Library.

MIDDLE EAR MECHANICS IN RESEARCH AND OTOLOGY

ISBN-13 978-981-270-737-6
ISBN-10 981-270-737-9

Printed in Singapore by World Scientific Printers (S) Pte Ltd

PREFACE

In summer 2006, the 4th International Symposium on Middle Ear Mechanics in Research and Otology was held at the University of Zurich, Switzerland. More than 250 participants from 33 countries of all five continents came together to present their newest results of research, to exchange their knowledge in practical applications, to discuss open questions and to discover new unsolved problems.

This book includes representative and selective articles of lectures and papers held during the symposium and thereby gives an overview of the ongoing research and current knowledge in function and mechanics of the normal, diseased and reconstructed middle ear. It covers basic research, engineering and clinical aspects of evaluation, diagnosis and surgery of the middle ear as well as implantable hearing devices. These subjects have been discussed in a very broad and interdisciplinary way between the participants. The 44 contributions went through a peer review process by the scientific committee.

After this fourth meeting of experts in a successful and developing series, this book follows the tradition of the organizers of the previous conferences to collect the contributions of the symposium. The 1st symposium was held 1996 in Dresden and was initiated by K. B. Hüttenbrink, the 2nd symposium was organized by S. N. Merchant and J. J. Rosowski 1999 in Boston and the 3rd symposium was held 2003 in Matsuyama, arranged by K. Gyo and H. Wada. We are proud to continue these series and to add a collection of current and interesting contributions presented and discussed intensively in Zurich during MEMRO 2006.

The meeting in Zurich took place in a very personal atmosphere; it has initialized and promoted many fruitful discussions with different points of view. The symposium gave good opportunities to maintain old friendships and to create new ones. We are very grateful to all helpers, institutions and sponsors that made this symposium so successful. Our special thanks go to “Baugarten Stiftung” in Zurich that generously funded the printing and distribution of this book.

The participants decided to continue the tradition of MEMRO and meet again 2009 in Stanford. We are sure that the next meeting will further improve the knowledge in understanding and treatment of the normal and the diseased middle ear.

Albrecht Eiber
Institute of Engineering and Computational Mechanics,
University of Stuttgart

Alexander Huber
Department of Otolaryngology Head and Neck Surgery,
University of Zurich

CONTENTS

OVERVIEW AND RECENT ADVANCES IN BONE CONDUCTION PHYSIOLOGY

Stefan Stenfelt, Department of Neuroscience and Locomotion,
Division of Technical Audiology, Linköping University, Linköping, Sweden
Email: stefan.stenfelt@inr.liu.se

During the mid 18th century it was found that sound could be transmitted through solids and in the 19th century it was generally accepted that a person can perceive sound by bone conduction (BC). Since then, the research community has tried to understand its fundamental mechanisms. This report provides an overview of the present state in BC physiology. Five factors contributing to BC hearing are identified: 1) sound radiated into the ear canal, 2) middle ear ossicle inertia, 3) inertia of the cochlear fluids, 4) alteration of the cochlear space, and 5) pressure transmission from the cerebrospinal fluid. Of these, inertia of the cochlear fluid seems most important. The vibration modes in the skull can be divided into three frequency ranges. At the lowest frequencies, approximately below 400 Hz, the skull moves as a whole with rigid body motion. At higher frequencies, up to 1 kHz, the skull motion can be modelled as a mass-spring system whereas at frequencies above 1 kHz, wave propagation dominates the skull vibration response. The wave propagation differs between the thin-boned cranial vault and the thick and dense bone of the skull base. Both vibration measurement of the cochlea and ear canal sound pressure can estimate BC perception changes caused by stimulation alterations for frequencies above 0.8 kHz; below 0.8 kHz measured hearing thresholds differ from skull vibration and ear canal sound pressure data.

1. Introduction

Bone conduction (BC) as a means for hearing stimulation has been used for nearly two centuries to distinguish between a sensorineural and a conductive hearing impairment. Although extensive research is reported in the literature, the interpretations are largely dependent on the knowledge of the normal hearing function. And as the knowledge increases in the field of hearing function and in areas as general acoustics and sound transmission in solids, the knowledge in the field of BC physiology increases as well. This report gives an overview of the present state in BC physiology.

Through history, different species of research animals (cats, guinea pigs, etc) as well as human specimens and live subjects have been used for the BC research. There is a potential problem comparing animal BC results with human BC results; one should be careful drawing general conclusions from animal data to the human. For example, animal skulls differ in geometry and composition from the human skull. This results in different vibration modes of the skull that can stimulate the inner ear differently. Further, in the human, the cochleae are positioned in the skull base surrounded by hard dense bone structure, whereas some animals have cochleae protruding out into the air-filled bulla.

One of the fundamental questions of BC sound was whether it was a cochlear stimulation or a stimulation of some other end organ. Another question was whether the BC transmission was linear or not. Several researchers have addressed these questions by cancelling one air conducted (AC) tone with one BC tone [1–3]. These studies are somewhat limited since they only use one single frequency and consequently only produce local basilar membrane stimulation. The concept of canceling a single AC tone with a BC tone was extended to include two tones; one of 0.7 and one of 1.1 kHz that was subjectively cancelled one at the time, simultaneously, and while a disturbing tone was present. These tests were conducted at three stimulation levels: 40, 50, and 60 dB HL. By comparing amplitude and phase settings for three test subjects at cancellation it was found that the deviations from a true linear response was less than 0.7 dB and 8 degrees at any of the test situations or levels used. The conclusion from these tests, together with previous reported cancellation tests, is that BC sound transmission is linear and a cochlear stimulation at frequencies and levels used for normal hearing.

2. Five contributing factors

Some researchers have identified one single main contributor for perceived BC sound [4,5] while others have reported it to be composed of several different contributors [6]. Here, five components are presented as contributing to BC hearing.

2.1 Part I. Outer ear

When the skull is vibrated by BC stimulation, sound is radiated into the ear canal that is subsequently transmitted to the cochlea by the ear drum and middle ear ossicles. With the BC stimulation applied at the mastoid and with the ear canal open, the outer ear part of the BC sound is 5 to 20 dB below other contributing parts and is not considered as a major contributing part to BC sound [7]. This may change when the stimulation is at another position, e.g. when the stimulation is at the forehead, the outer ear seems to contribute more at frequencies below 1 kHz.

When the ear canal is closed (e.g. by a finger or an ear plug) the BC sound in the ear canal is enhanced at the low frequencies; this is termed the occlusion effect. The exact frequency range and amount of elevation caused by the occlusion depends on the type and location of the occlusion device. However, the occlusion effect is determined by the acoustics of the ear canal and the resulting ear canal sound pressure alteration caused by the occlusion device can be estimated with good accuracy if the position and type of device is known. An estimate of the occlusion effect with ear plugs at two different depths and with one ear muff is shown in Fig 1.

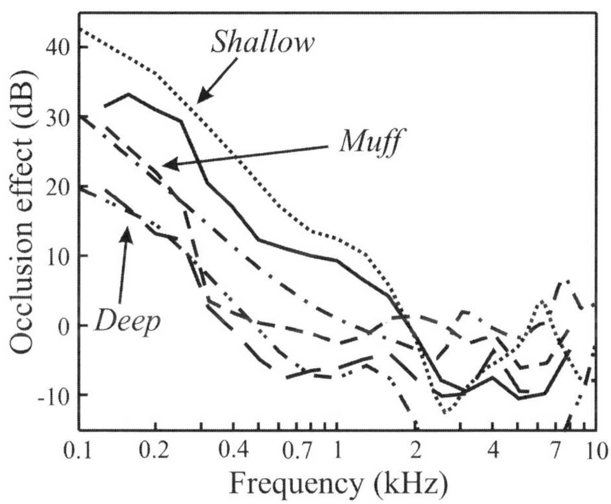

Fig. 1 The graph presents the measured ear canal sound pressure occlusion effect together with model prediction for ear plugs shallow and deeply inserted and with an ear muff of about 30 cm^3. Solid line: measured shallow inserted ear plug, dotted line: model estimated ditto, long-dashed line: measured deeply inserted earplug, dash-double dotted line: model estimated ditto, dashed line: measured ear muff, dash-dotted line: model estimated ditto.

2.2 Part II. Middle ear ossicle inertia

The three middle ear ossicles are suspended by several ligaments, the TM and two muscle tendons. This becomes a mechanical mass-spring system that, due to inertial forces on the masses, constitutes different vibration than the surrounding bone during BC stimulation. This difference motion between the stapedius footplate and the cochlear promontory provides a stimulation input to the cochlea [8]. The importance of the ossicle inertia component can be estimated by comparing the stapes footplate motion at threshold stimulation by AC and BC; this was done in [9] and some of those results are presented in Fig 2.

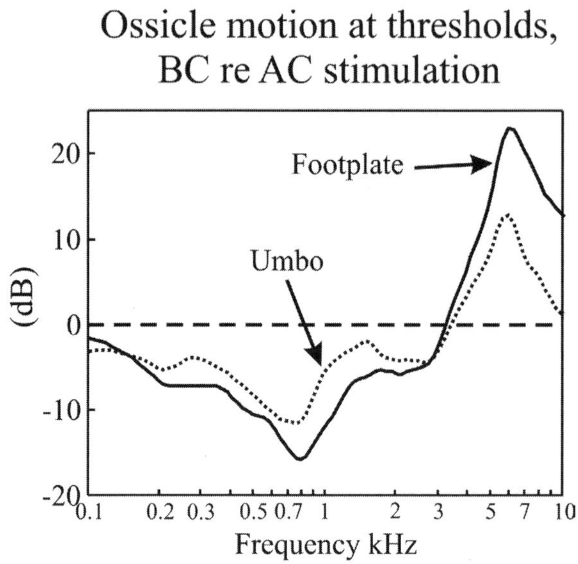

Fig. 2 Stapes footplate (solid line) and malleus umbo (dotted line) motion at BC threshold stimulation compared with the motion at AC threshold stimulation.

The vibration of the umbo and footplate at threshold vibration is 5 to 15 dB lower with BC stimulation compared with AC stimulation at frequencies between 0.2 and 1.5 kHz. This result indicates that middle ear inertia is not an important contribution to BC perception at these frequencies. At frequencies above 4 kHz, the comparison is not valid since the stimulation is probably no longer through the oval window. However, the similarity be-
4 tween the ossicle threshold motion between 1.5 and 3.5 kHz indicates that the inertial effects of the ossicles can contribute to BC sound perception within this frequency range. Also, lesions and manipulations of the ossicles provides results indicative of possible importance of ossicle inertia at the mid-frequency range [10].

2.3 Part III. Inertia of the cochlear fluids

As with the middle ear ossicles, inertial effects cause a relative motion between the cochlear fluids and the cochlear promontory bone. This type of motion relies on several compliant fluid in and outlets in the cochlea: the oval and round windows are two such fluid pathways, and others that can be of importance are the cochlear and vestibular aqueducts, nerve fibers, veins, and microchannels entering the cochlea. Since many BC threshold alterations with middle ear lesions corroborate the theory of fluid inertia it is believed to be the most important BC contributor for frequencies below 4 kHz [10].

2.4 Part IV. Alteration of the cochlear space

One of the first theories presented for BC perception was alteration of the cochlear space, often termed compression response. Since the cochlear fluids can be considered incompressible, any alteration of the cochlear space would force fluid to move and most probably cause a stimulation of the basilar membrane. First, alteration of the cochlear space requires wave propagation in the skull bone which begins at around 1 kHz [11]. Second, according to the theory a compression response would benefit from reduced fluid flow at the oval window (otosclerosis), and would be reduced by an opening at the vestibular side (fenestration operation or semicircular canal dehiscence). This is opposite to clinical findings for frequencies below 4 kHz. Compression may well be important at higher frequencies.

2.5 Part V. Pressure transmission from the CSF

A recent identified contributor to perception of BC sound is pressure set up in the cerebrospinal fluid surrounding the brain that is transmitted to the cochlea producing a traveling wave on the basilar membrane [12]. Although this mode does provide cochlear stimulation, it fails to explain several experimental findings, including BC threshold losses with certain lesions of the middle ear ossicles, lateralization of a BC tone, and transcranial attenuation. It is therefore unlikely that this contribution is significant for BC perception in the hearing frequency range.

3. BC transmission and skull vibration

When a BC stimulation is applied to the skull, the resulting skull motion depends on the position, direction, and frequency of the stimulation. The frequency response of the skull can roughly be divided into three response modes: (1) pure rigid body motion, (2) mechanical mass-spring system, and (3) wave propagation. The pure rigid body motion is at the lowest frequencies (up to 250 to 400 Hz). At these low frequencies the skull motion is solely determined by its geometry together with three translational and three rotational components. This vibration mode can be identified by investigation of the mechanical point impedance; it is the frequency range below the first impedance resonance where the impedance shows a mass-like behavior.

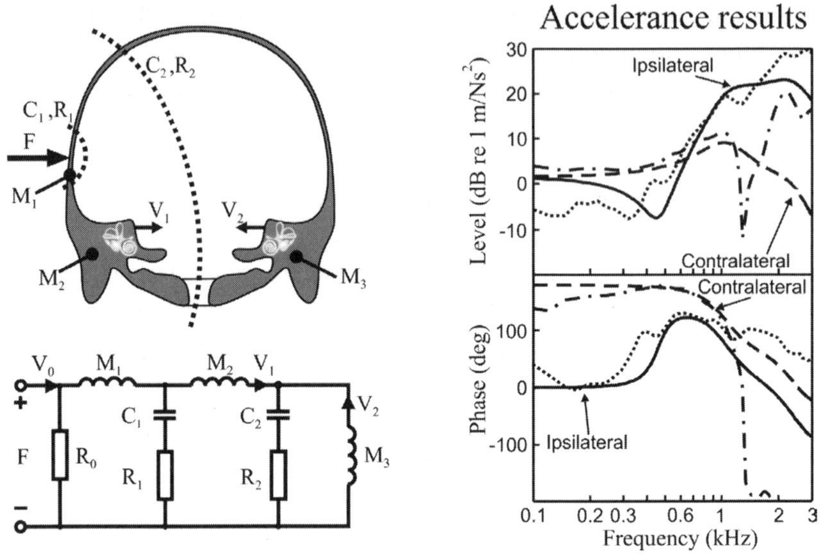

Fig. 3 The left part shows the anatomical structure and related lumped element model for estimation of the cochleae vibration during mastoid stimulation. The right part presents the level and phase of the accelerance transmission between the mastoid and cochlea. Solid line: modelled accelerance of the ipsilateral cochlea, dashed line: measured ditto, dashed line: modelled accelerance of the contralateral cochlea, dash-dotted line: measured ditto.

The next response mode, where the skull behaves as a mass-spring system, is at frequencies below the first skull resonance, which is approximately at 1 kHz [11]. In this frequency range, the motion of the skull can be approximated by three masses with springs in-between (see Fig 3). At higher frequencies, above the first skull resonance, the BC sound is transmitted by wave propagation. This wave propagation depends on type and size of the bone. At the cranial vault, where the skull bone is thin, the wave transmission is a mixture of bending, longitudinal, and transverse wave propagation. These waves are dispersive and the phase velocity increases from just above 200 m/s at 2 kHz to between 300 and 350 m/s at 10 kHz. In the skull base, where the cochleae are positioned, the bone is thicker and denser and the wave transmission is primarily by longitudinal wave propagation producing a constant wave speed of approximately 400 m/s. The different transmission modes and frequency ranges are depicted in Fig 4.

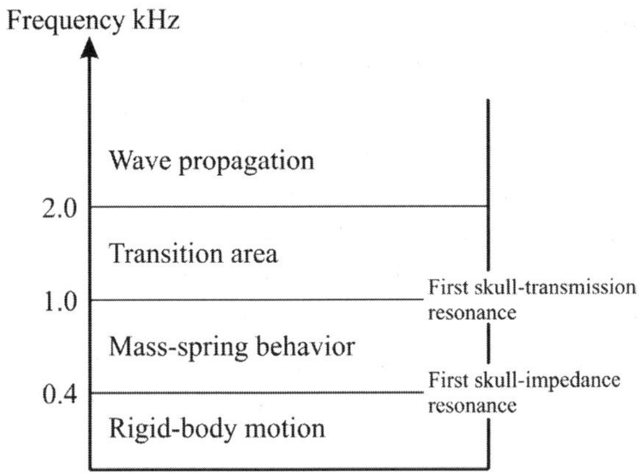

Fig. 4 Overview of the frequency ranges of the human heads' vibration modes.

The transcranial transmission, i.e. the sound transmitted from the mastoid to the contralateral cochlea compared with that transmitted to the ipsilateral cochlea was measured by three different methods; (1) mechanical vibration of the cochleaea obtained in cadaver heads [11], (2) ear canal sound pressure, and (3) hearing thresholds obtained in live humans. The results are presented in Fig. 5 where the three methods show similar results at frequencies above 0.8 kHz; almost monotonically decreasing transmission of −2 dB at 0.8 kHz to −15 dB at 8 kHz. At lower frequencies, the vibration and ear canal sound pressure data are similar whereas the threshold data are almost 7 dB lower at 0.5 kHz. This indicates that both vibration and ear canal sound pressure can be used to estimate changes in BC perception at frequencies at and above 1 kHz.

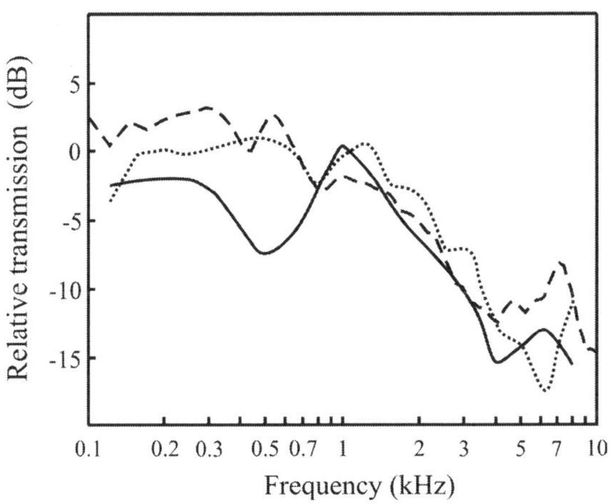

Fig. 5 The transcranial transmission with the stimulation at the mastoid estimated by three methods. Solid line: hearing thresholds, dotted line: ear canal sound pressure, dashed line: vibration of the cochlear promontory.

In another study, the ipsilateral vibration transmission was measured where the distance between the stimulation position and the ear canal opening increased by 10 mm for each new stimulation position. By comparing the decreased cochlear stimulation for each new stimulation position with the attenuation obtained when the stimulation position was moved over the sutura squamosa, the influence of the suture on BC transmission could be estimated. For frequencies below approximately 1.5 kHz, no significant difference was found while at frequencies above 1.5 kHz about 2 dB extra damping was caused by the suture. Hence, an extra high frequency loss of about 2 dB is found when the stimulation is behind this suture compared with in front of the same suture.

4. BC influence on hearing protectors

A hearing protection device (HPD) usually attenuates the sound field in (ear plugs) or just outside (ear muffs) the ear canal. In extremely noisy environments a combination of ear plugs and ear muffs can be used to obtain greater attenuation. The sound field is transmitted to the ear by three different routes: (1) the normal AC route, (2) by sound induced in the skull bone (BC), and (3) sound induced in the hard and soft tissues of the body that is transmitted to the cochlea by the skeleton and surrounding tissues (termed body conduction). For simplicity, the two latter are not separated but treated as a single entity termed BC.

The HPDs aims at reducing the AC transmission. However, due to the placement in or outside the ear canal, they cause an occlusion effect improving the BC sensitivity at low frequencies. The AC transmission from a sound field is 50 to 60 dB better than the BC transmission for frequencies up to 1 kHz, 40 to 50 dB greater around 2 kHz, improving to 50 to 60 dB at 4 kHz, to decrease again to 40 to 50 dB at 8 kHz. Hence, the maximal attenuation achievable with HPDs is 50 to 60 dB at low frequencies and 40 to 60 dB at higher frequencies; above these levels the BC transmission dominates and increasing the attenuation of the HPD does not increase the attenuation for the sound reaching the cochlea. However, due to the occlusion effect from the HPD, the achieved attenuation is often much lower than the theoretical limit. For example, at low frequencies an ear plug may produce up to 40 dB occlusion effect and with a theoretical limit for the BC sensitivity of 60 dB the resulting attenuation may be reduced to merely 20 dB.

References

1. von Békésy G., Zur Theorie des Hörens bei der Schallaufnahme durch Knochenleitung. *Ann Physik* **13** (1932) pp. 111–136
2. Wever E.G. and Lawrence M., *Physiological Acoustics* (Princeton University Press, Princeton 1954) pp. 240
3. Khanna S.M., Tonndorf J. and Queller J., Mechanical parameters of hearing by bone conduction. *J. Acoust. Soc. Am.* **60** (1976) pp. 139–154
4. Allen G. and Fernandez C., The mechanism of bone conduction. *Ann Otol. Rhinol. Laryngol.* **69** (1960) pp. 5–28
5. Brinkman W., Marres E. and Tolk J., The mechanism of bone conduction. *Acta Otolaryngol.* **59** (1965) pp. 109–115
6. Tonndorf J., Bone conduction: studies in experimental animals. *Acta Otolaryngol.* **Suppl. 213** (1966) pp. 1–132
7. Stenfelt S., Wild T., Hato N. and Goode R.L., Factors contributing to bone conduction: the outer ear. *J. Acoust. Soc. Am.* **113** (2003) pp. 902–913
8. Stenfelt S., Hato N. and Goode R.L., Factors contributing to bone conduction: the middle ear. *J. Acoust. Soc. Am.* **111** (2002) pp. 947–959
9. Stenfelt S., Middle ear ossicles motion at hearing thresholds with air conduction and bone conduction stimulation. *J. Acoust. Soc. Am.* **119** (2006) pp. 2848–2858
10. Stenfelt S. and Goode R.L., Bone conducted sound: Physiological and clinical aspects. *Otol. Neurotol.* **26** (2005) pp. 1245–1261
11. Stenfelt S. and Goode R.L., Transmission properties of bone conducted sound: Measurements in cadaver heads. *J. Acoust. Soc. Am.* **118** (2005) pp. 2373–2391
12. Freeman S., Sichel J.Y. and Sohmer H., Bone conduction experiments in animals: evidence for a non-osseous mechanism. *Hear. Res.* **146** (2000) pp. 72–80

MIDDLE EAR STATIC PRESSURE: MEASUREMENT, REGULATION AND EFFECTS ON MIDDLE EAR MECHANICS

J. J. J. Dirckx, Laboratory of Biomedical Physics, Department of Physics, University of Antwerp Groenenborgerlaan 171, B 2020 Antwerp, Belgium
Email: Joris.Dirckx@ua.ac.be

The middle ear is a semi-rigid biological gas pocket which is closed most of the time. It is believed that pressure in the middle ear (ME) is regulated by a complex combined action of the Eustachian tube muscles, eardrum deformation and gas exchange with the blood circulating in the mucosal lining. Sudden pressure variations of thousands of kPa occur in everyday situations and can be slow as well as fast. Both external pressure changes and ME gas exchange processes generate differences between the ME and ambient pressure. To understand the mechanisms and effects involved with quasi-static high amplitude pressure variations, we need to know how middle ear pressure varies in normal circumstances, investigate both fast and slow regulation mechanisms, and determine the effect of such pressures on middle ear mechanics. To measure the normal variations in middle ear pressure, we developed a monitoring system which is used in ambulant patients. We will show some results from direct measurements in intact ears. To investigate a possible fast regulation process, we performed measurements of eardrum deformation in gerbils. We found that volume displacement of the pars flaccida is small compared to middle ear volume, so that its fast pressure regulating function is limited to a very small pressure range. Finally, we will discuss some recent results, obtained in rabbits, of the effect of static pressure variations on middle ear ossicle motions. With heterodyne interferometry, we measured motions of umbo and stapes at pressure change rates between 200 Pa/s and 1.5 kPa/s. We will show that hysteresis in these motions increases as pressure change rate decreases, quite in opposite to the common notion that such hysteresis is mainly caused by visco-elasticity. We conclude that static and dynamic friction are important aspects of ossicle motion at slow pressure variations, new aspects which should be taken into account when trying to model quasi-static ossicle mechanics.

1. Introduction

The middle ear (ME) is a semi-rigid biological gas pocket, which is closed most of the time. The eardrum, and especially the pars flaccida (PF), are displaced if a pressure difference exists between the ME and ambient, making the gas filled cavity partly non-rigid. Under normal conditions, the Eustachian tube (ET) remains closed, but it will open spontaneously to equilibrate large pressure differences. During deglutition, the peristaltic movements of the ET walls regularly inject small boluses of air into the ME cavity. Gas exchange processes through the ME mucosa cause slow pressure variations, and external events such as blowing the nose or taking an elevator can cause sudden and large pressure changes.

At hearing threshold, the cochlea detects eardrum motions with amplitudes of less than 0.1 nm, while quasi-static pressures in everyday situations can generate eardrum motions a factor of millions larger. At 120 dB sound level, pressure amplitude is about 10 Pa, while quasi-static pressure variations of several kPa occur in everyday situations. The cochlea itself is protected from static overloads because for very low frequencies fluid can move freely at the helecotrema from the scala vestibule to the scala tympani. The large static loads however push the stapes far from its equilibrium position and cause large deformations of the round window. The fact that large static pressures are an inherent part of daily life, and that pressures up to at least 100Pa hardly influence hearing, suggests that ME mechanics protect the round window and the annular ligament of the stapes from these quasi-static pressure overloads. Although it is generally accepted that there is a correlation between ME pressure deregulation and important pathologies of the ME, the underlying basic processes still elude us, so more quantitative insight is needed in the several mechanisms of ME pressure regulation. To understand the mechanisms and effects involved with quasi-static high amplitude pressure variations, we need to know how ME pressure varies in normal circumstances, investigate both fast and slow regulation mechanisms, and determine the effect of such pressures on middle ear mechanics.

1.1 Pressure in the normal ME

To understand the effect and importance of the different regulatory mechanisms, it is first of all necessary to know how ME pressure varies over time, but little quantitative data are available. ME pressure can be assessed in two fundamentally different ways: indirect estimation from tympanometric recordings, and direct pressure measurements in the middle ear or the mastoid. The tympanometric approach is easy, and as it can be performed in any clinical setting with standard equipment, it has been used by many authors [1,2,3,4,5,6,7]. Indirect measurement has, however, several important drawbacks. First of all, a basic assumption is that the magnitude of the impedance of the ME mechanical system is at a minimum when ME pressure equals the ear canal pressure. This assumption is not necessarily true: it may well be that sound transfer is actually better when the ear is at a slight over or under pressure. Furthermore, recording a tympanogram takes at least several seconds, so the time resolution of the method is inherently very low, and in practice one can only perform the test a limited number of times without discomfort to the patient.

Short term direct measurements of ME pressure have been reported in several studies. The ME pressure can be accessed via a tympanic membrane perforation [5], or via the mastoid [8,9]. Attempts were also made to measure ME pressure via the Eustachian tube [10], but these measurements are done under general anaesthesia, which clearly may have an influence on the results.

Recently, a long term study was presented [11]. In this work, pressure was monitored over a period of 24 hours, with a sampling interval of 0.8 s and a pressure resolution of 3.9 daPa. The ME pressure was measured using an airtight stopper in the ear canal, and a small perforation of the eardrum.

To include the pressure regulation effect of the eardrum, it is, however, necessary to measure ME pressure with the eardrum intact. To detect changes in fast and small pressure buffering mechanisms, a good pressure measuring resolution, combined with a small sampling interval is necessary. We have developed a system which meets these requirements, and we will show preliminary results.

1.2 Pressure regulation by pars flaccida deformation

Deformation of the eardrum leads to changes of the ME volume and can therefore (partly) compensate the effect of external pressure changes. It is a very fast reacting mechanism and especially the soft PF may play an important role. The PF is commonly involved in many pathologies of the ME, but its actual function still remains unclear. Traditionally, the PF is seen as a regulator of static ME pressure: the easily bending membrane can reduce pressure by changing the ME volume. However, only few quantitative measurements of this deformation as a function of ME pressure are available. We have presented some results on PF volume displacement in healthy eardrums and in cases of induced pathology [12,13,14]. Tympanometric measurements may yield information on eardrum volume displacement as a whole, but they can not discriminate between the contributions of PF and pars tensa. We will show in-vitro quantitative data of PF volume displacement as a function of ME pressure, measured in Mongolian gerbil ears, to determine the possible role of the PF in ME pressure regulation.

1.3 Motion of ME ossicles under slow pressure variations

Few quantitative data exist on how the ossicles move in response to large quasi-static pressure changes and because of this lack of data only few efforts could be made to incorporate quasi-static behavior into models of ME mechanics. Some data are available on human cadaver temporal bones [15], but only at fixed pressure values. When designing ossicle prostheses and implantable ME hearing aids, the effects of large ossicle movements caused by quasi-static pressures should be taken into account. We investigated the response of the middle ear to slowly varying pressures by measuring the displacement of the umbo and the stapes in rabbits with a heterodyne interferometer.

2. Materials and Methods

2.1 Measurement of human ME pressure

To measure pressure in normal middle ears with intact eardrum, a surgical intervention is necessary to place a canulla in the mastoid, which is coupled to a pressure transducer. Subjects are chosen who have a normal middle ear, but who need surgery in a nearby area, such as the parotid gland. Initial measurements were made in four subjects at the Saint Augustine Hospital in Antwerp, Belgium. Recently, a new test site was set up at the ENT department of the Hospital Aalborg, Denmark, in collaboration with Dr. M. Gaihede and Dr. H. Jacobsen, and details of first results at this site are presented in a separate contribution in this volume.

The patient carries the small pressure transducer on the bandage on the head, and data are recorded in an electronic unit (carried in a pocket) at a rate of 10 measurements per second with a resolution of 1 Pa, during up to 48 hours. In the latest version of our system, readout is done over USB bus, and over this link incoming data can also be monitored on a laptop screen in real time, to perform acute experiments.

2.2 Deformation measurements of the gerbil eardrum

Gerbil temporal bones were collected immediately post mortem. The ME is then pressurized through a tube glued to a small hole through the bullar wall. The air pressure load was computer controlled so that it could be changed in small accurate steps. At each pressure step, the shape of the deformed membrane was measured with our opto-electronic moiré interferometer which we especially designed for research in otology [16].

2.3 Motion of ME ossicles under slow pressure variations

Temporal bones were removed from New Zealand rabbits, and the bulla was opened to expose the ossicles. Through a tube glued to the ear canal, pressures were applied with linear pressure change rates from 200 Pa/s to 1.5 kPa/s, and amplitude ±2.5 kPa. Motion of the stapes and umbo were measured with a heterodyne interferometer with position decoder.

3. Measurement Results

3.1 Measurement of human ME pressure

Fig. 1 presents the result of the 24 hour pressure recording in our first patient, and a 2 hour time detail in another patient. We see long periods of over and under pressure in the ME, the over pressure being present in periods where the patient was in recumbent position. Apart from the long term changes, we also see that pressure continuously varies. Although the magnitude of these fast variations is less than 10 daPa, they may be an important aspect of middle ear pressure variation.

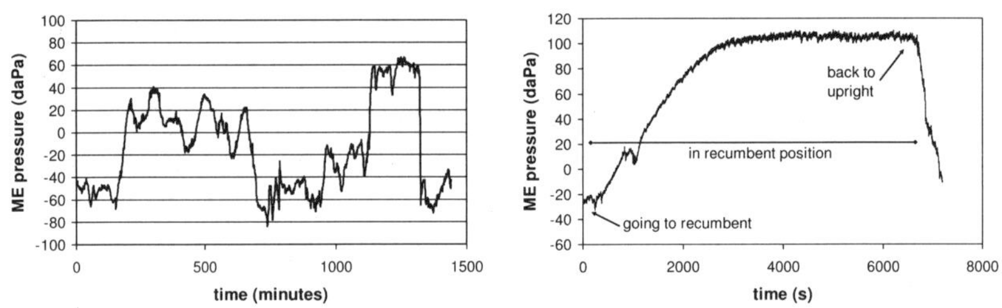

Fig. 1 24 hour recording of human middle ear pressure, and 2 hour time detail in an other patient.

We see how, in the recumbent position, there is a slow build up of positive pressure. Once the patient is upright again, the pressure drops quickly. The patient was in the bed, but NOT asleep, so pressure changes are not caused by a different gas composition during sleep, they are triggered by posture. Using our improved device with on-line monitoring capability, the Aalborg team is currently undertaking acute experiments on the effects of external pressure variations caused by, for instance, riding an elevator.

3.2 Deformation of the gerbil PF: volume displacement

The full-field deformation of the PF was measured with our optical technique in five gerbil ears, and volume displacement was determined at small pressure intervals in three sequential pressure cycles in the range ±200 daPa. Fig. 2 presents typical curves of volume displacement versus ME pressure (detailed results in [14]). The figure shows data obtained in two subsequent pressure cycles. Diamonds and triangles indicate the parts of the two curves where pressure is decreasing, squares and crosses are used in the parts where pressure is increasing. Starting from 0 Pa (pressure difference relative to ambient pressure), ME pressure is decreased to its maximal negative value. We then gradually let the pressure rise back to 0 Pa, followed by a further increase to its maximal positive value. The loop is completed by letting the pressure return to zero.

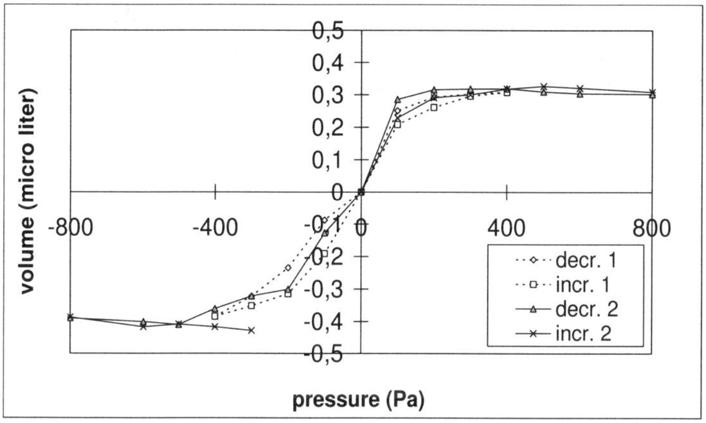

Fig. 2 Volume displacement of gerbil PF as function of pressure, recorded in a 40 daPa cycle and a subsequent 200 daPa cycle. Displacement does not change for pressures beyond 80 daPa, so we only plotted that part.

In all measured ears, volume displacement did not increase for pressures beyond 80 daPa (so we only plotted this part in Fig. 2) and the major part of the maximal volume displacement was reached in a very small pressure range of a few hundred Pa. Maximal volume displacement at –2kPa varied from –0.476 μl to –0.301 μl between ears, and maximal volume displacement at +2kPa ranged from 0.239 μl to 0.358 μl. The volumes of the ME cavities were also measured, and varied from 250 μl to 270 μl between ears. Maximal PF volume displacement is therefore smaller than 0.2% of the air volume enclosed in the ME. Following from Boyle's gas law, this implies that the PF can only compensate, at most, pressure changes of 0.2% of atmospheric pressure, or less than 20 daPa.

3.3 Motion of the ME ossicles under slow pressure variations

Both umbo motion and stapes motion show non-linear S-shaped curves as function of pressure (Fig. 3). Stapes displacement versus pressure curves are highly non-linear and become nearly horizontal for pressures beyond ±1 kPa, so higher pressure loads on the eardrum are not transduced to the cochlea. Stapes amplitude is independent of pressure change rate: (34 μm ± 3 μm, n = 6). At 1.5 kPa/s stapes shows no measurable hysteresis, which indicates that the annular ligament has little visco-elasticity. Hysteresis increases strongly at the lowest pressure change rates (Fig. 4). Umbo motion is also non-linear, yet less pronounced than stapes, and shows large hysteresis also at 1.5 kPa/s. The amplitude of umbo motion, produced by a ±2.5 kPa pressure change, decreases with increasing pressure change rate, from (165 μm ± 16 μm, n = 6) at 200 Pa/s to (118 μm ± 11 μm, n = 6) at 1.5 kPa/s. At 1.5 kPa/s, the ratio of stapes amplitude over umbo amplitude is 0.29. At 200 Pa/s the ratio decreases further to 0.21, which is three times the value previously reported in human cadaver ears [15].

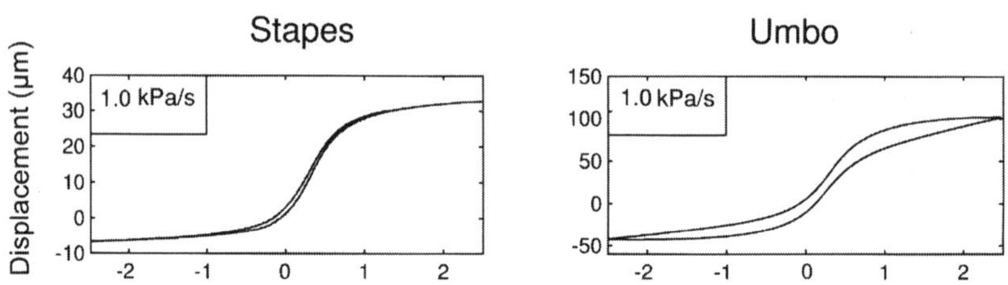

Fig. 3 Stapes and umbo positions as a function of pressure, measured at 1 kPa pressure change rate.

Umbo hysteresis increases with decreasing pressure change rate, as shown in Fig. 4. Using an estimate of eardrum surface area, we calculated an energy loss per pressure cycle (from −2.5 kPa to +2.5 kPa and back) of 1.3 μJ at 1.5 kPa/s increasing to 3.8 μJ at 200 Pa/s.

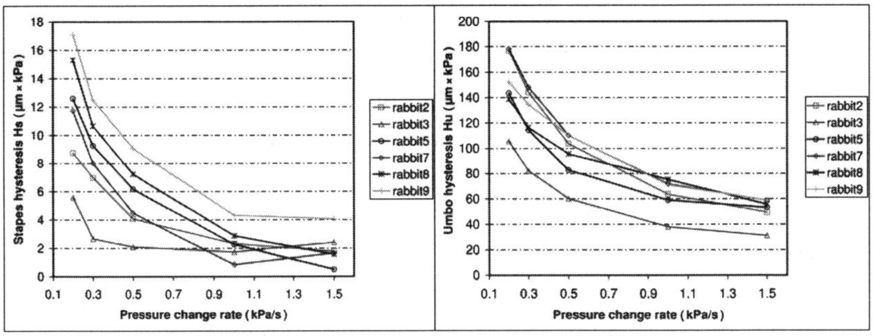

Fig. 4 Stapes hysteresis (Hs) and umbo hysteresis (Hu) as a function of pressure change rate. Hysteresis increases with decreasing pressure change rate, contrary to what is expected from a visco-elasticity governed system. Transition between dynamic and static friction may be an important additional mechanism in static-pressure middle ear mechanics.

4. Discussion and Conclusions

From our measurements of ME pressure in intact ears, we see that both rapid small variations and slower large variations are present, which both may need different regulatory mechanisms. We are currently gathering data to complete a normative set. Then, it will be particularly interesting to compare pressure fluctuations in ears with known ventilation problems to those found in normal ears.

Our measurements show that PF volume displacement in gerbils is a highly non-linear function of ME pressure. In previous work on human temporal bones, we also found very non-linear behavior of the PF [17]. Because maximal PF volume displacement is smaller than 0.2% of the ME volume, the deformation mechanism can not compensate for pressure changes greater than 0.2% of ambient pressure, or 20 daPa. At least all pressure changes beyond an initial 20 daPa will therefore result in loading of the pars tensa.

If the PF has a functionality as an ME pressure change buffer, the present results show that the effect is limited to a range of a few centimeter of water pressure. On the other hand, we see that even the tiniest changes in static ME pressure can make the PF move: a pressure change as small as 10 daPa results in a volume displacement of more than 50% of the maximal obtainable value. Small and fast pressure variations were constantly present in our recordings of ME pressure in humans and the PF may play an important role in reducing the magnitude of these fluctuations, and in detecting small pressure deviations. It has been proposed by other authors [18] that the PF may have a function as a very sensitive pressure detector. Our measurements show that the sensitivity of the membrane to extremely small static pressure changes is indeed high enough to fulfill this function.

In case of ventilation obstruction, the PF will not contribute to pressure regulation once a significant underpressure has developed due to the gas exchange processes. In a small ME volume, PF deformation will achieve more pressure regulation effect than in a large ME volume. This does not imply anything for a healthy ear with normal ventilation, but in a diseased ear it might mean that obliteration of the ME space can indeed help to reduce the effects of faulty ventilation. It has been suggested that diseased middle-ears tend to have smaller air volumes [19]. From those findings, one might tend to conclude that extending middle ear volume can reduce eardrum problems. While it may be true that smaller ME volume is correlated to higher incidence of TM pathology, our findings support the view that once pathology is present, the PF will regulate ME pressure better if middle-ear volume is reduced.

Apart from eardrum displacement, gas exchange and Eustachian tube function are the two main components in ME pressure regulation. Much work has been done in both fields [e.g. 20,21,22,23]. The ET is normally closed and will open only under large pressure differences, but also introduces very small quantities of air in a peristaltic motion triggered by swallowing. Gas exchange, on the other hand, is a slower process, yet recent investigations show that considerable amounts of gas can be removed from or added to the ME space on a time scale of minutes or even seconds [24].

The effect of static pressure on sound-induced vibration amplitudes has been investigated [25], but little knowledge exists on the quasi-static motions of the ossicles caused by slow pressure variations. To investigate the effect of quasi-static pressure variations, we performed high-resolution measurements of stapes and umbo displacements at different pressure change rates. Stapes peak-to-peak amplitude is independent of pressure change rate and does not show hysteresis for pressure change rates faster than 1 kPa/s. We conclude that the annular ligament possesses little visco-elastic properties. Stapes motion is limited to pressures of about ±1 kPa; for pressures beyond ±1 kPa, stapes position remains practically constant. Stapes motion and hysteresis are not just a lever ratio transformed mimic of umbo behavior, but are caused by very complex changes in ossicle joints and ossicle position.

Umbo hysteresis is present at 1.5 kPa/s, which may be the result of the visco-elastic properties of the eardrum and the ossicle joints. Umbo hysteresis however increases strongly as pressure change rate decreases. This finding is in direct contradiction with the notion that umbo and eardrum motion under static pressure is mainly governed by visco-elastic properties, in which case hysteresis should diminish at slower pressure change rates. We conclude that visco-elasticity is not the main source of the hysteresis at the lowest pressure change rates, and we put forward the hypothesis that static and dynamic friction in the joints play an important role as the static pressure situation is being approached. It will be of essential importance to take this into account to obtain realistic models of large quasi-static ossicle motions, by incorporating speed-dependent friction coefficients. More details are given in our recent publication on the subject [26].

References

1. Bylander A. K. H., Ivarsson A., Tjernström Ö., Andréasson L., Middle ear pressure variations during 24 hours in children. *Ann Otol Rhinol Laryngol.* **120** (1985) pp. 33–35
2. Grontved A., Kroch H.-J., Christensen P.-H., Jensen P. O., Schousboe H. H., Hentzer E., Monitoring middle ear pressure by tympanometry. *Acta Otolaryngol.* (Stockh) **108** (1989) pp. 101–106
3. Hergils L., Magnuson B., Morning pressure in the middle ear. *Arch Otolaryngol. Head Neck Surg.* **111** (1985) pp. 86–89
4. Knight L. C., Temporal changes in unilateral middle ear pressure under basal conditions. *Clin. Otolaryngol.* **16** (1991) pp. 543–546
5. Buckingham R. A., Ferrer J. L., Middle ear pressures in Eustachian tube malfunction: manometric studies. *Laryngoscope* **83** (1973) pp. 1585
6. Yee A.L., Cantekin E.I., Middle ear pressure changes in the steady state. *Acta Otolaryng. (Stockh)* **104** (1987) pp. 261–269
7. Alper C.M., Banks J.M., Philip K.D., Doyle W.J., Tympanometry accurately measures middle ear under pressure in monkeys. *Ann. Otol. Rhinol. Laryngol* **112**(10) (2003) pp. 877–884
8. Flisberg K. Ingelstedt S., Örtengren U., On middle ear pressure. *Acta Otolaryngol.* (Stockh) **182** (1961)
9. Hergils L., Magnuson B., Falk B., Different tympanometric procedures compared with direct pressure measurement in healthy ears. *Scand. Audiol.* **19** (1990) pp. 183–186
10. Takahashi H., Hayashi M., Honjo I., Direct measurement of middle ear pressure through the eustachain tube. *Arch Otorhinolaryngol* **243** (1987) pp. 378–381
11. Tideholm B., Jönsson S., Carlborg B., Welinder R., Grenner J., Continuous 24-hour measurement of middle ear pressure. *Acta Otolaryngol.* (Stockh) **116** (1996) pp. 581–588

12. Dirckx J.J.J Decraemer W.F. von Unge M. Larsson Ch. Measurement and modeling of boundary shape and surface deformation of the Mongolian gerbil pars flaccida. *Hear. Res.* **111** (1997) pp. 153–164
13. Larsson Ch. Dirckx J.J.J. Bagger-Sjöbäck D. von Unge M. Pars flaccida displacement patterns in purulent otitis media in the gerbil. *Otol. and Neurotol.* **24**(3) (2003) pp. 358–364
14. Dirckx J.J.J. Decraemer W.F. Larsson Ch. von Unge M., Volume displacement of the Mongolian gerbil pars flaccida as a function of pressure. *Hear. Res.* **118** (1998) pp. 35–46
15. Hüttenbrink K. B. The mechanics of the middle ear at static air pressures. *Acta. Otolaryngol.* (Stockh) **451** (1989) pp. 1–35
16. Dirckx J. J. J., Decraemer W. F., Opto-electronic moiré projector for real-time shape and deformation studies of the tympanic membrane. *J. Biomed. Opt.* **2** (1997) pp. 176–185.
17. Dirckx J. J. J., Decraemer W. F., Area change and volume displacement of the human tympanic membrane under static pressure. *Hear. Res.* **62** (1992) pp. 99–104
18. Hellström S., Stenfors L. E., The pressure equilibrating function of pars flaccida in middle ear mechanics. *Acta Physiol. Scand.* **118** (1983) pp. 337–341
19. Sadé J., Fuchs C. Secretory otitis media in adults: I. The role of the mastoid pneumatization as a risk factor. *Ann. Otol. Rhinol. Laryngol.* **105** (1996) pp. 643–647
20. Sadé J. and Ar A., Middle ear and auditory tube: Middle ear clearance, gas exchange and pressure regulation. *Otolaryngol. Head Neck Surg.* **116** (1997) pp. 499–524
21. Doyle W. J. and Seroky J. T., Middle ear gas exchange in rhesus monkeys. *Ann. Otol. Rhinol. Laryngol.* **103** (1994) pp. 636–645
22. Fink N., Ar A., Sadé J. and Barnea O. Mathematical analysis of atelectasis formation in middle ears with sealed ventilation tubes. *Acta Physiol. Scand.* **177** (2003) pp. 493–505
23. Doyle W. J., Seroky J. T. and Alper C. M., Gas exchange across the middle ear mucosa in monkeys. Estimation of exchange rate. *Arch Otolaryngol. Head Neck Surg.* **121** (1995) pp. 887–892
24. Yael Marcusohn, Joris J. J. Dirckx, Amos Ar, "High-Resolution measurements of middle ear gas volume changes in the rabbit enables estimation of its mucosal CO_2 conductance". *JARO* 7(2): 236–245 (2006) online May
25. Rosowski J. J., Lee Ch.-Y., The effect of immobilizing the gerbil's pars flaccida on the middle ear's response to static pressure. *Hear. Res.* **174** (2002) pp. 183–195
26. Dirckx J. J. J., Buytaert J. A. N., Decraemer W. F., "Quasi-static transfer function of the rabbit middle ear, measured with a heterodyne interferometer with high resolution position decoder". *JARO* 7(4): 339–351 (2006)

OSSICULAR MOTION DURING CHANGES IN STATIC PRESSURE IN THE AVIAN MIDDLE EAR

Robert Mills MS MPhil FRCS (Eng) (Ed), **Marek Zadrozniak** MD, **Zhang Jie** MD
Correspondence to: Dr R.P. Mills, Otolaryngology Unit, University of Edinburgh, Lauriston Building, Lauriston Place, Edinburgh EH3 9EN
Phone: (0)131-5363743, Email: r.mills@ed.ac.uk

The motion of the ossicle of the guillemot (*Uria aalge*) has been studied during changes in static pressure using digital video clips. The magnitude of the displacements in the medial to lateral plane have been measure by capturing digital still images and measuring the change in the distance between a fixed point on the oval window margin and a second point on the columella portion of the ossicle at different pressures, using the dimensioning tool of Corel Draw. The flexion of the ossicle at the junction of the columella and extracolumella which has been observed in other bird species is not so obvious in the guillemot, nor is the rocking motion of the stapes which occurs during variations in static pressure. The maximum medial movement of the ossicle when the pressure in the external auditory meatus was increased to 200 dPa was 0.1 mm. This species dives and swims under water and is therefore more likely to be exposed to significant changes in static pressure than other birds.

1. Introduction

The human middle ear appears to have a protective mechanism to prevent the possible adverse effects of static pressure on the inner ear. (1) Early human beings were probably not subjected to the large changes in static pressure which some modern humans experience during flying and diving. By contrast, birds evolved for flight and some species also dive under water to catch food. This led us to postulate that a similar protective mechanism might exist in the avian middle ear. Our initial studies, involving pheasants (*Phasianus colchicus*), the rock dove (*Columba livia*) and glaucous gull (*Larus hyperboreus*) demonstrated that there is flexion of the joint between the extracolumellar and columella of the ossicle, resulting in tilting of the footplate. (2) This initial study also included a gannet (*Morus basanus*). This species was of particular interest because these birds dive from considerable height, hitting the water at sixty miles an hour and descending to depths of up to sixty feet. (3) The pattern of ossicular motion observed in the other species was not as obvious in the gannet. More recently we have had the opportunity to study two specimens of another aquatic species, the guillemot (*Uria aalge*). These birds dive deeper that the gannet and spend longer periods under water, swimming with their wings.

2. Materials and Methods

The specimens studied were natural causalities collected from a beach on the east coast of Scotland. Their heads were removed and frozen until required. The middle ear was approached via a post-aural approach and bone removal was extended to expose the entire length of the ossicle. A spot of retro-relective paint was applied to the columella and a second to the margin of the oval window niche (Figure One). A tube was cemented into the external auditory meatus and connected to a manual impedance machine (Amlpaid Ltd, Italy). A side connection was connected to a digital pressure gauge (Testo 510, Testo Ltd, UK) so that the pressure in the external auditory meatus could be measured. The pressure in the ear canal was varied between + 200 and −200 dPa using the pump of the manual impedance meter. Digital video clips were recorded using a Dazzle DVC 80 capture device. This allowed examination of the pattern of motion of the ossicle during changes in static pressure. The pressure in the external auditory meatus was also altered in 50 dPa increments between −200 and +200 dPa. At each pressure a still image was captured using Corel Photopaint (Corel Corporation). The distance between the two spots of retro-reflective paint was measured in each image, using the dimensioning tool of Coreldraw (Corel Corporation) as previously described. (2,4) A small piece of titanium wire with a diameter of 0.5 mm was placed in the middle ear. Its diameter in the photographs was measured so that the size of the displacements could be calculated in millimetres. Each measurement was repeated three times, confirming the consistency of the measurements. This method has been used to measure displacements of the umbo in human temporal bones and yielded results comparable with those reported by Huttenbrink. (1)

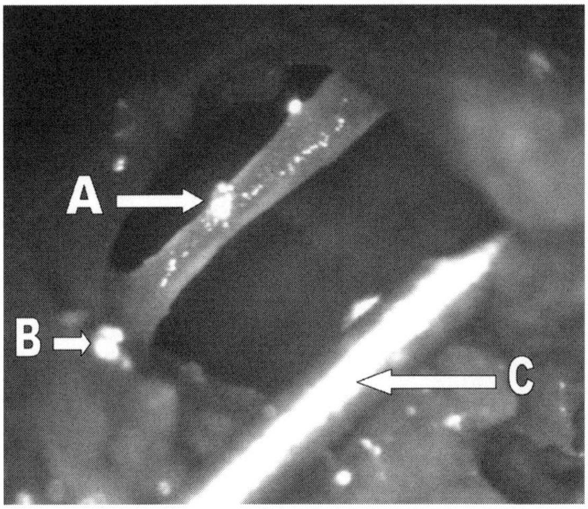

Fig. 1 Photograph of the middle ear anatomy of the guillemot (Uria aalge). The spots of retroreflective paint on the ossicle and oval window niche used for measuring displacements can be seen (A + B). A piece of 0.5 mm titanium wire (C) has been placed in the middle ear to allow the distance between A and B to be calculated.

3. Results

As in the case of the gannet, the footplate of the guillemot ossicle is relatively small. Analysis of the video clips indicated that the rocking motion of the footplate observed in the other species was much less obvious in the guillemot. It was more obvious in one specimen (guillemot 2) than the other (guillemot 1). Figure 2 shows the displacements of the ossicle in the medial to lateral plane for the two specimens. Larger displacements were recorded for guillemot 2. The maximum medial displacement of the osicle recorded was 0.1 millimetres.

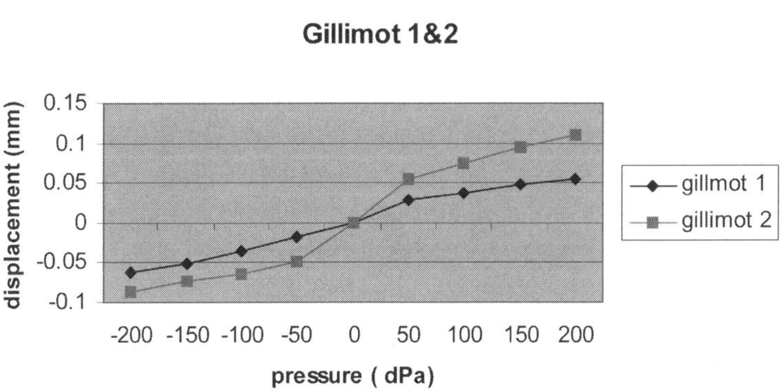

Fig. 2 Displacements of the ossicle in the medial to lateral plane in the guillemot (Uria aalge). N=2 specimens, mean of three measurements.

Figure 3 shows the mean displacements for the two guillemots with those for total ossicular replacement prostheses (TORPs) (Mills, Zadrozniak and Zhang; unpublished data). The mean values obtained are very similar.

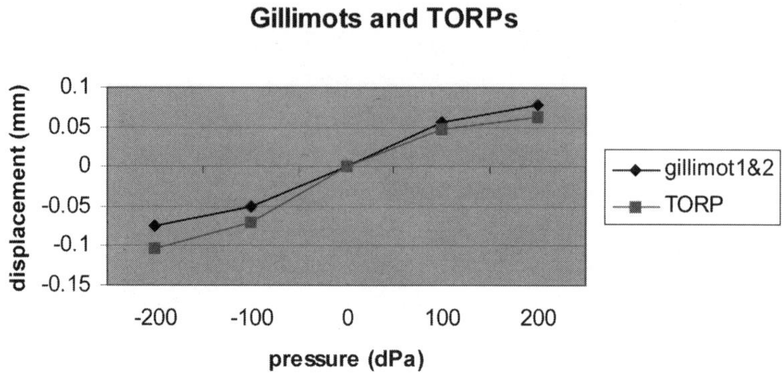

Fig. 3 Mean displacements for the guillemot ossicle (N= 6 sets of measurements) and TORPs in the human middle ear (N= 8 sets of measurements).

4. Discussion

Species of birds which dive under water are likely to be subjected to larger changes in static pressure than those which only fly. One might therefore have expected that the ossicular motion in the avian middle ear which we have previously described as a protective mechanism, analogous to the 'ossicular decoupling' described by Huttenbrink (1) in human ears, would be more obviously present in these birds. This has not proved to be the case. This in turn may mean that we were wrong to conclude that this is the significance of our previous observations. However, this element of the study is qualitative rather than quantitative and it may simply be that the motion is more obvious in species with a relatively large oval footplate, like the pheasant and rock dove. The gannet and the guillemot, by contrast, have small circular footplates and the attachment of the columella is more or less central, whereas in the other species it is markedly off-centre. We have only studied the motion of the avian ossicle over a limited range of pressure changes (–200 to + 200 dPa). In our human temporal experiments we found that a large proportion of the movement of the ossicular chain occurs during the first 200 dPa of the pressure change (4).

The difference in the magnitude of the ossicular displacements in the two specimens is of interest. It is possible that guillemot 1 was older than guillemot 2, or that the reduced motion of the ossicle was due to partial fixation by scar tissue resulting from previous inflammation. Alternatively the difference could be due to post mortem changes. The two birds were found together on the same area of beach and were in similar condition, suggesting that their deaths occurred at a similar time. So far we have only measured the displacements of the avian ossicle in this species and similar data from other birds' ears would be of interest.

It seems reasonable to assume that the displacements measured for the guillemot ossicles would be insufficient to cause inner ear damage. Given that the displacements measured for TORPs in human temporal bones are of the same order of magnitude, we conclude that this type of prosthesis in unlikely to cause inner ear damage during changes in static pressure within the range covered by theses experiments.

5. Conclusions

1) Changes in static pressure produce a combination of medial displacement and rocking motion of the footplate.

2) The maximum medial displacement of the ossicle of the guillemot recorded when a pressure of +200 dPa is applied is 0.01 millimetres.

3) Medial displacements of total ossicular replacement prostheses (TORPs) are of the same order of magnitude as those for the ossicle of the guillemot, over the same pressure range.

Acknowledgments
We thank the Polish Medical School Memorial Fund for financial support.

References

1. Hüttenbrink K-B., The mechanics of the middle ear at static pressures. Acta Otolaryngol.(Stockholm) (1988) Supplement **451**: pp. 1–35
2. Mills R.P. and Zhang Jie., Applied comparative physiology of the avian middle ear: the effect of static pressure changes in columellar ears. J. Laryngol. Otol. (in press)
3. Nelson B., Fishing techniques. In The Atlantic Gannet, Second Edition. Fenix Books Ltd. (2002) pp. 290–301
4. Mills R.P., Szymanski M. and Abel E.W., Movements of the intact and reconstructed ossicular chain during by changes in static pressure. Acta Otolaryngol. (Stockholm) (2004) **24**: pp. 26–29

DIRECT MEASUREMENTS AND MONITORING OF MIDDLE EAR PRESSURE

Henrik Jacobsen[1], Joris J.J. Dirckx[2], Michael Gaihede[1], Kjell. Tveterås[1]
Department of Otolaryngology, Head and Neck Surgery,
Aalborg University Hospital, Hobrovej 18–22, DK 9000 Aalborg,
Denmark[1] and Laboratory of Biomedical Physics, University of Antwerp,
Groenenborgerlaan 171, B 2020 Antwerp, Belgium[2]

Henrik Jacobsen: heja@rn.dk
Joris Dirckx: joris.dirckx@ua.ac.be
Michael Gaihede: mlg@rn.dk
Kjell Tveterås: kt@rn.dk

Corresponding author: Henrik Jacobsen

Keywords: middle ear pressure, direct measurements, monitoring, pressure equilibration, gas exchange

Purpose: The normal function of the middle ear depends on the maintenance of a pressure close to ambient pressure. However, deviation in middle ear pressure (MEP) is a common finding in otitis media and related sequelae, and hence, it is considered a major pathogenetic factor. Up till now, available data were either obtained from indirect measurements, resulting in limited accuracy, or from short term acute experiments, or from longer term measurements in ears with perforated eardrums. The purpose of the present study was to introduce a new improved method for direct accurate monitoring of MEP in ambulant humans with intact eardrums.

Materials and Methods: A new method is presented, where a catheter was inserted into the mastoid through a small hole drilled into its antero-lateral tip. Subjects included were patients admitted for parotidectomy, where this region is routinely exposed. The catheter was connected to a high accuracy pressure transducer (±1 Pa), and data were stored in a portable unit at a sampling rate of 10 Hz for up to 48 hours. Hence, MEP could be continuously monitored also after discharge from hospital for investigating pressure changes during daily life activities. The catheter was removed after 48 hours

similarly to an ordinary drainage tube, and data transferred to a PC. The patients were considered normal subjects, since they all had no previous middle ear complaints.
Results: Preliminary findings demonstrated a reliable system, where the effects of various pressure related phenomena could be demonstrated. Valsalva maneuver produced pressure peaks of 3 to 4 kPa, and pressure changes related to changes in altitude were found with subsequent counter regulation, where the MEP approached 0 Pa. Counter regulation was found both in a stepwise pattern explained by openings of the Eustachian tube, but also as a slower gradual equilibration with constant slope likely to be explained by gas exchange. Moreover, periodic high frequency pressure changes explained by pulsation of the mucosa were found. The amplitude of these pressure alterations varied from around 4 to 20 Pa.
Conclusions: The method showed high accuracy and demonstrated detailed description of a variety of pressure changes. Such data provide new information on the exact pressure variations of the normal human middle ear and possibly of its regulation both in terms of the overall pressure changes, but also in terms of changes in mucosa perfusion. Such improvement in basic knowledge on the overall MEP regulation in normal ears is also likely to improve the understanding of dysregulation in pathological ears as well as treatment strategies.

1. Introduction

Negative middle ear pressure (MEP) is frequent in children with secretory otitis media [1], where the insertion of ventilation tubes into the tympanic membrane (TM) is a very common procedure performed in up to 28 % of children before the age of 6 years [2]. Moreover, a large spectrum of sequelae to otitis media is related to the presence of negative middle ear pressure and constitutes the major parts of indications for ear surgery (retraction pockets, atelectasis of the TM, cholesteatoma formation) [3]. Hence, MEP is a significant factor in the pathogenesis of middle ear disorders [2,3].

Consequently, measurements of MEP are highly relevant from both clinical and basic points of view. Methods applied to determine MEP are direct and indirect. *Indirect* determination by tympanometry is by far the most widespread method. However, it was early pointed out that the procedural volume displacement of the TM affects the MEP itself, and thus, results in inaccuracies especially in cases of a small middle ear volume (V_m) and a flaccid TM [4]. This concern has obtained more recent attention in studies investigating tympanometric accuracy of MEP in mechanical [5,6] and animal models [7]. *Direct* methods include puncturing of the mastoid [4,8], puncturing the TM [9,10], insertion of a transducer through the Eustachian tube (ET) [11], and measuring the pressure in an occluded ear canal with a TM perforation or a VT [12]. While these direct methods may have advantages compared to tympanometry, there are still various methodological and ethical limitations.

In continuation of improving these methods a new approach has previously been introduced, where a transducer is connected directly to the mastoid cavity in human subjects [13]. This method has the advantage of recording the MEP behind an intact TM, and hence, also avoiding the additional volume of the ear canal [12]. Preliminary results have been reported, and the current study describes further improvements of this method and extends the preliminary findings illustrating its various possibilities.

2. Materials and Methods

2.1 Instrumentation

A pressure transducer including a sampling unit was connected to the mastoid cavity by a catheter in human adult volunteers. Pressure was measured with an ultra-small high resolution transducer (2mm diameter, Endevco 8507C1), which was equipped with temperature compensating electronics, so that absolute accuracy is better than 5Pa over 24 hours. Pressure range was ±4 kPa, and data were sampled at 10 Hz by the sampling unit with a resolution of 1Pa. The transducer was mounted in a small brass cylinder (9×30 mm) carried close to the bandage. The catheter connecting to the mastoid was 15 cm long with an outer/inner diameter of 3.5/2.0 mm.

Data from the sampling unit were sent to a PC over USB bus using a custom made program (Matlab 7.0), which also allowed to store patient data and to perform a first analysis. Acquisition was possible both directly on-line as well as from a data storage of up to 48 hours of pressure monitoring. The sampling unit measured 28×65×138 mm and was carried in a breast pocket.

2.2 Subjects and procedure

The study included results from 5 patients, who were referred to our department for parotidectomy, where the antero-lateral aspect of the mastoid is routinely exposed in order to identify the facial nerve. Hence, this area for accessing the mastoid was readily available, and a small hole could be drilled through the compact bone layer into the mastoid. The catheter was inserted and by suturing the connective tissue above the bone tightly, air tightness was ensured. Finally, the functioning of the system was checked under the otomicroscope by tapping gently on the tympanic membrane with a cotton stick resulting in recordable pressure peaks.

The subjects were otherwise healthy with no history of previous middle ear disorders and presented with normal otomicroscopy, tympanometry and pure tone audiometry. The day after surgery the patient could be discharged with the equipment for monitoring at home being mobilized and in daily surroundings; on the second day the catheter was removed similarly to an ordinary drainage tube and the returning of the pressure to 0 Pa was observed. The experiment was approved by our Ethical Committee (2005/50).

3. Results

In Fig. 1 the functioning of the system is illustrated by immediate synchronous pressure peaks up to 950 Pa resulting from tapping the TM. In Fig. 2 the results from a Valsalva procedure are depicted also illustrating the correct function by the system. An immediate steep pressure increase up to 3 kPa was found; in some cases pressure peaks obtained were out of range, i.e. >4 kPa.

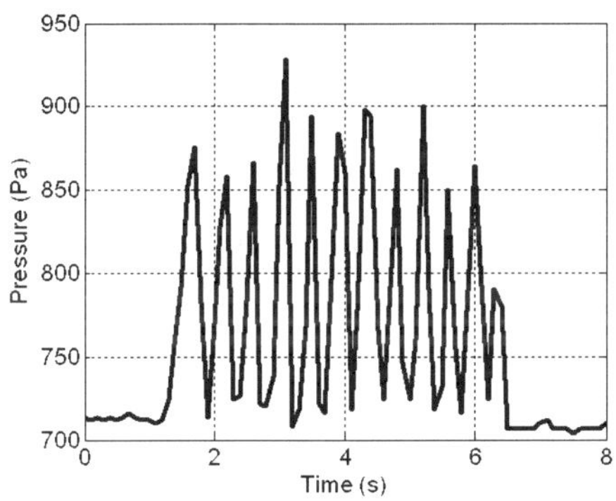

Fig. 1 Repeated synchronous pressure peaks recorded in response to tapping the TM after the pressure recording system has been mounted.

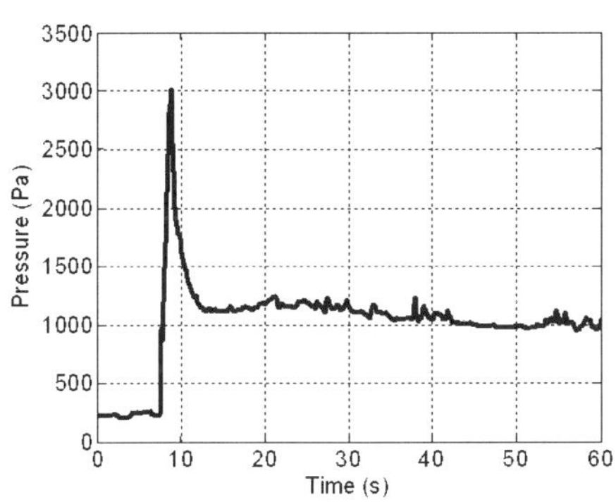

Fig. 2 Rapid pressure increase in response to Valsalva manoeuvre.

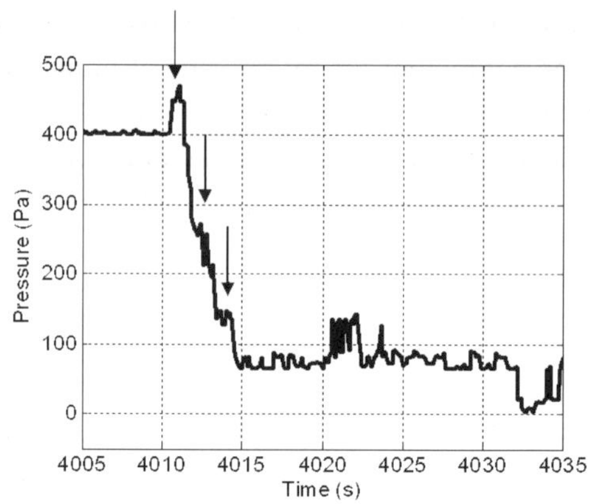

Fig. 3 Pressure equilibration of positive MEP in a step-wise pattern; arrows indicate swallowing followed by steeper decreases towards 0 Pa.

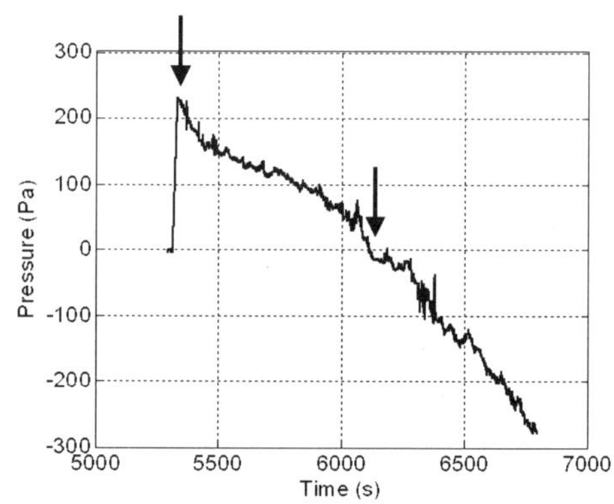

Fig. 4 Pressure equilibration of positive MEP with a constant slow decrease in pressure; left arrow indicate start of pressure decrease, while the right arrow indicate MEP becoming negative.

In Fig. 3 equilibration of a positive MEP in a stepwise pattern is illustrated. Three distinct points with an M-shaped form characteristic for swallowing are found (not clearly seen at this time resolution) followed by subsequent steep pressure decreases. The MEP approaches to almost 0 Pa. This pattern is different from equilibration of a similar positive pressure found in Fig. 4. The increased pressure seen initially resulted from an up-going elevator trip (31 m), which is followed by a constant pressure decrease; after 15 min the MEP becomes negative and decreases further on.

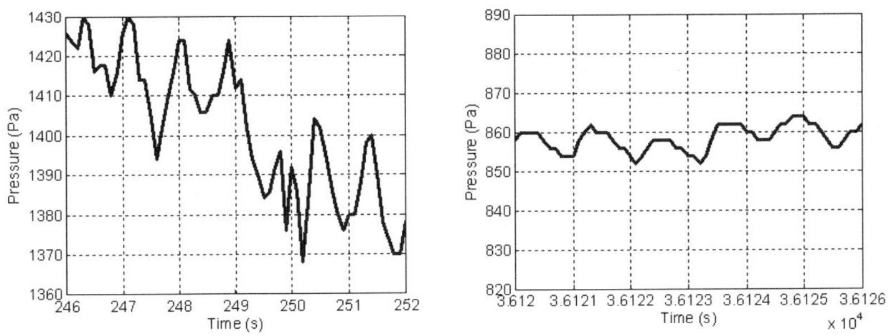

Fig. 5 In both graphs periodic pressure fluctuations at high resolution are illustrated. In the left graph the pressure amplitude is high around 20 Pa after Valsalva, while in the right graph the amplitude is only around 4 Pa during sleep (note identical ranges on axes in both graphs).

Fig. 5 demonstrates small pressure fluctuations seen at the high resolution in time and pressure. These fluctuations are explained by pulsatile pressure changes in the mucosa of the middle ear and mastoid. Hence, the heart rate can be calculated; in both graphs, 5–6 peaks appear during 6 s, and hence, the heart rate was 50 to 60 beats per min. The pressure amplitude of the left graph amounts to around 20 Pa occurring after a Valsalva maneuver; in the right graph the amplitude is only around 6 Pa occurring during sleep at night.

4. Discussion

The initial experiment by touching the TM repeatedly at the end of surgery ensured the correct function of the system, since pressure increments were immediately recorded by the transducer. Further, the prompt pressure increase seen related to the Valsalva maneuver also confirms its correct function. Moreover, at the end of the experiment, when the catheter was removed from the mastoid cavity, the pressure returned to 0 Pa. These observations were made in all subjects.

The preliminary results from our 5 subjects included many data on various situations, but only a few of these have been illustrated here. The positive pressure equilibration seen in Figs. 3 and 4 showed two different ways of counter regulation of a positive MEP towards 0 Pa. In one case a stepwise pattern was found, where three steep decreases were preceded by M-shaped patterns characteristic for swallowing (Fig. 3). Hence, this could be attributed to swallowing with openings of the ET resulting in MEP approaching to ambient pressure. It should be noted that the M-shaped pattern was always found in relation to swallowing, but it was not consequently related to the equilibration of a deviating MEP, and hence, to an actual ET opening.

In the other case the equilibration of a positive MEP was found to be gradual with a constant slope (Fig. 4). Hence, in this situation there were no apparent ET openings involved in the pressure decrease, and it seemed likely that gas exchange was taking place with a net absorption of gas. After 15 min the MEP became negative. This phenomenon also confirmed the tightness of the measuring system, since a pressure decrease explained by leakage would not show subsequent development of a negative MEP.

These observations suggest that pressure equilibration took place in two different ways: stepwise with ET openings and gradual due to gas exchange. The magnitude of the positive pressures is higher around 400 Pa in Fig. 3, while only 200 Pa in Fig. 4. It can be speculated that a more deviating MEP elicit counter regulation by more efficient ET openings, whereas smaller pressures are only regulated by gas exchange. However, individual differences in ET and mastoid function may also play a role. The counter regulation of negative MEP is also interesting especially from a clinical point of view, and our current results have also shown such examples, which will be described in future studies.

The small periodic pressure changes seen at high resolution in time and pressure (Fig. 5) were found throughout all recordings; since their frequency was found to correspond to the heart rate, these changes have been attributed to pulsation in the mucosa [13]. Generally the amplitude was only 3–6 Pa, but in some cases it was higher up to 20 Pa (Fig. 5). Changes in the pulsation amplitude are likely to reflect alterations in the perfusion of the mucosa. Hence, the high amplitude found after Valsalva in Fig. 5 may be explained by a high perfusion rate resulting in increased gas absorption, and thus, an overall decreasing MEP as seen on the graph. Contrary, the smaller amplitude found during sleep (Fig. 5) may reflect a low perfusion rate and hence lower gas exchange rate. Further, the MEP is rather stable in this case, which corresponds to the low exchange rate.

The issue of an active role of the mastoid in MEP control has been questioned [14], but the current observations may imply the existence of an active counter regulation represented by controlled changes in the perfusion of the mastoid. Hence, the phenomenon is interesting for further investigations submitting the middle ear to various pressure challenges and recording the subsequent pressure changes including the high frequency signals explained by mucosa pulsation.

The overall monitoring of the MEP was successful in terms of the acquisition of large amounts of data, but the analysis of these is hampered at this stage, since we need to analyze in more detail distinct well defined experiments in order to recognize the various pressure-related phenomena. Hence, we have not gone into a detailed description of this issue. Future experiments may include an automated pattern recognition analysis for a detailed detection of events related to the various phenomena.

Previous methods used for detailed long-term monitoring of MEP included subjects with either a TM perforation or a ventilation tube inserted, since the pressure is measured at the ear canal [12]. Our present approach accessing the mastoid included the buffering effect of the TM, which is important in its own passive way [15], but also may be very important, if afferent input from mechano-receptors in the TM plays a role in a central neural feedback control of the MEP [16]. Limitations of our method included its current application only in normal ears, and that patients with diseased ears often have sclerotic mastoids, which will complicate the accessibility of the mastoid. Further, damping of pressure changes between the compartments (middle ear and mastoid) could theoretically influence our results, but pressure gradients have been found to dissipate quickly in model experiments [17].

5. Conclusions

Preliminary results showed that our method demonstrated a high accuracy and detailed recordings of MEP and its changes in response to various pressure stimuli. These have to be corroborated and described in more detail, and methods for describing full monitoring of the MEP have to be worked out. On this basis, our method is likely to provide new information which is valuable for understanding the variations in MEP and its counter regulation. This is a prerequisite for the overall description of pressure regulation and the improvement of treatments for patients. The method was found safe, since no side effects were observed.

Acknowledgments

A grant from "Speciallæge Heinrich Kopp's legat" made it possible to compensate our patients for any discomfort in participating in the experiments.

References

1. Zielhuis G. A., Rach G. H. and van-den-Broek P., The occurrence of otitis media with effusion in Dutch pre-school children. *Clinical Otolaryngol* **15** (1990) pp. 147–153
2. Gaihede M., Hald K., Nørgaard M., Wogelius P., Buck D. and Tveterås K., Epidemiology of pressure regulation. Incidence of ventilation tube treatments and its correlation to subsequent ear surgery. *Proceedings of the 4th International Symposium on Middle Ear Mechanics in Research and Otology*
3. Sadé J., Ar A., Middle ear and auditory tube: Middle ear clearance, gas exchange, and pressure regulation. *Otolaryngol Head Neck Surg* **116** (1997) pp. 499–524
4. Flisberg K., Ingelstedt S. and Örtegren U., On middle ear pressure. *Acta Otolaryngol (Stochk)* **Suppl 182** (1963) pp. 43–56
5. Gaihede M., Middle ear volume and pressure effects on tympanometric middle ear pressure determination: Model experiments with special reference to secretory otitis media. *ANL* **27** (2000) pp 231–239
6. Cinamon U. and Sadé J., Tympanometry versus direct middle ear pressure measurement in an artificial model: is tympanometry an accurate method to measure middle ear pressure? *Otol Neurotol* **24** (2003) pp. 850–853
7. Alper C. M., Banks J. M., Philp K. D. and Doyle W. J., Tympanometry accurately measures middle ear underpressures in monkeys. *Ann Otol Rhinol Laryngol* **112** (2003) pp. 877–884
8. Hergils L. G., Magnuson B. and Falk B., Different tympanometric procedures compared with direct pressure measurements in healthy ears. *Scand Audiol* **19** (1990) pp. 183–186
9. Buckingham R. A. and Ferrer J.L., Middle ear pressures in eustachian tube malfunction: manometric studies. *Laryngoscope* **83** (1973) pp. 1585–1593
10. Sadé J., Halevy A. and Hadas E., Clearance of middle ear effusions and middle ear pressures. *Ann Otol Rhinol Laryngol Suppl* **25** (1976) pp. 58–62
11. Takahashi H., Hayashi M. and Honjo I., Direct measurement of the middle ear pressure through the eustachian tube. *Arch Otolaryngol* **243** (1987) pp. 378–381
12. Tideholm B., Jönsson S., Carlborg B., Welinder R. and Grenner J., Continuous 24-hour measurement of middle ear pressure. *Acta Otolaryngol (Stockh)* **116** (1996) pp. 581–588
13. Dirckx J.J.J., Somers Th., Decraemer W.F., Govaerts P., Offeciers E., Continuous pressure monitoring in the intact middle ear. In P. Magnan and A. Chays (eds.)

Cholesteatoma and ear surgery. (Label Production, Marseilles, France 2001) pp. 41–47

14. Doyle W. J., Middle ear pressure regulation. In J. J. Rosowski and S. N. Merchant (eds) *The function and mechanics of normal, diseased and reconstructed middle ears.* (Kugler, The Hague, the Netherlands 2000) pp. 3–21
15. Dirckx J. J. and Sadé J., Middle ear pressure regulation: basic research and clinical observation. *Otol Neurotol* **26** (2005) pp. 300–309
16. Sami S., Gaihede M., Nielsen L. G., and Drewes A. M., Dynamic versus static pressure evoked potentials. Indications of central middle ear pressure regulation in humans. *Proceedings of the 4th International Symposium on Middle Ear Mechanics in Research and Otology*
17. Felding U. N., Banks J. M. and Doyle W. J., Middle ear gas exchange in the air phase. Acta Otolaryngol **123** (2003) pp. 808–811

DYNAMIC VERSUS STATIC PRESSURE EVOKED POTENTIALS. INDICATIONS OF CENTRAL MIDDLE EAR PRESSURE CONTROL IN HUMANS

Saber A.K. Sami[1,2], **Michael Gaihede**[1], **Lars-Gustav Nielsen**[1], **Asbjørn M. Drewes**[2,3]
Department of Otolaryngology, Head and Neck Surgery[1], Center of Excellence in Visceral Biomechanics and Pain, Department of Gastroenterology[2], Aalborg University Hospital, Hobrovej 18–22, DK 9000 Aalborg and Center for Sensory-Motor Interactions (SMI)[3], Aalborg University, Frederiks Bajersvej 7D, DK 9220 Aalborg Ø, Denmark

Saber Sami A. K.: saber@smi.auc.dk
Michael Gaihede: mlg@rn.dk
Lars-Gustav Nielsen: lgn@dadlnet.dk
Asbjørn M. Drewes: drewes@smi.auc.dk

Corresponding author: Saber A. K. Sami

Keywords: auditory brainstem, middle ear pressure regulation, electroencephalography, signal analysis, source analysis

Purpose: In clinical practice, the presence of negative middle ear pressure (MEP) is very common and most often related to secretory otitis media. Although pathological changes in the tympanic membrane may be associated with impaired baroreceptor function, little is known about the middle ear's active regulation of pressure. New information on these aspects would be of major significance in otological research. On this background we have designed a new experimental method for conducting pressure stimuli to the ear canal and investigated the corresponding multi-channel pressure-related evoked potentials (PREP) in humans. This was then compared with multi-channel auditory evoked potentials for the same subjects.

Materials and Methods: The experiments were conducted by stimulating the tympanic membrane initially with acoustic rarefaction click stimuli and afterwards with a novel computer controlled pressure triggering system for rapid synchronized pressure loads (≈3 kPa). In seven adult subjects the resulting brain evoked responses were recorded from 64 surface electrodes using a standard EEG cap. A full band EEG acquisition

method was adopted, signals were sampled at 20,000 Hz, and band-pass filtered between 150 and 3000 Hz.
Results: The study compared early multi-channel auditory evoked potentials to pressure-related evoked potentials. Although these waveforms are given in the same time scale, they differed significantly. Source localization was adopted on a realistic head model to show the location of these early neural generators. The same time interval with the highest signal to noise ratio was investigated for each condition. The acoustic condition showed activation of the lateral lemniscus while the pressure condition showed activation in medulla followed by the activity, which was generated by the cerebellum.
Conclusions: In agreement with earlier studies in primates, our current findings showed an early activation of the brainstem in response to pressure stimulation of the TM and the middle ear. The additional activation of the cerebellum was assumed to play a role in controlling the activity of the Eustachian tube. Further studies along this line are likely to provide basic knowledge on the possible role of an overall neural control of the MEP.

1. Introduction

Despite much research, especially during the last decade, many of the central mechanisms of the human ear's functions for both dynamic and quasi static pressures loads remains unknown. Due to its' obvious pertinent role, dynamic pressure loads (i.e acoustic) and the subsequent neurophysiological mechanisms have been widely investigated. Among the well known methods are auditory evoked potentials (AEPs), which can be obtained by recording the electrical brain activity from the human scalp following an acoustic stimulus. The earliest AEPs, which arise within the first 10 ms following stimulus onset, were initially described by Jewett as auditory brainstem responses (ABR) [1].

Of the different latency scalp-recorded AEPs, most attention has focussed on refining the origins of the ABR, presumably because of its value in otoneurological investigations [2]. Although the ABR was first described more than a quarter of a century ago, the nature and location of the generators of its waveforms are still not definitively understood [3]. The human ABR consists of a series of up to seven waveforms, which have been standardized in the International Federation of Clinical Neurophysiology guidelines. Although ABRs have been extensively studied in animals, there is a great lack of functional data on the human brainstem origin of these waveforms.

Even though recordings of electrical brainstem activity have excellent temporal resolution, they have poor spatial resolution. Traditionally, ABR recordings have been limited to a maximum of three channels, owing to previous trivial technical limitations. However, recording the full, physiologically relevant range of frequencies in a multi-channel setting is currently readily attained with commercially available EEG amplifiers, which have a wide dynamic range and a high sampling rate. Furthermore, over the past decades, source localization algorithms have been developed to improve spatial localization by determining the position and strength of electrical sources associated with surface recorded electrical potentials [4,5]. The afore-mentioned developments lend the opportunity to investigate deep brain structures in real-time.

While it is generally accepted that the auditory system is influenced by all three regions of the ear in terms of anatomical and functional divisions of the ear, little is known about the quasi-static pressure regulatory mechanisms in the middle ear. Because the middle ear is isolated from the direct communication with the environment, the functional prerequisite of pressure equilibrium is maintained intermittently through a pressure regulation mechanism. Similarly to the circumstances following dynamic pressure loads, the brainstem's possible involvement in quasi-static pressure regulation has also been put forward by Eden et al [6]. Their experiments in primates have demonstrated anatomical and physiological connections between the tympanic plexus of the middle ear cavity, respiratory centres in the brainstem (nucleus of the solitary tract) and the muscles of the ET [6,7]. The extent of similar connections in humans, although likely is still not known.

It is known that the occurrence of acoustic stimuli received by the human ear gives rise to afferent neural activity, which is reflected by changes in AEPs. Similarly, afferent neural activity related to the brainstem in response to quasi-static pressure changes of the middle ear seems to be a prerequisite, if a central control mechanism of MEP regulation exists. Multichannel EEG configurations, together with advanced methods of source analysis, may elucidate these plausible neural pathways and centres related to quasi-static pressure stimulus. Thus, this methodology seems useful to investigate the possible brainstem mechanisms for the dynamic as well as for the alleged quasi-static role in the human ear. New information on the differences of these aspects could be of major significance in otological research. Hence, the objective of this study was to compare the differences in waveform and location of deep brain sources following both dynamic and quasi-static load stimulation of the tympanic membrane on the same time scale.

2. Materials and Methods

Seven subjects (three females and four males) without any history of otological or neurological problems participated. They were aged between 32 and 44 (mean 37.7) years. Routine pure tone audiometry, tympanometry and otomicroscopy were in all cases normal. In addition, one 38-year old deaf subject was included as a control subject in order to differentiate between auditory and pressure responses that may arise from audible pressure stimuli conducted in the experiment. His tympanometry and otomicroscopy were also normal. Informed and written consent was obtained from all participants, and the study was approved by our Ethical Committee (Ref No 2004/51).

For the acoustic stimulation, rarefaction click stimuli were produced by applying rectangular voltage pulses of 100 μs duration to insert earphones in an Eclipse EP25 (Interacoustics A/S, Assens , Denmark). The time interval between the onsets of two successive stimuli was fixed, yielding a constant stimulation rate of 10 Hz. Monaural stimulus conditions were tested with right stimulation. The monaural clicks were presented at a level of 80 dB HL in order to produce constant wave VI responses [8].

For quasi-static pressure stimulation the experiments were conducted by stimulating the tympanic membrane with a novel computer controlled pressure triggering system for rapid 1 Hz synchronized pressure loads (+3 kPa). The pressure control system was connected to the ear via a tube system and an ear probe, and hence, pressure stimuli were transmitted to the ear canal and the TM.

The EEG was recorded from 64 surface electrodes using a standard EEG cap (Quick-Cap International, Neuroscan, El Paso, Texas, USA) following the extended international 10–20 system. The impedance at all 64 electrodes was below 3 kΩ. In addition, two electrodes were placed at the right upper brow and the left external canthus to monitor eye movements. A linked-ears reference was used. EEG signals were sampled at 20,000 Hz for a high resolution, and band-pass filtered between 150 and 3500 Hz (SynAmps2, Neuroscan, El Paso, Texas, USA). The event related potentials (ERPs) were gathered separately and sampled from 2 ms before and 15 ms after the onset of the stimulus.

In order to investigate which latencies provided a major contribution to source activity, the Global Field Power (GFP) measure was used. The objective of the GFP measure is to quantify the immediate global activity across the spatial potential field sampled over the scalp. The result of this analysis is a waveform that represents the temporal changes in GFP. The method of Multiple Signal Classification (MUSIC) fits dipoles to potential dipolar locations in the regions of interest. The underlying process is a singular value decomposition assigned to separate the signal space [5]. The commercially available MUSIC algorithm (ANT ASA, Enschede, Netherlands) was used here to confirm the anatomic localization of the dipole in the brainstem.

3. Results

Table 1a depicts the normal ABR responses of the subjects in accordance to the International Federation of Clinical Neurophysiology (IFCN) guidelines [9], while Figure 1 illustrates a common pattern of neuro-electrical activity detected in all seven subjects, but with some inter-individual differences. In order to compare the most robust acoustic signal (i.e signal with highest signal to noise ratio) on the same time scale as that of pressure evoked response we considered the localization of the acoustic brainstem wave VI response. The monaural stimuli produced a dipole fit found in the contra-lateral hemisphere. In the average over subjects, the mean distance in x-direction between dipoles corresponding to monaural right stimuli is only 1.2 cm. Figure 2 also shows that wave VI was likely located in the lateral lemniscus.

Table 1a Distributions of latencies for ABR responses: interpeak intervals of (I–III), (III–V) and (I–V) for all subjects (N=7).

Peak	I-III	III-V	I-V
Time	ms	ms	ms
Mean	2.22	2.12	4.32
SD	0.09	0.18	0.17

Table 1b Distributions of PREP peaks N1 to P3 showing average latency for all subjects.

Peak	N1	P1	N2	P2	N3	P3
Time	ms	ms	ms	ms	ms	ms
Mean	4.3	6.5	7.7	9.7	14.0	16.9
SD	0.7	0.9	0,8	1.0	0.9	0.7

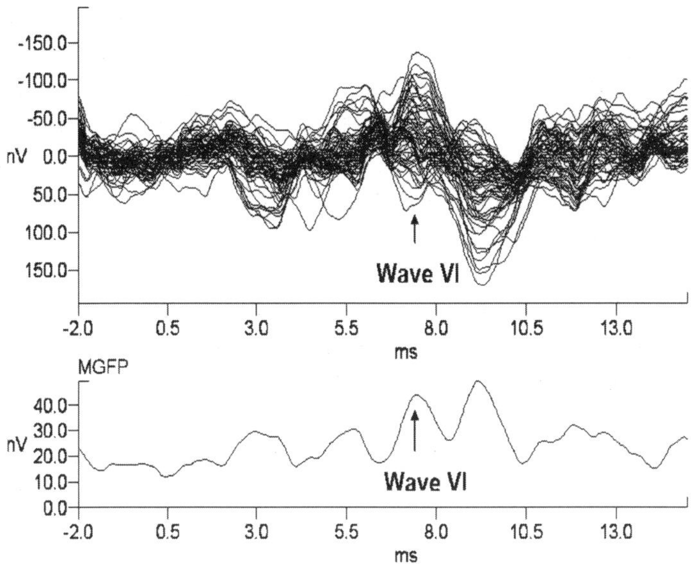

Fig. 1 Shows the ABRs of one subject for all 64 measured channels (upper part) with linked-ears reference as well as the mean global field power MGFP (lower part) showing the clear activity of wave VI.

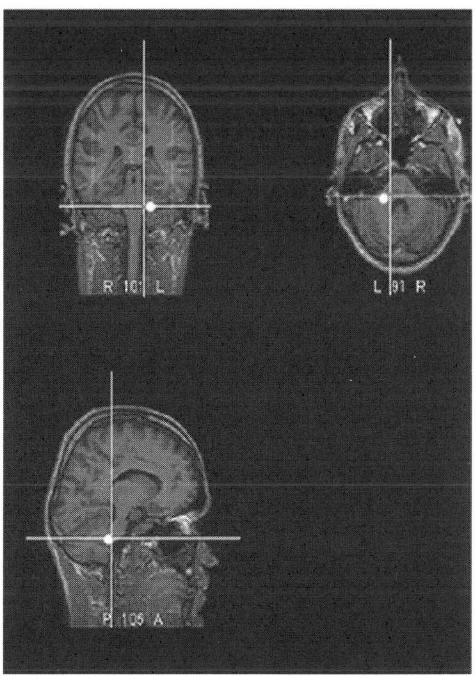

Fig. 2 Locations of a rotating dipole and topography following right monaural acoustic activation in a representative subject after MUSIC source localization on wave VI.

For a relative examination with AEPs the study demonstrates the early pressure related event potentials (PREP) following the quasi-static pressure loads of the tympanic membrane. Figure 3 shows the common PREP pattern detected in all the normal subjects; a similar pattern was found in the deaf subject. Table 1b depicts the normal PREP responses including the individual variation of the subjects for comparative purposes following the methodology outlined in the International Federation of Clinical Neurophysiology guidelines for evoked brain responses [9]. Although these waveforms are given in the same time scale as the auditory brainstem potentials, they differ significantly ($p>0.05$) from those based on the standard features. Changes were seen in the latency response times and the amplitude responses were approximately twice in magnitude.

As in the case of AEP, source localization was also adopted on a realistic head model for PREPs to show the location of these early neural generators on a similar time scale. The dipole model showed a residual variance lower than 5%, and therefore it could be reliably applied to the individual data. Figure 4 shows that the earliest dipolar activities were observed in the medulla followed by the activity that was generated by the cerebellum.

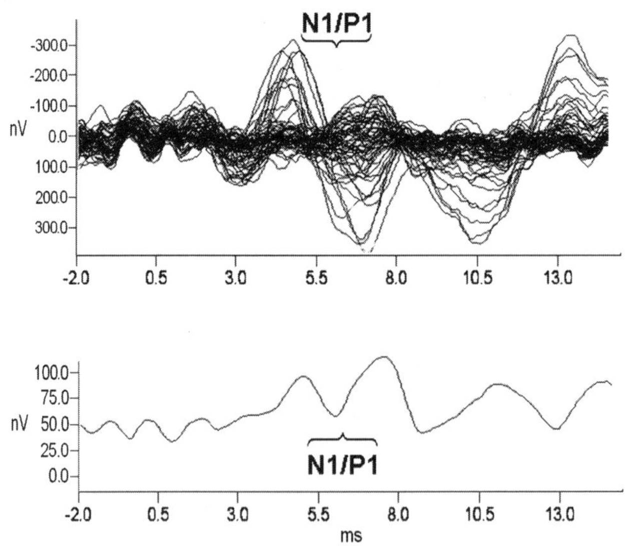

Fig. 3 The early PEPs from –2 to 15 ms, which includes activity of an individual healthy subject from N1 to P3 in a butterfly plot arrangement (this superimposes all 64 channels together) (upper part), while the lower part shows the mean global field power.

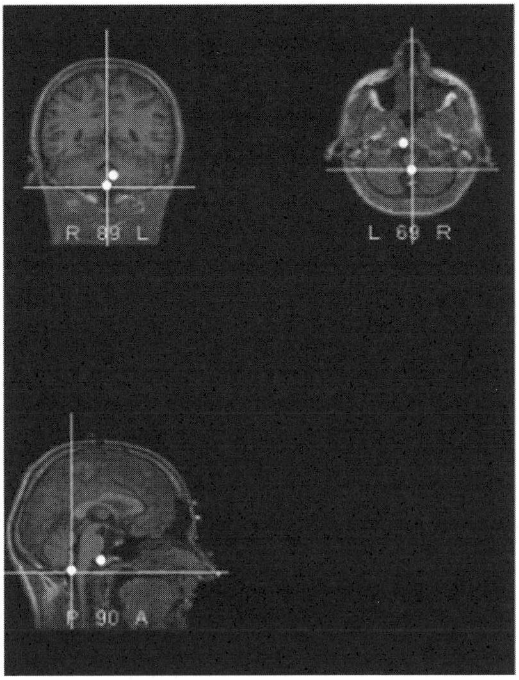

Fig. 4 The two earliest sources from the N1/P1 complex for the same individual subject as in Fig. 1 in the brainstem and cerebellum (left) superimposed on MNI standard MRI head model.

4. Discussion

Accurate non-invasive techniques for determining the neuro-electrical activity in human brainstem structures are needed for functional localization of electrophysiological signals. The present study attempted to address this issue by investigating the spatio-temporal activity in human brainstem structures through the use of a multi-channel EEG method. The approach focused on the source analysis of monaurally evoked auditory late brainstem potentials and compared it to quasi-static pressure related event potentials. The results showed a significant difference in both latency and amplitude of the two waveforms, while the source analysis indicated that the subsequent localization of activation for the acoustic and quasi-static pressure stimuli were different. The pump delivering the quasi-static pressure stimuli inherently also resulted in a small acoustic stimulus due to the valve, which could influence the PREP's. However, our deaf subject showed PREP responses similar to the normal group. Hence, this also indicated a distinct pattern related to pressure stimuli, since acoustic responses were not possible in this case.

Whereas the previous neuro-tracer results have been based on animal studies and have shown respiratory centers in the medullary parts of the brainstem (nucleus of the solitary tract) [6], a feedback mechanism controlling the MEP pressure is most likely to be present in humans also, and a few studies have been corroborating this hypothesis: the presence of mechanoreceptor-like corpuscles in the human TM [10], the pressure sensivity of the human TM including neural adaptation and its decreased sensitivity in pathological ears [11], and the effects of local anaesthetics of the human TM resulting in a decreased ET function [12]. Hence, our current results confirm the afferent components of these results, but additionally suggest a role of the cerebellum, which might be explained by its motoric control of the Eustachain tube function.

However it should be noted that in practical applications, attempts to localize deep brain activity are confounded by numerous sources for errors due to insufficient spatial sampling, too low number of electrodes, inaccurate models, as well as noise. In order to overcome these limitations, EEG was recorded from 64 surface electrodes using a standard EEG cap. We used the realistic head model to avoid localization errors caused by the spherical approximation, which is known to deteriorate with deeper sources. Additionally, the good signal to noise ratio which was maintained following the pressure stimulation makes these deep sources as robust as their cortical counterparts [13]. Therefore this technique may also be used in future experiments along this line and may prove useful in more detailed descriptions of components in MEP feedback control.

Acknowledgments
Oda Petersens Fund and ENT specialist Poul Traun-Petersens Fund contributed financially to our study. Jackie Eriksen, Medical Equipment ApS, Denmark, kindly provided the NeuroScan Amplifyiers used.

References

1. Jewett D.L., Romano M.N., Williston J.S., Human auditory evoked potentials: possible brain stem components detected on the scalp. *Science* **167** (924) (1970) pp. 1517–1518
2. Chiappa K.H., *Evoked potentials in clinical neurology,* 3rd ed. New York: Raven Press; 1997
3. Biacabe B., Chevallier J.M., Avan P., Bonfils P., Functional anatomy of auditory brainstem nuclei: application to the anatomical basis of brainstem auditory evoked potentials *ANL* **28** (2001) pp. 85–94

4. Scherg M., Fundamentals of dipole source potential analysis. In: F. Grandori, M. Hoke, G. L. Romani (Eds.): *Auditory Evoked Magnetic Fields and Electric Potentials.* Karger, Basel, vol. 6. (1990) pp. 40–69
5. Mosher J.C., Lewis P.S. and Leahy R.M., Multiple dipole modeling and localization from spatio-temporal MEG data. *IEEE Trans. Biomed. Eng* **39** (1992) pp. 541–557
6. Eden AR, Gannon PJ. Neural control of middle ear aeration. *Arch Otolaryngol Head Neck Surg* **113** (1987) pp. 133–137
7. Eden AR, Laitman JT, Gannon PJ. Mechanisms of middle ear aeration: Anatomic and physiologic evidence in primates. *Laryngoscope* **100** (1990) pp. 67–75
8. Maurer K., Uncertainties of topodiagnosis of auditory nerve and brain-stem auditory evoked potentials due to rarefaction and condensation stimuli. *Electroencepalogr. Clin Neuro-physiol;* **62** (1985) pp. 135–140
9. Nuwer M., Aminoff M., Goodin D., Matsuoka S., Maugiere F., Starr A. and Vibert J.-F., IFCN recommended standards for brainstem auditory evoked potentials. *EEG & CN* **91** (1994) pp. 12–17
10. Nagai T, Tono T. Encapsulated nerve corpuscles in the human tympanic membrane. *Arch Otorhinolaryngol* **246** (1989) pp. 169–172
11. Rockley TJ, Hawke WM. The middle ear as a baroreceptor. *Acta Otolaryngol.* **112**(5) (1992) pp. 816–823
12. Nagai T, Nagai M, Nagata Y, Morimitsu T. The effects of anesthesia of the tympanic membrane on the Eustachian tube function. *Arch Otorhinolaryngol* **246** (1989) pp. 210–212
13. Whittingstall K., Stroink G., Gates L., Connolly J.F. and Finley A., Effects of dipole position, orientation and noise on the accuracy of EEG source localization. *Biomed Eng Online* **6** (2003) pp. 2–14

SUBANNULAR VENTILATION TUBES IN TREATMENT OF CHRONIC TUBAL DYSFUNCTION – RESULTS IN 85 CONSECUTIVE CASES

Martin Glümer Jensen, Henrik Jacobsen, Michael Lyhne Gaihede, Jørn Rosborg
Department of Otolaryngology, Head and Neck Surgery,
Aalborg University Hospital, Hobrovej 18–22, DK 9000 Aalborg, Denmark

Martin Glümer Jensen: dmgj@rn.dk, Phone +45 9932 2911, Fax +45 9932 2938
Henrik Jacobsen: heja@rn.dk, Phone +45 9932 2911, Fax +45 9932 2938
Michael Lyhne Gaihede: mlg@rn.dk, Phone +45 9932 2911, Fax +45 9932 2938
Jørn Rosborg: jornrosborg@yahoo.dk, Phone +45 9932 2911, Fax +45 9932 2938

Corresponding author: Martin Glümer Jensen

Key words: Long term ventilation, subannular ventilation tube, middle ear pressure, chronic Eustachian tube dysfunction

Purpose: The appearance of a negative middle ear pressure is well-known during the course of secretory otitis media, occasionally leading to complications like tympanic membrane retraction, atelectasis or cholesteatoma. The usual treatment is insertion of ventilation tubes into the tympanic membrane (TM), a procedure that often has to be performed several times, perhaps with insertion of long-term T-tubes. However, repeated tube insertions increase the risk of persisting TM perforations, and for T-tubes the risk may amount to 33%. Hence, there is an obvious need for methods of long-term ventilation with lower risk of persisting perforation. The objective of the present study was to describe the clinical course including the life-time of subannular ventilation tubes (SVT) for long-term middle ear ventilation.

Material and methods: A retrospective study of patient records was performed in a consecutive series of 85 patients, who had an SVT inserted during the period from 1979 to 2004. A tympanotomy was performed and a small groove was drilled in the bony annulus of the floor of the external ear canal. A SVT (Per-Lee© 60.-angle) was fitted and inserted into the groove, and the tympanomeatal flap repositioned. Hence,

the tube was placed peripherally to the tympanic membrane itself. The life-time was determined for the SVT as well as the improvement in hearing levels and complications during the course of treatment.
Results: The group included 85 SVT's in 58 patients. The mean life-time was 58 months (range 1.5 to 168). The mean hearing improvement was 17 dB (PTA)(range −15 to 41). The average number of out-patient visits was 6 per year, and the rate of subsequent TM perforations was 9% after extrusion or removal of the SVT.
Conclusions: The duration of the SVT was considerably longer than both conventional ventilation tubes (mean 9 months) and long-term T-tubes (mean 20 months). Maintaining its function required regular out-patient visits with removal of crusts, treatment of occasional episodes of plugging, otorrhoea, and granulation. The rate of persisting perforation after extrusion or removal was smaller than for T-tubes.

1. Introduction

The appearance of a negative middle ear pressure is well-known during the course of chronic secretory otitis media and related sequelae like tympanic membrane (TM) retraction, atelectasis, and development of cholesteatoma [1]. These conditions are explained by a chronic dysfunction of the Eustachian tube and decreased ventilation of the middle ear [1,2]. The usual treatment is often insertion of a ventilation tube into the tympanic membrane, but in many cases long-term ventilation is required [2], which may result in either repeated insertions of conventional tubes or long-term T-tubes. However, both these approaches increase the risk of persisting TM perforations, and with regard to T-tubes the rate varies between 19 and 33% [3–5]. Hence, the search for a method for lasting aeration of the middle ear with low complication rates is still ongoing. The objective of the present study was to describe the in situ lifetime of subannular ventilation tubes (SVT) of the Per-Lee© type, its effects on hearing and complication rates in a series of patients with chronic Eustachian tube dysfunction.

2. Materials and Methods

The study included a consecutive series of patients treated with SVT in our department from 1979 to 2004. All patients showed chronic tubal dysfunction in a variety of conditions: chronic secretory otitis media, severe retraction or atelectasis; in some cases cholesteatoma was included. The patient records were retrospectively reviewed for information about the life time of the SVT, which was determined by the time difference in months between insertion of the tube and the first date of control, where the tube was found non-functioning. Further, hearing levels before and after surgery (3 to 12 months), the number of complications, and number of out-patient controls were recorded. The setting was a tertiary referral centre.

The insertions of the SVT included a tympanotomy performed under general anaesthesia exposing the bony annulus of TM, and a small groove around 0.7 mm long was drilled at its postero-inferior margin. The SVT was a silicone Per-Lee© 60° flange ventilation tube (Richards/Gyrus ENT, USA/UK) (Fig. 1). The tube was fitted in length and at its medial diameter, and hence inserted into the groove. Subsequently, the tympanomeatal flap was replaced, and thus, the SVT was positioned peripherally to the TM. Finally, the ear canal was dressed in usual manner with gauze. Surgery often included additional procedures depending on the pathology, i.e. grafting of perforations or atrophic TM's, tympanoplasty type II or III.

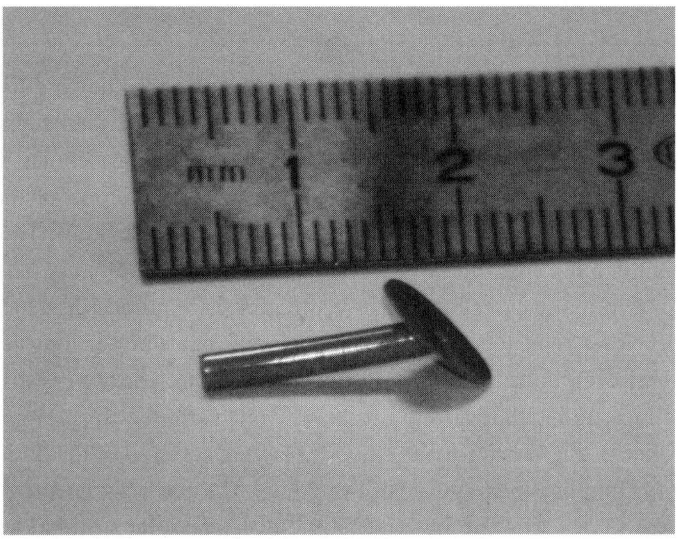

Fig. 1 Per-Lee© 60° flange silicone ventilation tube.

3. Results

The study group included 58 patients with 85 SVT insertions. In 13 patients, bilateral SVT's were employed, whereas in 14 cases re-operations were reported; in two of these patients 3 insertions were performed. The mean age was 19 years (range 4 to 70). All patients had a follow-up period of at least one year after tube insertion. During the study period 3 patients were lost from follow-up, leaving 82 cases for analysis.

The mean life time was 58 months (range = 1.5 to 168; SD = 7; 95% confidence interval = 45 to 72; median 35 months). The duration of the SVT's has been illustrated by a Kaplan-Meier survival plot (Fig. 2) At the time of reviewing the clinical data 25 (31%) SVT's were still in function, 37 (45%) had been removed surgically, and spontaneous extrusion was reported in 20 cases (24%).

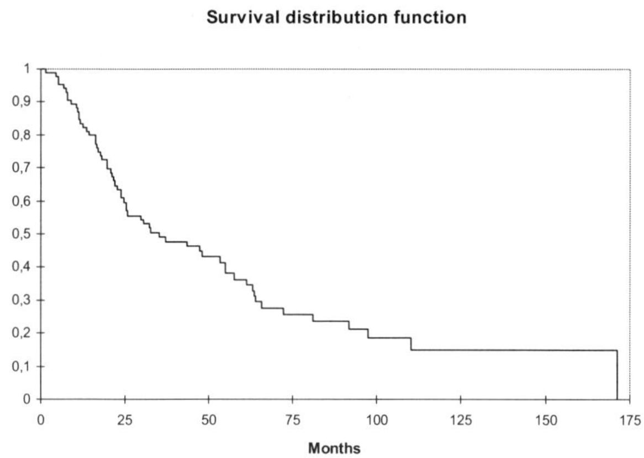

Fig. 2 Kaplan-Meier survival plot of the SVT life time.

The mean hearing gain was 17 dB (range –15 to 41 dB) measured as an average of pure tone audiometry at 500, 1000, 2000 and 4000 Hz. The mean number of out-patient controls was 6 per year (range 1.4 to 36.6), i.e. once in every two months. During the course of these control visits, the number of complications were recorded and referred to as early complications, i.e. during the tube life time. The most common early complications were intermittent crusts, plugging, otorrhoea and granulations as shown in Table 1. Furthermore, the usage of ear drops was registered.

Table 1 Distribution of early complications.

Early complications	(%)
Crusts	86
Plugging	49
Otorrhoea	39
Granulations	33
Ear drops	62
Other	11

After the extrusion or removal of the SVT, various complications were also recorded as late complications. These included persisting TM perforation in 9% of cases, decreased hearing compared to the pre-operative level in 9%, and cholesteatoma in 2%.

4. Discussion

4.1 SVT duration

The mean life time of the current method was 58 months, i.e. almost 5 years. In comparison, T-tubes inserted into the TM have been reported to maintain function between 32 and 38 months on average [3,4]. Recently, similar T-tubes with a subannular insertion technique have been reported with a mean duration of 24 months [6]. Our study showed a gap between the mean life time (58 months) and median (35 months). This indicates an early segregation with some SVTs being extruded relatively fast, whereas in other cases the tubes tend to remain in situ for a very long time (up to 14 years). At the time of review 31% of the SVT's were still functional, whereas 45% had been removed, predominantly due to recurrent otorrhoea, plugging and granulations. In 24% of the cases the SVT was spontaneously extruded.

4.2 Hearing level

The improvement in hearing level was on average 17 dB, but ranged between –15 to 41. Negative values were obtained in cases with concomitant pathology that also affected the hearing level; detailed analysis of the hearing gain related to these different other pathological conditions as well as related surgery awaits future studies. However, our current gain compares well to 15 dB reported for conventional T-tubes by Heerbeek et al. [3], and 13 dB reported for subannular T-tubes by Croutier et al. [6].

4.3 Early complications

Crusts were common findings appearing in 86% of all control visits and considered a minor and inevitable complication (Table 1). Various degrees of plugging were found in 49% of the visits explained by crusts, otorrhoea (39%), or granulations (33%), and hence, these conditions were often found together. Similar complications are also found in other tubes, and thus, otorrhoea has overall been reported in 18 to 33% of cases in T-tubes and subannular tubes [7]. One should bear in mind that the current group consisted of chronically diseased ears, where even T-tubes had been used earlier on more occasions, and complications would be expected. Ear drops were employed on many occasions (62%) for inflammation, but frequently also for the resolution of crusts.

The frequent out-patient control visits were important in order to maintain the function of the SVT and amounted to a mean of 6 per year. One extreme case with 36.6 controls per year was explained by a short complicated course of post-operative infection with 5 visits within 1.5 months, after which the SVT was removed. Further analysis of our data is likely to demonstrate that the majority of these early or "in course" complications are related to cases with the shorter duration of the SVT; in some cases with long duration remarkably few complications were found, and these cases needed only 1 to 2 control visits per year.

4.4 Late complications

Persisting perforation of the TM after removal or extrusion of the SVT was found in 9% of the cases. In comparison, Croutier found 8% perforations using T-tubes inserted subannularly [6]. However, for T-tubes inserted into the TM, perforation rates are significantly higher between 16 and 33 % [3–5,7]. Decreased hearing compared to pre-operative level was reported in 9% of the cases due to less successful late results of ossicular reconstruction. Cholesteatoma was found in 2 cases (2%).

In summary, the treatment of chronic tubal dysfunction can be repeated conventional ventilation tubes or long-term T-tubes. Our method offers an alternative with longer duration and low perforation rates. Alternatively, some surgeons may favour grafting the TM with cartilage, and hence, enhancing the stiffness of the TM resulting in a greater pressure resistance, but the acoustic properties can be hampered by this method [8]. Furthermore, increasing the TM stiffness may prevent retractions, but negative pressure and transudation in the middle ear may still occur without ventilation. In addition, the current method could be performed with other concomitant otosurgery depending on pathology. The patients included in this group were all under general anaesthesia due to either young age or the extent of pathology, but in fact, insertion of the SVT could be done under local anaesthesia as well.

5. Conclusions

The study showed that our method was suitable for lasting aeration of the middle ear with the longest mean lifetime of 58 months reported in the literature. The occurrence of early complications during the course of the SVT life time was inevitable in these chronically diseased ears, thus necessitating frequent controls in order to maintain the tube functionality. The hearing improvement of 17 dB and perforation rate of 9% was comparable to other studies using a subannular approach. The procedure was safe and could be performed in combination with other otosurgical procedures. Overall, we find this technique to be a worthy alternative in the treatment of chronic tubal dysfunction, though it should obviously be remembered that a TM perforation is not necessarily a problem, unless accompanied by larger hearing deficits or repeated infections.

References

1. Sadé J., Ar A., Middle ear and auditory tube: Middle ear clearance, gas exchange, and pressure regulation. *Otolaryngol Head Neck Surg* **116** (1997) pp. 499–524.
2. Avraham S., Luntz M. and Sadé J., The influence of ventilating tubes on the surgical treatment of atelectatic ears. *Eur Arch Otorhinolaryngol.* **248** (1991) pp. 259–261
3. Van Heerbeek N., De Saar G. M. A. C. and Mulder J. J. S., Long-term ventilation tubes: results of 726 insertions. *Clin Otolaryngol* **27** (2002) pp. 378–383
4. Strachan D., Hope G. and Hussain M., Long-term follow-up of children inserted with T-tubes as a primary procedure for otitis media with effusion. *Clin Otolaryngol Allied Sci.* **21** (1996) pp. 537–541
5. Mangat K. S., Morrison G. A. J. and Ganniwalla T. M., T-tubes: a retrospective review of 1274 insertions over a 4-year period. *International Journal of Pediatric otorhinolaryngology* **25** (1993) pp.119–125.
6. Cloutier J.F., Arcand P., Martinez J., Abela A., Quintal M.C. and Guerguerian A.J., Subannular Ventilation Tubes: Retrospective Study. *The Journal of Otolaryngology,* **34** (5) (2005) pp. 312–316
7. Kay D. J., Nelson M. and Rosenfeld R. M., Meta-analysis of tympanostomy tube sequelae. *Otolaryngol Head Neck Surg,* **124** (2001) pp. 374–380.
8. Murbe D., Zahnert T., Bornitz M. and Hüttenbrink K. B., Acoustic properties of different cartilage reconstruction techniques of the tympanic membrane. *Laryngoscope* **112** (2002) pp. 1769–1776

ON THE WAY TO DIFFERENTIALLY DIAGNOSING MIDDLE-EAR AND INNER-EAR DISORDERS

Diana Ţurcanu, Ernst Dalhoff, Hans-Peter Zenner, Anthony W. Gummer
University Tübingen, Department Otolaryngology, Tübingen Hearing Research Centre
Section Physiological Acoustics and Communication, Elfriede-Aulhorn-Str. 5,
72076 Tübingen, Germany, Phone: +49 7071 29 88191, Fax: +49 7071 29 4174
Email addresses: diana.turcanu@uni-tuebingen.de, ernst.dalhoff@web.de,
anthony.gummer@uni-tuebingen.de
Homepage: http://www.uni-tuebingen.de/cochlea

Laser Doppler vibrometry has proved to be very useful in diagnosing ossicular chain disorders by measuring umbo velocity. Although it has been supposed that these measurements contain information about both the middle ear and the inner ear, it has not been possible to separate the information, nor to provide information about the inner ear.

Here, we propose a method to provide information about the inner ear, separating it from middle-ear components, in records of vibration measurements on the human umbo. For this purpose, distortion product otoacoustic emissions (DPOAEs) were measured on the human eardrum using a very sensitive laser Doppler vibrometer. Besides providing valuable information about cochlear status, especially at low level stimulation, velocity-DPOAEs allowed us to objectively estimate the hearing threshold. Thresholds were predicted with a standard deviation of only 8 dB. Moreover, the DPOAEs can provide information about the input and output impedances of the eardrum, opening perspectives for characterising and diagnosing middle- and inner-ear function.

We propose that vibration measurements of DPOAEs on the human eardrum could become a new tool for separating middle-ear from inner-ear disorders and for objective assessment of hearing threshold.

1. Introduction

Laser Doppler vibrometry is a non-contacting optical measurement technique that allows measurement of instantaneous velocity of a vibrating object. The technique is valuable for the evaluation of eardrum vibration in response to sound. From its first use on the cat eardrum [1], it has proved capable of detecting middle-ear disorders. Subsequent experiments on other animals, human temporal bones and finally living humans certified this ability and showed a high sensitivity in diagnosing ossicular chain disorders.

Since its first employment in living humans [2], efforts were made to diagnose also inner-ear disorders and subsequently to perform a differential diagnosis between middle and inner-ear disorders [3]. However, in the meantime no statistical difference was observed between normal subjects and subjects with sensorineural hearing loss [4,5]. Remembering that cochlear amplification occurs at sound pressure levels (SPL) of less than 60 dB [6], the reason for this negative finding might be the lack of sensitivity of the available LDVs – they are limited to measurements above 60 dB SPL. Also, there is a paucity of algorithms to separate middle-ear from inner-ear components.

In this study we propose a method for characterising and diagnosing middle and inner-ear function in records of vibration measurements on the human umbo. For this purpose, we developed a very sensitive LDV which allowed measurements of the distortion product otoacoustic emissions (DPOAEs) as vibration of the human umbo. Using features of these velocity-DPOAEs, we were able to evaluate cochlear status, objectively estimate the hearing threshold and provide perspectives for separating middle and inner-ear components.

2. Materials and Methods

The study was performed in 20 ears from 20 volunteer subjects (age 20–30 years), selected to have a normal eardrum and DPOAEs present at the cubic difference frequency, $2f_1-f_2$. Classic audiometric tests indicated "normal" hearing in all subjects.

Using the new LDV, the experiment concentrated on measuring DPOAEs, especially $2f_1-f_2$ DPOAE input-output (I/O) functions. For comparison purposes, DPOAE I/O functions were also measured acoustically.

The vibration-measurement set-up consisted of a custom-built LDV capable of measuring picometer-sized umbo vibrations in the presence of extraneous movements of the human body (e.g. swallowing, heart beat). The light source was a laser diode emitting in the near infrared (λ =

810 nm) and the interferometer was a conventional heterodyne type. The object beam (0.43 mW) was coupled into the imaging path of an ENT-operational microscope and focused to a 1/e-diameter of 23 μm in the object plane of the microscope.

Stimulus generation and data acquisition were performed using custom software, running on a computer equipped with a 16-bit AD/DA card. Acoustic stimuli were delivered free-field by separate channels using DT 48 earphones, coupled with acoustically damped plastic tubes to the tip of a modified standard aural speculum, fitted into the subject's ear canal during the experiments. Sound pressure in the ear canal was controlled with a probe-tube microphone ER-7C, whose tube was advanced 2–4 mm from the eardrum. A small piece of reflecting material (0.5x0.5 mm^2, 40–50 μg) was placed on the umbo of the subject using a suction needle, in order to enhance signal-to-noise ratio (SNR). The SNR improvement due to the reflector was up to 30 dB. Some experiments were also conducted without introducing a reflector. Control experiments with direct focussing on the unloaded eardrum gave no indication of artefacts in the frequency spectra or I/O functions up to at least 7 kHz.

Vibration measurements were performed in open-field. Microphone and laser signals were low-pass filtered, sampled by the A/D converter and analysed with a 2048-point Fast Fourier Transform, resulting in a 25-Hz frequency resolution. Raw data were saved for off-line processing.

The stimulus parameters were: f_2 = 4–9.5 kHz, f_2/f_1 = 1.2, L_2 = 25–65 dB SPL, in 10 dB steps, and $L_1 = 0.4\ L_2 + 39$ dB. For a single DPOAE measurement, 200–500 data blocks were required.

For the analysis, the whole time signal of one DPOAE measurement was divided into three equal length parts. Each part was first separately averaged in the time domain and finally the three spectra were RMS-averaged.

Sound-field measurements of DPOAE I/O functions were made
closed-field with a clinical measurement system (DP 2000, Starkey, Eden Prairie, MN, USA), using the same stimulus parameters.

Pure-tone threshold was measured in each subject immediately after the DPOAE measurements using Békésy audiometry. The threshold was measured for the f_2 frequencies where vibration-DPOAEs were obtained. The frequency was swept in 100-Hz steps and the sound pressure level was changed in 1-dB steps, with a speed of 5 dB/s.

3. Results

3.1 DPOAEs measured as vibration on the human eardrum

DPOAEs were measured as vibration of the human umbo. They are called velocity-DPOAEs. In all subjects, we were able to obtain velocity-DPOAEs at the cubic distortion level $2f_1–f_2$. The number of velocity-DPOAEs we could measure in one subject varied between 5 and 24 (mean: 15 DPOAEs per subject). The time required to measure one velocity-DPOAE was 1–3 minutes. The amplitudes for the velocity-DPOAEs across subjects varied between 1 and 8 pm; the noise level for the vibration measurements was better than 1 pm.

3.2 Hearing threshold estimation using DPOAEs measured as vibration on the human eardrum

A linear dependency was found between the amplitude of DPOAE-velocity (v_{DP}) and the logarithm of the velocity amplitude at f_2 (v_2). This corresponds to the same behaviour obtained for the acoustically measured I/O functions (in closed sound field) by Boege and Janssen [7] and confirmed by Gorga *et al.* [8] and by our sound field measurements (136 acoustically measured I/O functions).

Extrapolation of the linear regression line fitted to the I/O function gives the estimated DPOAE threshold (EDPT). For the vibration measurements, the EDPT represents the value of v_2 for which v_{DP} is zero and is denoted as v_{EDPT}. Using the measured relation between L_2 and v_2 on the eardrum, we calculated the sound pressure which would be necessary to yield v_{EDPT}, and called it p_{EDPT}. By comparison, the EDPT derived from the acoustically measured I/O functions represents the value of L_2 for which the level of the DPOAE (L_{DP}) is zero and is denoted as L_{EDPT} [7]. The importance of EDPT lies in its ability to estimate objectively the hearing threshold at f_2.

In order to be included in the analysis, each velocity-DPOAE I/O function was required to satisfy certain criteria: i) for the regression line: $r^2 \geq 0.8$ and slope ≥ 0.2 μPa/dB, ii) standard deviation of the EDPT < 10 dB and iii) SNR for the velocity-DPOAE > 4 dB; if the SNR ≤ 4 dB, the data were accepted if the average value of S/N and S/σ_s (σ_s = unbiased estimate of the standard deviation of S derived from the three equal length parts of one measurement – see Material and Methods) was > 1.58 (i.e. > 4 dB). For the acoustically measured DPOAE I/O functions, the criteria were similar excepting for the SNR, which was required to be > 6 dB.

Thirty velocity-DPOAE I/O functions fulfilled the criteria and were accepted for the threshold estimation. Békésy threshold was compared with p_{EDPT} using linear regression analysis with a fixed slope of 1.18 dB/dB (originally reported by Boege and Janssen [7]). The standard deviation from the regression line was only 8.6 dB SPL. For comparison, the same analysis was performed for an identical data set selected from the acoustically-measured DPOAE I/O functions; this yielded a standard deviation of 16.7 dB SPL – this is much larger than the one obtained from the vibration of the umbo.

From the 136 acoustically-measured DPOAE I/O functions, 116 were accepted for the threshold estimation and yielded a standard deviation of 11.2 dB SPL, comparable to the standard deviation reported by Boege and Janssen [7] for a large number of I/O functions (N = 4236).

4. Discussion

The results show that measurement of eardrum vibration near auditory threshold is possible in human subjects up to high frequencies. This allowed us to evaluate the mechanical status of the cochlea, especially at low sound pressure levels, and to perform an objective estimation of the hearing threshold. The standard deviation of the auditory thresholds derived from the vibration measurements was 8 dB smaller than that derived from acoustical measurements. The success of this estimator is probably due to smaller sound-field calibration errors for an open ear-canal condition for the vibration measurements, compared with those for the closed ear-canal condition used for conventional acoustic DPOAEs.

Measurement of velocity-DPOAEs on the eardrum also opens perspectives for better characterising and diagnosing middle and inner-ear function. Since the output and input impedances of the umbo can now be obtained in vivo, manipulating middle-ear impedances could provide information for differentially diagnosing middle-ear and cochlear disorders.

Acknowledgments

This work was supported mainly by the German Research Council, DFG Gu 194/6–1 and partially by the European Commission, Marie Curie Training Site, HEARING (QLG3-CT-2001-60009) and Wilhelm Schuler-Stiftung.

References

1. Tonndorf J. and Khanna S. M., Submicroscopic displacement amplitudes of the tympanic membrane (cat) measured by a laser interferometer. *J. Acoust. Soc. Am.* **44** (1968) pp. 1546–1554
2. Goode R. L., Ball G. and Nishihara S., Measurement of umbo vibration in human subjects – method and possible clinical applications. *Am. J. Otol.* **14** (1993) pp. 247–251
3. Rodriguez Jorge J., Zenner H.-P., Hemmert W., Burkhardt C. and Gummer A. W., Laservibrometrie. Ein Mittelohr- und Kochleaanalysator zur nicht-invasiven Untersuchung von Mittel- und Innenohrfunktionsstörungen. *HNO* **45** (1997) pp. 997–1007
4. Huber A. M., Schwab C., Linder T., Stoeckli S. J., Ferrazzini M., Dillier N. and Fisch U., Evaluation of eardrum laser doppler interferometry as a diagnostic tool. *Laryngoscope* **111** (2001) pp. 501–507
5. Whittemore K. R. Jr., Merchant S. N., Poon B. B. and Rosowski J. J., A normative study of tympanic membrane motion in humans using a laser Doppler vibrometer (LDV). *Hear. Res.* **187** (2004) pp. 85–104
6. Robles L. and Ruggero M. A., Mechanics of the mammalian cochlea. *Physiol. Rev.* **81** (2001) pp. 1305–1352
7. Boege P. and Janssen T., Pure-tone threshold estimation from extrapolated distortion product otoacoustic emission I/O-functions in normal and cochlear hearing loss ears. *J. Acoust. Soc. Am.* **111** (2002) pp. 1810–1818
8. Gorga M. P., Neely S. T., Dorn P. A. and Hoover B. M., Further efforts to predict pure-tone thresholds from distortion product otoacoustic emission input/output functions. *J. Acoust. Soc. Am.* **113** (2003) pp. 3275–3284

TOWARD AN UNDERSTANDING OF MIDDLE EAR MECHANICS USING OTOREFLECTANCE: THE CHARACTERISTICS OF ENERGY REFLECTANCES

Fei Zhao[1], Rhys Meredith[2], Natasha Wotherspoon[1], Andrew Rhodes[1]
[1] School of Health Science, University of Wales Swansea, Singleton Park, Swansea, SA2 8PP, Wales
[2] Audiology Department, Singleton Hospital, Sketty, Swansea, SA2 8QA, Wales

Address for Correspondence: Dr Fei Zhao, School of Health Science, University of Wales Swansea, Singleton Park, Swansea SA2 8PP, UK
Phone: +44 1792 295276, Fax: +44 1792 295487, Email: f.zhao@swan.ac.uk

Otoreflectance (OR) is a newly developed hearing-test instrument utilizing acoustic signals, which are presented and recorded in the ear canal. It provides an objective measurement of the middle ear transfer function for a frequency range of 0.25 to 8 kHz. In the present study, reflectance measurements were performed in 25 subjects (50 ears) using an experimental OR system. The energy reflectance (ER) was recorded and plotted against each 1/6th octave frequencies from 0.25 to 8.0 kHz. Three types of the ER-plot configurations were found in subject with normal middle ear function using the OR test, which may represent different stiffness conditions in the normal middle ear. Notches found at around 1.1 kHz are close to the middle ear resonant frequency region, whereas notches around 3.4 kHz indicate another frequency region of the middle ear that functions efficiently. This may be associated with a number of factors to be found in the ear transmission system. The central frequency of ER-plot notches in both low to mid and the high frequency bands correlated significantly with the frequencies in the corresponding sound pressure variations obtained in the SPL-plots.

1. Introduction

Measurements of acoustic immittance are used to investigate normal middle ear mechanics and to detect mechanical disturbances resulting from middle ear disease. Conventional tympanometry with a single, low-frequency (usually 220 or 226 Hz) probe tone is used as a routine procedure in audiological and otological assessment. It measures how the acoustic immittance of the middle ear system changes as air pressure is varied in the external ear canal [1–3]. It is a useful diagnostic tool for detecting certain types of middle ear pathologies associated with changes in tympanometric patterns. However, when a low frequency probe tone is applied, the tympanogram obtained reflects mainly stiffness-controlled components and provides little information on mass-controlled components such as the ossicular chain. Therefore, it is less sensitive to some middle ear pathologies and provides limited information about middle ear mechanics.

Various studies have shown that multi-frequency tympanometry appears to be a useful method for determining the effects of middle ear pathologies on the mechano-acoustical status of the middle ear system [4–7]. For example, a system has been developed to measure the middle ear dynamic characteristics using a high resolution, sweep-frequency impedance meter (SFI). This records sound pressure in dB SPL across a frequency range rather than immittance measures in the conventional impedance meter [6,7]. It provides information on middle ear dynamic characteristics, including the resonance frequency and the sound pressure change (ΔSPL). This reflects the magnitude of the tympanic membrane volume displacement at the resonance frequency and represents an index of middle ear mobility.

Otoreflectance (OR) is a newly developed hearing-test instrument utilizing acoustic signals presented and recorded in the ear canal. The loudspeaker delivers a sound signal to the ear canal that travels to the tympanic membrane. Some of the sound energy is transmitted into the middle ear but a proportion is reflected back to the probe. A microphone measures this reflected response along with the incident signal from the loudspeaker. The acoustic reflectance characterizes the ratio of the reflected pressure signal to the incident pressure signal. A number of studies have shown that measuring reflectance has several advantages [8–13], for example, 1] it provides calibrated measurements of the transfer function over a wide frequency range (0.25 to 8 kHz); 2] it is more closely related to hearing sensitivity than measures of input immittance, and 3] it is less sensitive than immittance to probe position and standing waves in the ear canal.

Because OR measurement is simple, fast, objective, reproducible and non-invasive, and some changes of energy reflectance are associated with certain types of middle ear pathologies, it has great potential for use in the audiology clinic. The aim of this study was to investigate the characteristics of energy reflectance at ambient pressure in normally hearing subjects using the OR system. It would provide further insight into the middle ear mechanics and thus contribute to the clinical application of OR and facilitate further research.

2. Materials and Methods

2.1 Subjects

In this study, a total of 25 subjects with normal hearing were recruited from the School of Health Science, University of Wales Swansea. The inclusion criteria for "normality" were:

(1) No recent hearing disability nor any aural symptoms;

(2) Otoscopically normal;

(3) Normal middle ear function: the normal range of middle ear pressure adopted was within −50 to +50 mm H_2O. The normal range of peak compliance ranged from 0.3 to 1.6 ml [14]. Individuals who complied with the above criteria but who had a previous history of ear infections in childhood were included in the study.

The mean age of the subjects with normal hearing was 29.64 years (SD 9.4). Their ages ranged from 21 to 47 years. There were 16 males and 19 females.

2.2 Methods

All subjects followed a clinical protocol, which consisted of an otoscopic examination and middle ear function measurements. These included admittance and Otoreflectance (OR) testing.

2.2.1 Tympanometry

Conventional tympanometry with a probe tone of 226 Hz was carried out with a GSI-33 Middle Ear Analyser. Meatal pressure was varied between −200 and +200 daPa. Middle ear pressure and maximum compliance were measured.

2.2.2 OR testing

The OR measuring system is designed to measure wideband acoustic transfer functions at ambient static pressure. The hardware consists of a Windows XP personal computer, a CardDeluxe sound card manufactured by Digital Audio Labs, and an Etymotic ER10C probe assembly. The software called 'ReflWin' was developed and distributed by Dr Douglas Keefe, Acoustic

Physics Laboratory, Boys Town National Research Hospital, Omaha, NE, USA.

Data acquisition was performed at a sample rate of 22.05 kHz per channel using the CardDeluxe sound card with 24-bit resolution in an analogue-to-digital converter (ADC1) and a pair of digital-to-analogue converters (DAC1 and DAC2). A more detailed description of the calibration theory and signal processing algorithms of OR testing were presented in the previous publications [8,9]. The click signal was repetitively synthesized by one of the digital-to-analog converts in a 1024-sample buffer, corresponding to an inter-click interval of 46.4 ms. The bandwidth was from 0.25 to 8.0 kHz.

The energy reflectance (ER) was recorded and the results were presented as an ER-plot, i.e., the ER was plotted for each $1/6^{th}$ octave from 0.25 to 8.0 kHz. The ER data were scaled from 1.0 (all of the sound energy reflected by the middle ear) to 0.0 (all of the sound energy absorbed by the middle ear). Results from other acoustic immittance measurements were also recorded, such as the acoustic admittance and sound pressure in dB SPL.

2.3 Working definition of an Energy Reflectance (ER) notch:

The term "ER notch" in the context of this study was defined as a localised sharp decrease in the ER value, followed by a recovery. A significant notch should extend over at least ½ octave and the deepest point of the notch must have an ER of less than 0.7. Following this definition, most of the ER-plots demonstrated the presence of two notches in the low to mid and high frequency bands. It thus seems reasonable to subdivide our results into these two frequency bands, i.e., ER notches situated between 0.25 Hz to 2.0 kHz were defined as low to mid frequency and notches between 2.0 kHz and 8.0 kHz were defined as high frequency (e.g. Figure 1).

2.4 Analysis of OR notches:

The parameters of ER notch measurements were defined as follows:
The ***Centre Frequency*** **(Fa):** corresponds to the frequency of the deepest point of the notch;
The Depth **(Ra):** represents the absolute value of the notch lower extremity expressed as the ER value measured at Fa;

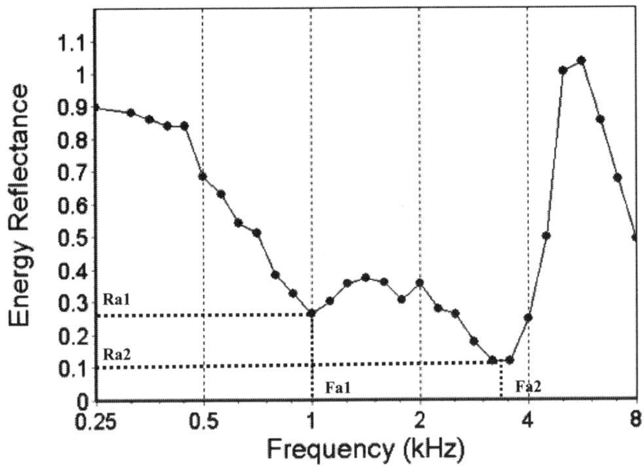

- Fa1: Central frequency of the low to mid frequency notch
- Fa2: Central frequency of the high frequency notch
- Ra1: Energy reflectance corresponding to the low to mid frequency notch
- Ra2: Energy reflectance corresponding to the high frequency notch

Fig. 1 The parameters of ER notch measurement in the Otoreflectance.

3. Results

The ER-plot configuration was analysed on the basis of the notch definition and the characteristics were as described above. Three different types of ER-plot were found, i.e.,

Type I: Symmetric 'W' shape: A notch is present in both the low to mid and high frequency bands with similar depths (*Ra*) ($|Ra1-Ra2| \leq 0.1$). The central frequency (*Fa*) of each notch is around 1.0 kHz and 4.0 kHz respectively (Figure 2a, top).

Type II: Asymmetric 'W' shape: A notch is present in both the low to mid and high frequency bands, but the *Ra* of the notch in the low to mid frequency band is shallower than that of the notch in the high frequency band ($|Ra1-Ra2|>0.1$) (Figure 2b, top).

Type III: 'U' shape: A single, deep notch is present with the *Fa* shifted toward the high frequency band between 2.0 and 5.0 kHz (Figure 2c, top).

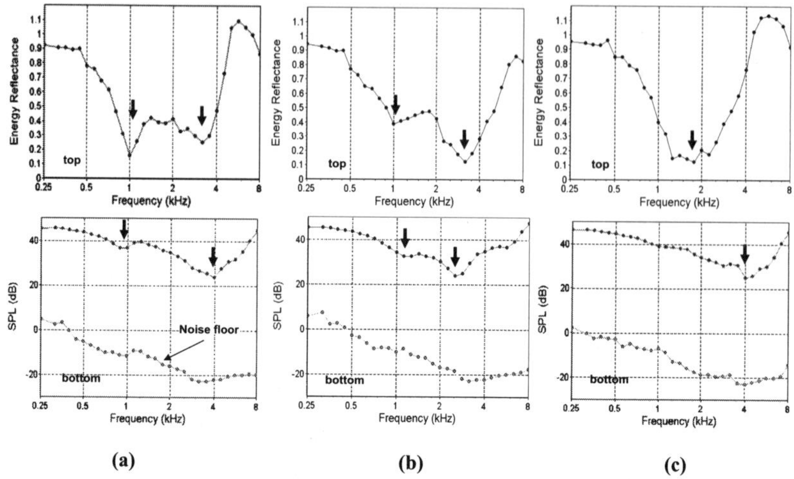

Fig. 2 Three different types of ER-plot configurations were found as shown in Figures 2a, 2b and 2c, i.e.,
2a (top): an example of Type I ER-plot showing a symmetric 'W' shape
2a (bottom): the corresponding SPL-plot to Type I ER-plot
2b (top): an example of Type II ER-plot showing an asymmetric 'W' shape
2b (bottom): the corresponding SPL-plot to Type II ER-plot
2c (top): an example of Type III ER-plot showing a 'U' shape
2c (bottom): the corresponding SPL-plot to Type III ER-plot.

In this study, 23 out of 50 (46.0%) ears showed a type I ER-plot, 19 ears (38.0%) had a type II ER-plot and 8 (16.0%) ears showed a type III ER plot. The characteristics of ER notches were analysed in terms of the main parameters, i.e. the *Fa* and the *Ra*. Table 1 shows the main parameters of the ER notches for the three different types of ER configurations.

Table 1 The averaged central frequency and energy reflectance of the notches in three type ER-plots.

	Central Frequency (kHz) (Mean ± 1 SD)		Energy Reflectance (%) (Mean ± 1 SD)	
	Low to mid frequency notch	High frequency notch	Low to mid frequency notch	High frequency notch
Type I	1.1±0.3	3.5±1.2	16.5±11.0*	23.1±20.0
Type II	1.1±0.3	3.3±0.9	42.0±13.4	13.0±11.0#
Type III		3.4±1.4		23.0±8.9

*: The mean ER of the low to mid frequency notch in Type I plot vs. the mean ER of the low to mid frequency notch in Type II plot, $p<0.0005$;

#: The mean ER of the low to mid frequency notch vs. the mean ER of the high frequency notch in Type II plot, $p<0.0005$.

A comparison of the mean parameters of notches in the separate frequency regions was performed using one-way ANOVA. This showed that neither the *Fa* nor the *Ra* of the notches in the high frequency region differed significantly between the three types of ER-plot ($F_{freq2}=0.21$, $F_{refl2}=2.5$, $p>0.05$). For the notches in the low to mid frequency band, although there was no significant difference in the *Fa* of the Type I and Type II notches ($F_{freq1}=0.05$ $p>0.05$), the mean *Ra* obtained in Type II ER-plots was significantly lower than those obtained in Type I ER-plot ($t=-6.8$, $df=40$, $p<0.0005$). Moreover, the mean Ra for type II ER-plots was significantly lower for notches in the low to mid frequency region than those found in the high frequency region ($t= 9.9$, $df=18$, $p<0.0005$).

The sound pressure change (ΔSPL) in the ear canal reflects the magnitude of the tympanic membrane volume displacement at the resonance frequency (a detailed description of this measurement has been provided in references 6, 7, 16). The ΔSPL was also measured using the OR system in order to be compared with the corresponding ER notches. As marked in Figures 2a and 2b (bottom), the frequencies corresponding to the ΔSPLs (i.e., the lowest inflection points on the SPL-plots) were consistent with the central frequencies of the ER notches in types I and II configurations. However, this was not the case with the notches in type III ER-plots (Figure 2c, bottom).

The central frequency of ER-plot notches in both low to mid and high frequency bands correlated significantly with the frequencies in the corresponding ΔSPLs obtained in SPL-plot (Figures 3a and 3b). Their correlation coefficients were 0.87 ($p < 0.0005$) and 0.33 ($p < 0.05$), respectively.

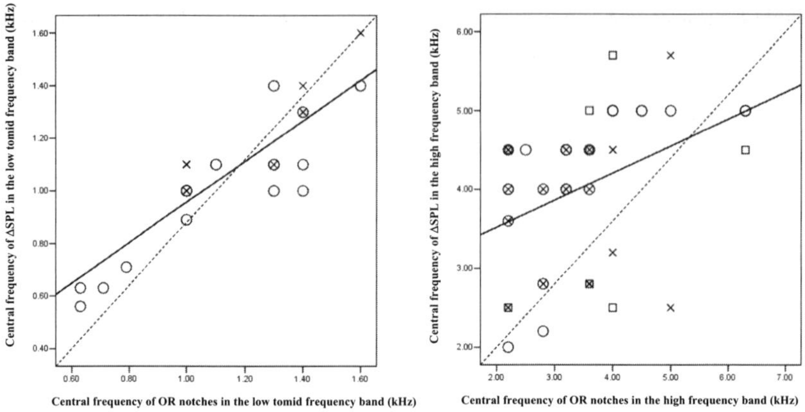

(a) **(b)**

O : Central frequencies obtained in Type I ER-plot
X : Central frequencies obtained in Type II ER-plot
□ : Central frequencies obtained in Type III ER-plot

Fig. 3 Correlation between the central frequencies of ER notches in low to mid and high frequency regions and frequency regions of sound pressure variations.

4. Discussion

Previous studies have shown ER variations as a function of frequency, i.e., high ER in the low frequencies, a decrease to a minimum in the mid frequencies, followed by an increase at higher frequencies [10–13]. By definition, a decrease of the ER represents a frequency where a large proportion of energy is absorbed by the middle ear, whereas an increase in the ER indicates a frequency where a large proportion of energy is reflected by the middle ear. ER variations at different frequency regions are affected by several different factors, e.g., middle ear resonance, external ear canal resonance and influences from the middle ear cavity and mastoid air cell system.

In this study, the new term of ER "notch" was defined to describe the characteristics of ER in order to investigate ER-plot configurations. The presence of notches in the ER-plot appears in frequencies related to the resonances in the middle ear system. This is where sound energy entering the external ear canal is transmitted most efficiently into the cochlea. For example, the mean central frequency of the notches in the low frequency region (1.1 kHz) in this study appears very close to the middle ear resonant frequency (between 1.0 and 1.2 kHz) reported by previous studies [9,15]. Therefore, the presence of the notches in the low frequency region is most likely to be associated with the resonance of the middle ear.

Furthermore, the mean central frequency of the notches in the high frequency region (3.4 kHz) found in this study indicates another frequency region of efficient middle ear function that reduces the reflected sound, and hence results in more efficient transmission into the middle ear. This may be associated with many factors in the transmission system, e.g., external ear canal resonance, vibration of tympanic membrane, mass of the ossicles, and the middle ear cavity [13]. This is an area worthy of further study.

Acknowledgments

We are grateful for helpful suggestions and technical support provided by Drs Douglas Keefe and Denis Fitzpatrick, Acoustic Physics Laboratory, Boys Town National Research Hospital, Omaha, NE, USA. Dr Fei Zhao was supported to attend the 4th Middle Ear Mechanics in Research and Otology (MEMRO) by Royal Society Conference Grant.

References

1. Colletti V., Tympanometry from 200 to 2000 Hz probe tone. *Audiology* **15** (1976) pp. 106–119
2. Funasaka S., Funai H. and Kumakawa K., Sweep frequency tympanometry: its development and diagnostic value. *Audiology* **23** (1984) pp. 366–379
3. Lilly D.J., Multiple frequency, multiple component tympanometry: new approaches to an old diagnostic problem. *Ear and Hearing* **5** (1984) pp. 300–308
4. Muchnik C., Hildesheimer M., Rubinstein M. and Gleitman Y., Validity of tympanometry in cases of confirmed otosclerosis. *Journal of Laryngology and Otology* **103** (1989) pp. 36–38
5. Colletti V., Fiorino F., Sittoni V. and Policante Z., Mechanics of the middle ear in otosclerosis and stapedoplasty. *Acta Otolaryngologica* (Stockholm) **113** (1993) pp. 637–641
6. Wada H., Kobayashi T., Suekate M. and Tachizaki H., Dynamic behaviour of the middle ear based on sweep frequency tympanometry. *Audiology* **28** (1989) pp. 127–134
7. Wada H., Koike T. and Kobayashi K., Clinical application of the sweep frequency measuring apparatus for diagnosis of middle ear diseases. *Ear and Hearing.* **19** (1998) pp. 240–249
8. Keefe D.H., Ling R. and Bulen J.C., Method to measure acoustic impedance and reflection coefficient. *J. Acoust. Soc. Am.* **91** (1992) pp. 470–485
9. Keefe D. H., Bulen J. C., Arehart K.H. And Burns E.M., Ear-canal impedance and reflection coefficient in human infants and adults. *J Acoust. Soc. Am.* **94** (1993) pp. 2617–2638

10. Margolis R.H., Saly G.L. and Keefe D.H., Wideband reflectance tympanometry in normal adults. *Acoust. Soc. Am.,* **106** (1999) pp. 265–280
11. Keefe D.H., Folsom R., Gorga M.P., Vohr B.R., Bulen J.C. and Norton S., Identification of neonatal hearing impairment: Ear-canal measurements of acoustic admittance and reflectance in neonates. *Ear Hear.* **21** (2000) pp. 443–461
12. Keefe D.H. and Simmons J.L., Energy transmittance predicts conductive hearing loss in older children and adults. *J. Acoust. Soc. Am.* **114** (2003) pp. 3217–3238
13. Feeney M.P., Grant I.L. and Marryott L.P. Wideband energy reflectance measurements in adults with middle-ear disorders. *J. Speech, Language, and Hear. Res.* **46** (2003) pp. 901–911
14. Margolis R.H. and Hunter L.L., Tympanometry – Basic Principles and Clinical Application. In Rintlemann, W. F. and Musiek F. eds. *Contemporary Perspectives on Hearing Assessment.* Boston: Allyn & Bacon
15. Valvik B.R., Valvik B.R., Johnsen M. and Laukli E., Multifrequency tympanometry. *Audiology* **33** (1994) pp. 245–253
16. Zhao F., Wada H., Koike H., Ohyama K., Kawase T. and Stephens D. Middle ear dynamic characteristics in patients with otosclerosis. *Ear Hear* **23** (2002) pp. 150–158

A NEW DIAGNOSTIC APPARATUS FOR OSSICULAR FIXATION: EVALUATION OF USABILITY THROUGH MEASUREMENTS IN HUMAN TEMPORAL BONES AND IN PATIENTS

Takuji Koike[1], Shinji Hamanishi[2], Yu Yuasa[3], Ryo Yuasa[3], Toshimitsu Kobayashi[4], Hideko H. Nakajima[5], Wade Chien[5], Michael E. Ravicz[5], Saumil N. Merchant[5], John J. Rosowski[5], Richard L. Goode[6], Hiroshi Wada[2]

[1] Department of Mechanical Engineering and Intelligent Systems, The University of Electro-Communications, 1-5-1 Chofugaoka, Chofu, Tokyo 182-8585, Japan
Email: koike@mce.uec.ac.jp
[2] Department of Bioengineering and Robotics, Tohoku University, Sendai 980-8579, Japan
[3] Sendai Ear Surgicenter, Sendai, Japan
[4] Department of Otorhinolaryngology – Head and Neck Surgery, Tohoku University Graduate School of Medicine, Sendai 980-8574, Japan
[5] Department of Otology and Laryngology, Harvard Medical School, and Eaton-Peabody Laboratory, MA 02114, USA
[6] Stanford University Palo Alto VA Medical Center Palo Alto, CA 94304, USA

To evaluate ossicular mobility in surgery, an apparatus that quasi-statically measures the load and displacement of the ossicles has been developed. This apparatus was used to measure the ossicular mobility in human temporal bones before and after the ossicles were artificially fixed. These results were compared with simultaneous estimates of ossicular mobility obtained with a laser Doppler velocimeter (LDV). In addition, the ossicular mobility of three patients with otosclerosis or chronic otitis media was also measured to evaluate the usability of the apparatus. The apparatus could make estimating the change of mobility between pre and post-treatments for ossicular fixation possible, and positive correlation was seen between ossicular mobility and hearing level. These results suggest that our apparatus has the ability to detect the difference in ossicular mobility quantitatively between fixed and normal ears, and shows that our apparatus could be a useful tool in the surgical estimate of ossicular disorders.

1. Introduction

The middle ear consists of the tympanic membrane (TM) and the ossicles, i.e., the malleus, incus, and stapes. This tiny structure performs the important function of transmitting sound efficiently from the ear canal to the cochlea. Therefore, if the mobility of the ossicular chain becomes worse because of disorders of the middle ear such as otosclerosis or tympanosclerosis, conductive hearing loss occurs. This kind of impairment is usually treated with surgery, i.e., tympanoplasty. The evaluation of ossicular mobility during tympanoplasty is an important parameter in decisions regarding surgical repairs of diseased ears as well as for post-surgical improvement in hearing level. In most cases of tympanoplasty, the mobility of the ossicles is intraoperatively detected by palpation with a hook. However, the result of this inspection depends on the surgeon's ability to use a hook to determine whether the ossicles are fixed or not; therefore, quantitative evaluation of ossicular mobility has been difficult to date.

To evaluate ossicular mobility in surgery, direct measurement of mobility has been investigated using a laser Doppler velocimeter [1] and by using a piezoelectric ceramic device that directly vibrates the stapes [2]. Hand-guided devices for measuring ossicular mobility [3, 4, 5] have also been developed. These devices measure ossicular impedance at frequencies of more than 1 kHz. However, the impedance measured at a high frequency of more than 1 kHz contains not only the stiffness component, but also the mass and damping components of the ossicles and the cochlea [1, 6, 7, 8]. In the case of ossicular fixation, measuring the stiffness component of the impedance of the ligaments and tendons, which is greater than that in the normal ear, is important. A low frequency or static measurement is therefore advantageous for detecting a slight change in the stiffness component due to fixation of the ossicles.

We have developed an apparatus that quasi-statically measures the load and displacement of the ossicles, where the stiffness defined by the slope of the load-displacement curve has been used as an index of ossicular mobility. In a pilot study, this apparatus was used to measure the ossicular mobility in human temporal bones before and after the ossicles were artificially fixed. These results were compared with simultaneous estimates of ossicular mobility obtained with a laser Doppler velocimeter (LDV). In addition, ossicular mobility in patients was measured during tympanoplasty using this apparatus to confirm the possibility of a quantitative evaluation of ossicular mobility in humans.

2. Methods

2.1 Measurement system

A schema of an apparatus for measuring ossicular mobility is shown in Fig. 1. This apparatus consists of a probe and control devices. The probe is developed by combining a small-sized force sensor and a high-precision hydraulic actuator. The force sensor with a push rod is installed at the end of the guide tube of the probe and connected to the hydraulic actuator by wires. When the tip of the push rod contacts an object like an ossicle, the actuator moves the tip out 50 microns. The reaction force from the ossicles, in other words, the load applied to the ossicles (F) is detected by the force sensor as the tip advances (X). An ossicle that is fixed is expected to generate a greater load (reaction force) than one that is mobile. The relationship between the load and displacement of the tip is displayed on the computer screen. Each measurement takes 0.25 seconds. The measurement time was determined experimentally to reduce the effect of hand trembling.

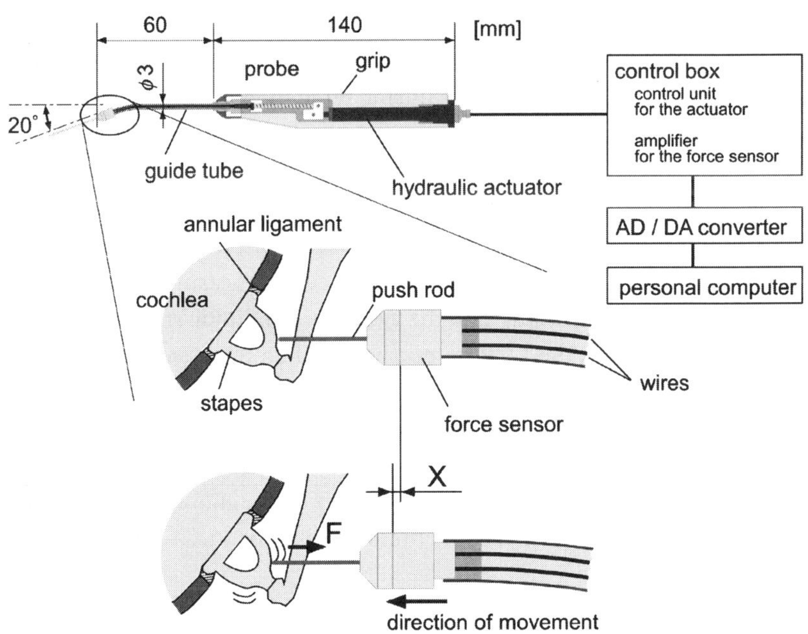

Fig. 1 Probe of the apparatus for measuring ossicular mobility.

2.2 Human temporal bones

Four fresh temporal bones were used in this study. A posterior tympanotomy and superior atticotomy were performed to give access to the stapes and malleus head. The stapes footplate or/and malleus head were artificially fixed. The stapes footplate fixation was made with either dental cement or gel-type cyanoacrylic glue, and the malleus fixation was made with a dental-cement bar between the malleus head and the tegmen. The ossicular mobility was measured with our apparatus at the crus of the stapes, the malleus head, and the long process of the incus before and after the ossicles were artificially fixed. The vibration amplitude at the crus of the stapes when sound pressure was applied to the tympanic membrane by a microphone (ER-4C, Etymotic Research) coupled to the entrance of the bony ear canal was also measured with a laser Doppler velocimeter (LDV, HLV-1000, Polytec).

2.3 Patients

The relationship between the load and displacement of the normal and fixed ossicles in patients was measured with our apparatus during surgery. Measurements were performed in three patients who had disorders of the middle ear. The transmeatal approach was selected. After the external auditory canal skin was elevated, atticotomy with a small chisel was performed to observe the ossicles. A clear view of the stapes was provided by this approach. The tympanic membrane and ossicles were left intact. The tip of the probe was inserted into the tympanic cavity, and measurements were performed at the crus of the stapes during tympanoplasty.

3. Results

3.1 Comparison of the mobility and vibration amplitude

Figures 2(a) and (b) show load-displacement curves measured at the crus of the stapes with our apparatus, and the vibration amplitude at the crus of the stapes measured with the LDV, respectively. When the ossicles were fixed, the stiffness of the ossicles, i.e., the slope of the load-displacement curve, was larger than that of the normal ear. Because the reciprocal of the stiffness (= slope of the curves) represents the mobility of the ossicles, ossicular mobility is evaluated by 1 / (Slope). The ratio of the mobility of the fixed ossicles to that of the normal ear is therefore obtained using the following equation:

$$\text{Mobility change (dB)} = 20 \log (\text{Mobility}_{\text{fixed}}) / (\text{Mobility}_{\text{normal}}) \\ -20 \log (\text{Slope}_{\text{fixed}}) / (\text{Slope}_{\text{normal}})$$

In the same way, the changes in the amplitude at 500 Hz were quantified using the equation:

$$\text{Amplitude change at 500 Hz (dB)} = 20 \log (\text{Amplitude}_{\text{fixed}}) / (\text{Amplitude}_{\text{normal}}).$$

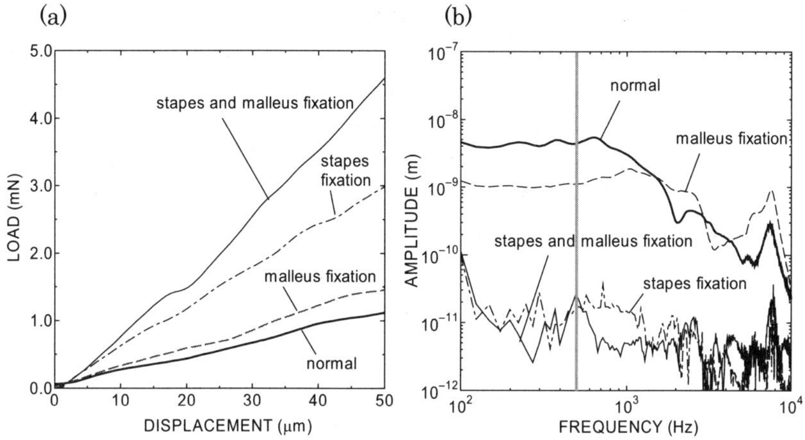

Fig. 2 Measurement results obtained from a temporal bone
(a) Load-displacement curves measured at the crus of the stapes with our device.
(b) Vibration amplitude at the crus of the stapes measured with the LDV.

Figure 3 shows the relationship between the change in mobility and the change in amplitude measured at the crus of the stapes. Although the number of the data was not sufficient and the plots concentrated at one domain, the correlation between mobility and amplitude was detected.

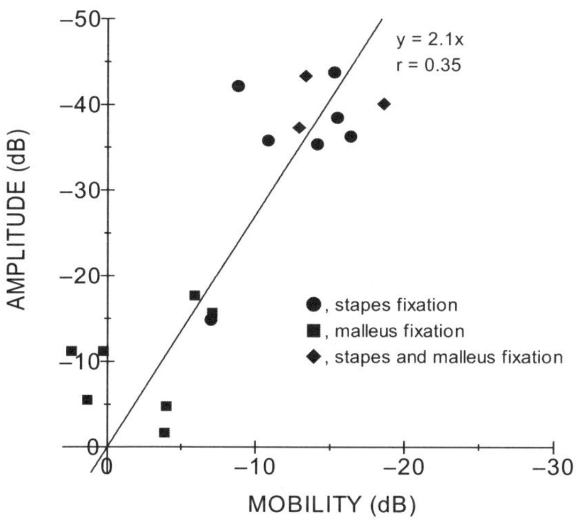

Fig. 3 Relationship between the change in mobility measured at the stapes and the change in the amplitude measured at the stapes.

3.2 Mobility measurement in patients

Figure 4 shows one example of the relationship between the load and displacement measured at the crus of the stapes in a patient with chronic otitis media. The measurements were performed before a treatment and after the stapes was mobilized and the stapedial muscle tendon cut off. The slope of the curve obtained from pre-treatment increased steeply and that of post-treatment rose gently. The hearing level after the treatment was improved by 25.0 dB.

To clarify the relationship between ossicular mobility measured by our apparatus and hearing level in patients, attention was paid to the relationships between mobility and the air-bone gap. In this case, since the load-displacement curves showed good repeatability within a load range less than 5 mN, the displacement of the ossicles when the applied load reached 5 mN was defined as the index of ossicular mobility, i.e., a large displacement indicates a good mobility of the ossicles. Figure 5 shows the relationship between the air-bone gap and the values of the displacement of the ossicles when the applied load was 5 mN. The number of the data was too little to analyze statistically, but correlation was seen between the displacement and air-bone gap.

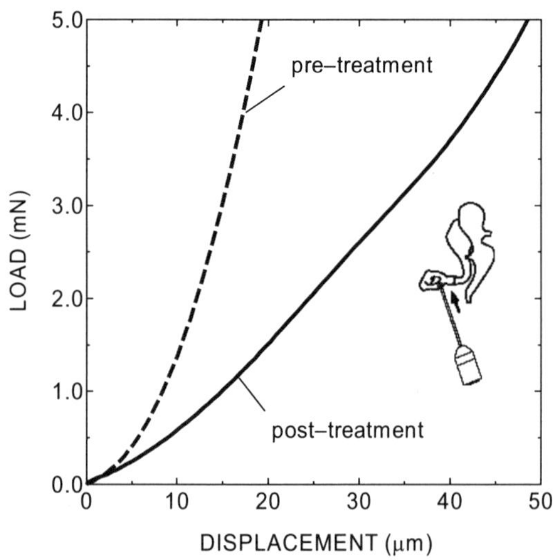

Fig. 4 Relationship between the load and the displacement of the ossicles in a patient Measurements were performed at the crus of the stapes. The patient (a 58-year-old female) suffered from chronic otitis media and ossicular mobility seemed to be slightly disturbed. Measurements were performed before the ossicle mobilization and cutting of the stapedial muscle tendon, and after the operation at the crus of the stapes, respectively. The ossicular chain was kept physiologic.

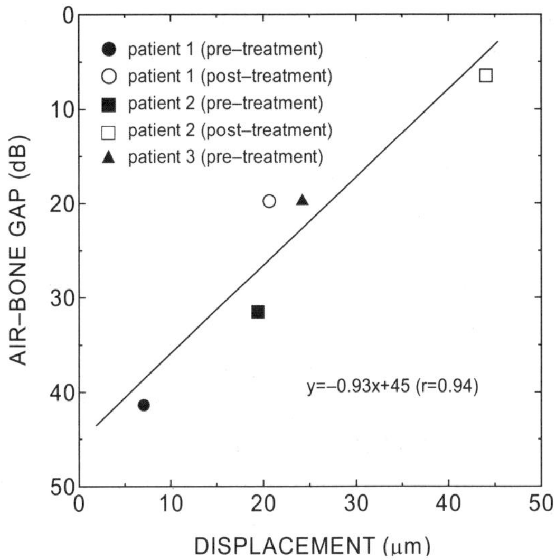

Fig. 5 Relationship between air-bone gap and the displacement of the ossicles when the applied load was 5 mN.

4. Discussion

Figure 3 suggests the possibility that the change in the vibration amplitude of the ossicles caused by sound can be quantitatively evaluated by statically measuring the mobility of the ossicles in micrometer order although the vibration of the middle ear caused by the sound we usually hear is in nanometer order [9, 10].

Regarding the measurements in patients, the slope of the curve obtained after treatment was significantly smaller than that obtained before treatment as shown in Fig. 4. This result suggests that our newly developed system has the ability to detect the difference in ossicular mobility between pre and post-treatment.

Hearing gain, defined as the difference between hearing level checked before treatment and the hearing level after treatment, is one of the most important factors in diagnosing the hearing condition of patients. However, performing the hearing test during surgery is generally difficult because fitting sound devices to the patient under surgery is time consuming and sterilization of a receiver is troublesome. If the hearing gain can be estimated by a simple method during surgery, the effect of the surgery will be improved. As shown in Fig. 5, a correlation between the air-bone gap and the values of the displacement of the ossicles was found. When the mobility of the ossicles becomes worse due to fixation, the transmitting mechanism of sound is inhibited and this pathological change then causes conductive hearing loss. From this point of view, it seems reasonable to suppose that there are some correlations between ossicular mobility and hearing level. The prognosis of recovery of post-operative hearing level therefore may be attained during surgery. However, collection of further data and analysis will be required for these detailed relations in the future.

5. Conclusions

Although the data set is small, the ossicular mobility measured with our apparatus correlates with the vibration amplitude of the ossicles and air-bone gap. This result suggests that our apparatus has the ability to detect the difference in mobility quantitatively between pre and post-treatments for ossicular fixation during surgery, and supports the idea that our device could be a useful tool in the surgical estimate of ossicular disorders and post-surgical improvement in hearing level.

References

1. Merchant S.N., Ravicz M.E. and Rossowski J.J., Acoustic input impedance of the stapes and cochlea in human temporal bones. *Hearing Research* **97** (1996) pp. 30–45
2. Gyo K., Sato H., Yumoto E. and Yanagihara N., Assessment of stapes mobility by use of a newly developed piezoelectric ceramic device. *Ann Otol Rhinol Laryngol* **109** (2000) pp. 473–477
3. Hofmann G., Zahnert T., Vogel U., Offergeld C. and Hüttembrink K.B., Hand-guided electromagnetic sensor for measurement of stapes mobility. In *Abstract of the Second International Symposium on Middle-ear Mechanics in Research and Otosurgery.* (Boston, MA, USA, Oct 21–24, 1999) p. 64
4. Zahnert T., Hüttenbrink K.B., Bornitz M. and Hofmann G., Intraoperative measurement of stapes mobility using a hand-guided electromagnetic probe [in German]. *Laryngo Rhino Otologie* **80** (2001) pp. 71–77
5. Iwakura T., Fujioka H., Tateno M., Eng M., Kohno H., Hato N., Sato H. and Gyo K., Development of a handheld ossicular vibration tester for surgery, In Kiyofumi Gyo and Hiroshi Wada (eds.) *Proceedings of the 3rd Symposium on Middle ear mechanics in research and otology.* (World Scientific, Singapore 2003) pp. 324–327
6. Zwislocki J., Analysis of the middle-ear function. I. Input impedance. *J Acoust Soc Am* **34** (1962) pp. 1514–1523
7. Shanks J.E., Tympanometry. *Ear Hear* **5** (1984) pp. 268–280
8. Nishihara S., Aritomo H. and Goode R.L., Effect of changes in mass on middle ear function. *Otolaryngol Head Neck Surg.* **109** (1993) pp. 899–910

9. Wada H., Ando M., Takeuchi M., Sugawara H., Koike T., Kobayashi T., Hozawa K., Gemma T. and Nara M., Vibration measurement of the tympanic membrane of guinea pig temporal bones using time-averaged speckle pattern interferometry. *J Acoust Soc Am* **111** (2002) pp. 2189–2199
10. Huber A., Koike T., Wada H., Nandapalan V. and Fisch U., Fixation of the anterior mallear ligament: diagnosis and consequences for hearing results in stapes surgery. *Ann Otol Rhinol Laryngol* **112** (2003) pp. 348–55.

SOURCES OF VARIABILITY IN REFLECTANCE MEASUREMENTS ON NORMAL HUMAN EARS

Susan E. Voss, Picker Engineering Program, Smith College, Northampton, MA, USA
51 College Lane, Northampton, MA 01063, USA, Email: svoss@email.smith.edu
Nicholas J. Horton, Department of Mathematics and Statistics, Smith College, Northampton, MA, USA, Email: nhorton@email.smith.edu
Rebecca R. Woodbury, Picker Engineering Program, Smith College, Northampton, MA, USA, Email: rwoodbur@email.smith.edu
Caitlyn A. Shea, Picker Engineering Program, Smith College, Northampton, MA, USA
Email: cshea1@nd.edu
Ashley H. Smith, Department of Mathematics and Statistics, Smith College, Northampton, MA, USA, Email: ahsmith@email.smith.edu

The development of acoustic reflectance measurements to augment middle-ear diagnostic testing may lead to noninvasive tests that provide information currently unavailable from standard audiometric testing. Reflectance measurements were made on both live-human and human-cadaver ears to quantify inter-subject variability relative to intra-subject variability due to temporal changes in either an individual ear or the measurement system, methodological issues including estimates of ear-canal area, and measurement location within the ear canal. To compare intra-subject versus inter-subject variability, multiple reflectance measurements were made on five live human subjects (10 ears). The variability among ears from different subjects was greater than the variability within repeated measurements on a single ear at all frequencies except from 2000 to 4000 Hz, where inter-subject variability was smaller. Reflectance measurements in human-cadaver ears demonstrate that reflectance depends on both the ear-canal location and variations in the ear-canal area. However, these variations are also small relative to inter-subject variations.

1. Introduction

Objective tests do not exist for many middle-ear pathologies and many middle-ear lesions remain unconfirmed unless surgical intervention occurs. An objective test of middle-ear function such as reflectance would be significant for (1) determining a range of middle-ear lesions for all ages, (2) following the duration of fluid in the ears of children prone to otitis media, and (3) differentiating between conductive and sensory-neural hearing loss in newborn hearing screening programs. In order to differentiate between reflectance measurements on normal and abnormal middle ears, the reflectance in a normal ear must be well defined and understood. One factor currently limiting the development of diagnostic tests that rely on ear-canal reflectance measurements is that normal-hearing human ears show inter-subject variations [1], which are up to 10 dB between 100 and 4000 Hz and up to 25 dB between 4000 and 10000 Hz [2]. To quantify how normal variations affect the reflectance of normal ears, the effects of three sources of variability are characterized in this work: (1) intra-subject versus inter-subject variability, (2) effect of ear-canal measurement location, and (3) effect of ear-canal cross-sectional area.

2. Methods

2.1 What is reflectance?

When sound waves vibrate the tympanic membrane, some acoustic energy is reflected back into the ear canal and some is transmitted to the cochlea where it is transduced to a neural signal and sent to the brain. The ratio between the reflected pressure wave and the incident pressure wave is described quantitatively as the reflectance R, with $0 \le |R| \le 1$. Similarly, the fraction of energy that is reflected can be described quantitatively by the energy reflection coefficient $\mathcal{R} = |R|^2$, such that $\mathcal{R} = 1$ indicates all energy is reflected and $\mathcal{R} = 0$ indicates that all energy is transmitted.

To measure reflectance, sounds are generated and sensed by an ear-canal probe system. The reflectance is commonly computed from measurements of the acoustic impedance in the ear canal Z_{EC}, where Z_{EC} can be computed from a pressure measurement in the ear canal and the Thévenin equivalent of the sound-delivery system [2, 3, 4]. Reflectance R is related to the impedance by the equation:

$$R(f) = \frac{Z_{EC}^N(f) - 1}{Z_{EC}^N(f) + 1} \tag{1}$$

where f is frequency and Z_{EC}^N is the ear-canal impedance normalized by its characteristic impedance z_o, with $z_o = \rho c/A$ where ρ is the density of air, c is the speed of sound in air, and A is the cross-sectional area of the ear canal in the plane of the measurement. Energy reflectance $\mathcal{R}$ is calculated as $(f) = |R(f)|^2$.

2.2 Human Subjects

The measurement protocol was approved by the Smith College Institutional Review Board (IRB). Measurements were made on ten ears from five subjects. Each ear was free of wax as indicated via otoscopic examination and each ear had normal hearing (i.e., < 20 dB HL at standard audiometric frequencies). Tympanometry was performed on every ear before each measurement; in all cases, the tympanometric results were normal. The transducer was positioned about 13 mm into the ear canal, which suggests it sat about 10 to 17 mm from the tympanic membrane, as average ear canal lengths range from about 23 to 30 mm [5]. All measurements were repeated approximately weekly for three to five weeks, and comparisons were made to determine how the energy reflectance measurements vary in the same ear. A constant ear-canal area of 0.43 cm^3 was assumed for all calculations of reflectance.

2.3 Cadaver ears

2.3.1 Ear acquisition and preparation

Five cadaver ears were obtained through the nonprofit group Life Legacy and included the complete outer ear, middle ear, and inner ear. The donors had no known history of ear disease, and each ear appeared normal when examined with an otologic operating microscope. The ears were shipped on dry ice and kept frozen until measurements were made. The middle ear air space was vented through the Eustachian tube using tygon tubing so that no static pressure difference would accumulate across the tympanic membrane. The tympanic membrane and middle ear were moistened periodically with saline, which was suctioned before measurements were taken.

2.3.2 Transducer positioning

At each measurement location, the distance from the end of the yellow foam tip that pointed outwards to the most protruding part of the anterior side of the ear canal was measured with a measuring stick. This distance was later compared to a mold of the ear canal to determine the corresponding distance from the end of the transducer to the most medial portion of the tympanic membrane.

2.3.3 Ear canal cross-sectional area

The reflectance depends on the cross-sectional area of the ear canal, A (Eq. 1). To estimate the cross-sectional area of the ear canal, a silicone-based mold of each ear canal was made. The mold was cut into cross-sections with a razor blade, and the cross-sectional area at each measurement location was determined using a microscope camera and digital analysis software

(ImageJ). The estimate of the area found using this technique is referred to as the measured area.

In order to determine the sensitivity of the reflectance to the estimate of the cross-sectional area, two additional measures of cross-sectional area were used: acoustic and constant. The acoustic estimate of the area is based on the impedance measurements from 500 to 5000 Hz [6, 7]. The constant cross-sectional area is 0.43 cm^3 at all positions in all ears [2].

2.4 Measurement system

For both the live human and cadaver ears, ear-canal pressures were generated and sensed with an Etymotic ER-10c earphone/microphone system controlled by a computer running SysID and Matlab software. The sound stimulus was a broad-band chirp containing frequencies from 25 Hz to 24 kHz and an input voltage of 0.1 V. Response magnitudes and angles were calculated from a 2048-point DFT of the time domain average of 500 responses sampled at 48 kHz.

The middle-ear input impedance at the measurement location, Z_{EC}, was calculated from the measured ear-canal pressure and the Thévenin-equivalent of the transducer [2, 3, 4, 8]. Pressure measurements made in four cylindrical tubes provided four complex equations for the two unknown Thévenin equivalents. Acoustic estimates of the tube lengths were obtained by minimizing the error function in the over-determined system of four equations [2, 3, 4], and the optimized lengths were used to compute the two unknown Thévenin equivalents. Results were checked by comparing measured and theoretical impedances in five additional tubes. Energy reflectance was calculated by squaring the magnitude of the pressure reflectance (Eq. 1).

3. Results

3.1 Intra-subject versus inter-subject variability: repeated measurements on live human ears

Repeated measurements of energy reflectance were made on ten live human ears (left and right ears of five subjects). Figure 1 summarizes these results. In the left plot, five measurements on both the left and the right ears of subject 1 are plotted. Features of these measurements include: (1) the left and right ears appear similar and (2) the measurements show little variability except in the frequency range of 2000–4000 Hz. These measurements on subject 1 are typical of all five subjects.

The right side of Fig. 1 plots the means from all subjects. At frequencies outside the range 2000–4000 Hz, the variability that results from a session (intra-subject variability) appears to be substantially smaller than the variability that results from a subject (inter-subject variability). For the frequency range 2000 to 4000 Hz, the inter-subject variability is smaller than at other frequencies and the effects of repeated measurements are larger than the effects of subject.

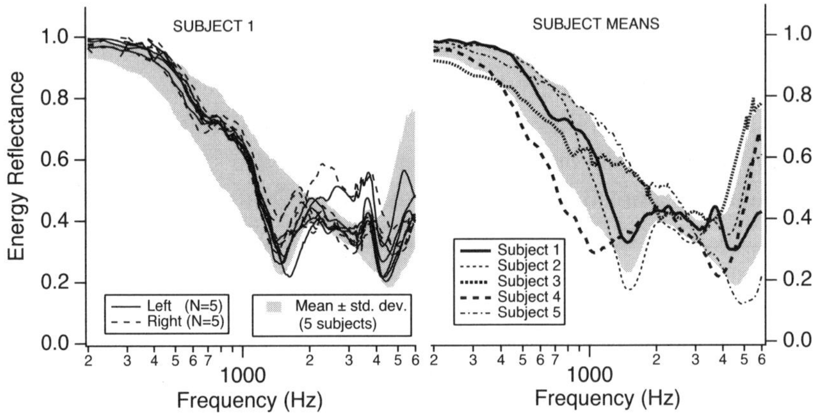

Fig. 1 Energy reflectance measurements made on live human ears. LEFT: Measurements made on the left and right ear of subject 1. A total of five measurements were made on each ear with one measurement session once per week over a five week period. RIGHT: Mean measurements on each of the five subjects. Measurements on the left and right ears of each subject were combined to compute the mean. BOTH: The gray shaded region indicates the mean plus and minus the standard deviation of the mean measurements made on the five subjects (left and right ears were combined for each subject).

3.2 Effects of measurement location on energy reflectance: measurements on cadaver ears

Figure 2 shows the energy reflectance measured at seven ear-canal locations for an example ear (LL7 Left). In general, the magnitude of the reflectance decreases systematically as the distance from the tympanic membrane increases. The difference in magnitudes becomes more pronounced as the distance from the tympanic membrane increases; in this example, the location-induced differences in energy reflectance are relatively small for distances within 20 mm of the tympanic membrane.

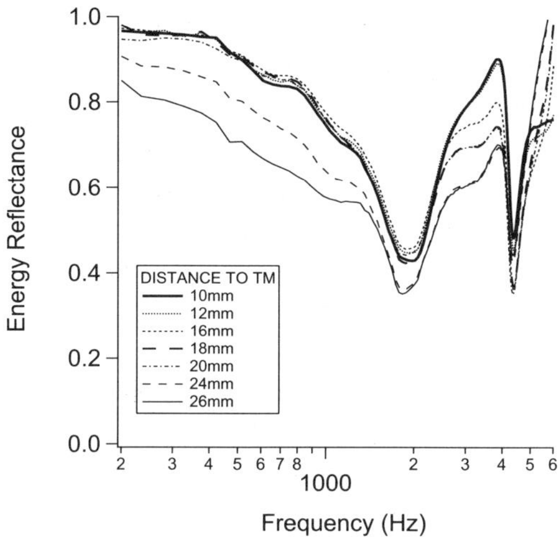

Fig. 2 Energy reflectance measured on cadaver ear LL7 (Left) with ear-canal measurement location the parameter. The legend indicates each measurement location in terms of distance from the tympanic membrane.

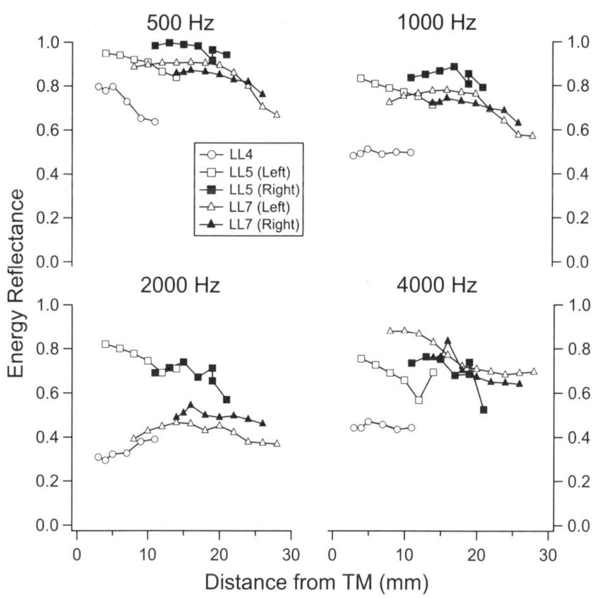

Fig. 3 Plots showing the energy reflectance at 500, 1000, 2000, and 4000 Hz for each of the five ears (from three cadaver donors) at each measurement location. These plots show that the changes in energy reflectance within each ear due to measurement location are generally not as great as the inter-subject variability in reflectance magnitude for different measurement locations. In addition, the left and right ears from the same person are more similar to each other than to ears from a different person.

To compare the effects of measurement location with inter-subject variability, Fig. 3 plots the energy reflectance as a function of measurement location for each ear at the discrete frequencies of 500, 1000, 2000, and 4000 Hz. The results from the left and the right ear of the same subject are generally more similar than the results between ears from different subjects. Additionally, the variations in energy reflectance within a given subject that result with different measurement locations are generally smaller than the inter-subject variations.

3.3 Effects of ear-canal cross-sectional area on energy reflectance: measurements on cadaver ears

For each ear, the cross-sectional area of the ear canal at each measurement location was estimated using a silicone-based mold, an acoustic estimate [6, 7], and a constant area of 0.43 cm^2 [2]. For all five ears and all ear-canal locations, the error between the mold-estimated and the acoustically measured area is generally less than 30%, and the error between the mold-estimated and the constant area is generally less than 40%. In order to examine the sensitivity of the energy reflectance to cross-sectional area, energy reflectance was calculated using all three area estimates for measurements made closest and furthest from the tympanic membrane. Figure 4 plots the energy reflectance for two ears [LL4 and LL7 (left)] at the closest and furthest locations from the tympanic membrane, using each of the three area estimates at each location. The effects of the cross-sectional area on the energy reflectance are generally smaller than the effects of measurement location, as the three energy reflectance plots at the closest location are generally distinct from the three energy reflectance plots at the furthest location (Fig. 4).

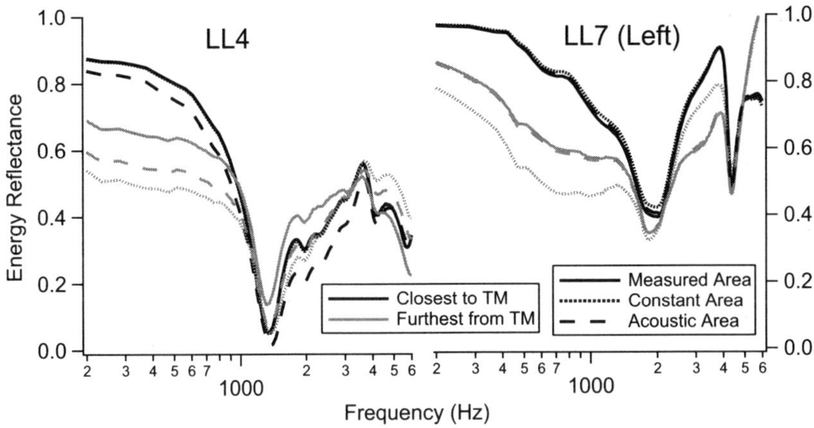

Fig. 4 Plots showing the effect of the cross-sectional area estimate on the energy reflectance. The measurements made closest to the tympanic membrane are plotted in black and those made furthest from the tympanic membrane are plotted in gray. The energy reflectance calculated using the measured area is shown with a solid line, the energy reflectance calculated using the acoustic estimate is shown with a dashed line, and the energy reflectance calculated using the constant estimate is shown with a dotted line.

4. Discussion

Three specific sources of intra-subject variations in energy reflectance measurements were studied: (1) effects of intra-subject variability over repeated measurement sessions, (2) effects of ear-canal measurement location, and (3) effects of the ear-canal cross-sectional area estimate. In general, all of these effects were small relative to inter-subject variations, with the exception of intra-subject variability over repeated measurement sessions in the frequency range of 2000–4000 Hz.

Repeated measurements on an individual ear demonstrated smaller variations than measurements made on a population of live ears (Fig. 1) except at frequencies from 2000–4000 Hz. In the frequency band of 2000–4000 Hz, these repeated measurements showed relatively little inter-subject variability as compared to other frequencies. Assuming that normal and abnormal ears have energy reflectances that differ in this band, then this observation suggests that the development of an energy-reflectance based diagnostic test might emphasize the frequency region of 2000–4000 Hz to distinguish between normal and abnormal ears. We note this observation is on a small number of ears and that the results on the cadaver ears have a larger range of energy-reflectance values from 2000–4000 Hz; future work might examine the responses in this frequency range on a larger population of ears.

Acknowledgments
This work was supported by grant NIH 1 R15 DC007615-01 from the NIDCD, National Institutes of Health and a grant from the Ford Motor Company. We thank Meghan Taugher for helping to make the measurements and John Rosowski for helpful discussions.

References

1. H. Hudde., Measurement of the eardrum impedance of human ears. *J. Acoust. Soc. Am.,* **73**: 242–247, 1983
2. S.E. Voss and J. B. Allen. Measurement of acoustic impedance and reflectance in the human ear canal. *J. Acoust. Soc. Am.,* **95**: 372–384, 1994
3. J. B. Allen. Measurement of eardrum acoustic impedance. In J. B. Allen, J. L. Hall, A. Hubbard, S. T. Neely, and A. Tubis, editors, *Peripheral Auditory Mechanisms,* pages 44–51. Springer-Verlag, 1986
4. D. H. Keefe, R. Ling, and J. C. Bulen. Method to measure acoustic impedance and reflection coefficient. *J. Acoust. Soc. Am.,* **91** (1): 470–485, 1992
5. E. G. Wever and M. Lawrence. *Physiological Acoustics.* Princeton University Press, 1954
6. D. H. Keefe, J. C. Bulen, K. H. Arehart, and E. M. Burns. Ear-canal impedance and reflection coefficient in human infants and adults. *J. Acoust. Soc. Am.,* **94** (5): 2617–2638, 1993
7. G. T. Huang, J. J. Rosowski, S. Puria, and W. T. Peake. A noninvasive method for estimating acoustic admittance at the tympanic membrane. *J. Acoust. Soc. Am.,* **108**: 1128–1146, 2000
8. S. T. Neely and M. P. Gorga. Comparison between intensity and pressure as measures of sound level in the ear canal. *J. Acoust. Soc. Am.,* **104**: 2925–2934, 1998.

OCCLUSION OF THE EAR CANAL AND ITS EFFECTS ON HEARING TESTS

Kiyofumi Gyo, Toshiki Maetani, Naoto Hato, Masamitsu Hyodo

Address: Kiyofumi Gyo, MD, Department of Otolaryngology, Ehime University
Toon, Shizukawa, Ehime, 791-0295, Japan, Email: kiyofumi@m.ehime-u.ac.jp

Keywords: ear canal resonance, bone conduction, tinnitus, loudness matching

Objective: Three issues concerning occlusion of the ear canal were investigated. 1) What is the nature of a sound induced by occluding the ear canal? 2) Does wearing an air-conduction (AC) receiver affect on tinnitus matching test? 3) How far is a sound emitted into the ear canal during bone conduction (BC) hearing test? Does wearing an AC receiver affect on the results?

Methods: 1) Effects of ear canal occlusion were studied in 10 ears of 5 normal volunteers. The ear canal was occluded by the following three procedures; inserting the index finger, filling water into the ear canal, and wearing an AC receiver. The subjects were asked to match a sound induced by ear canal occlusion to a reference sound which was provided by an AC receiver on the contralateral ear. 2) Effects of wearing AC receiver on tinnitus matching test were investigated in 25 patients suffering from unilateral tinnitus. Pitch and loudness of the tinnitus were matched by presenting comparative sounds to the contralateral ear, with and without wearing an AC receiver on the involved ear. 3) Twenty-two ears of 11 normal volunteers were the subjects of BC study. BC sound was presented on the forehead and the sound pressures emitted in the ear canal were measured with and without wearing an AC receiver on the test ear.

Results: 1) Occlusion of the ear canal with the index finger or filling water in it caused a sound similar to roaring tinnitus, which resembled 125 Hz band-pass noise. The intensity of the sound was 17.2±4.5dB and 9.4±2.2dB, respectively. In contrast, wearing an AC receiver did not induce such sound. 2) Pitch of the tinnitus was differently perceived by wearing an AC receiver in 9 of 25 patients (36%), while that of loudness in 15 patients (60%). Most of them heard the tinnitus louder by wearing an AC receiver. 3) Sound pressure emitted in the ear canal was enhanced by wearing an AC receiver at most 17.9±4.9dB at 0.8 kHz, although it decreased slightly at 2–4 kHz.

Conclusion: Occlusion of the ear canal affects variously on the audiological testing. The effects are minor, however, care should be taken in interpreting the results, since wearing an AC receiver may modify them.

1. Introduction

Occlusion of the ear canal induces a sound similar to a roaring tinnitus [1]. The origin remains controversial, but the sound is supposed to be a sum of various vital noises that are transmitted or emitted in the ear canal. We seldom care about this phenomenon since the sound is soft and does not bother our lives. In audiological testings, however, such sound may modify the results since most of the tests are undergone with the ear canals closed with air conduction (AC) receivers bilaterally [2]. In this paper, three issues concerning closure of the ear canal are presented; 1) What is the nature of a sound induced by occluding the ear canal? 2) Does wearing of an AC receiver affect on loudness balancing test that is undergone to evaluate nature of tinnitus? 3) How far does the sound radiate into the ear canal during bone conduction hearing test? Does wearing an AC receiver affect on the results? All the following tests were conducted in our audiometry room where the noise level was below 30 dB(A).

2. Nature of a Sound Induced by Occluding the Ear Canal

2.1 Materials and methods

The subjects were 10 normal ears of 5 volunteers, the age ranging from 24 to 39 years old. They belonged to our clinic and were instructed in their tasks before testing. The ear canal was occluded by the following three procedures; 1) inserting the index finger in the ear canal, 2) filling the ear canal with water (physiological saline), and 3) wearing an AC receiver. Comparative sound (reference sound) was given to the contralateral ear (non-test ear) via an AC receiver. The subjects were asked to manipulate the dial of an audiometer (Rion AA–70) to adjust pitch and loudness of a reference sound, when they noticed a noise by closure of the ear canal. In loudness balance test, a comparative sound was adjusted in 1 dB step. Pitch of the test sound was fixed to 125 Hz, since a sound induced by closure of the ear canal resembled a band pass noise around 125 Hz.

2.2 Results

All the subjects mentioned that the sound heard by closure of the ear canal resembled low-pitched roaring noise and was close to 125 Hz band-pass noise, the pitch ranging from 82 to 134 Hz. When the ear canal was occluded by inserting the index finger, loudness of the induced sound was 17.2±4.5dB. When the ear canal was filled with water, it was 9.4±2.2dB. In contrast, such sound was not heard when wearing an AC receiver.

3. Effect of Wearing an Air Conduction Receiver on Tinnitus Matching Test

3.1 Materials and methods

This study was undergone by 25 patients suffering from unilateral tinnitus. Original diseases were chronic otitis media in 12 cases, unknown sensorineural hearing loss in 10 cases, tinnitus without hearing loss in 2 cases and sudden deafness in 1 case. Pitch and loudness matching were done by presenting a comparative sound to the uninvolved ear, with or without wearing an AC receiver on the involved ear. Comparative sounds were adjusted by 1/2 octave step in pitch matching, and by 5 dB step in loudness balancing.

3.2 Results

Pitch of the tinnitus was differently perceived when wearing a receiver in 9 of 25 patients (36%), while that of loudness in 15 patients (60%). As shown in Fig. 1, loudness of tinnitus may be overestimated when tested by wearing an AC receiver on the involved ear.

		loudness			(ears)
		weaker	unchanged	larger	total
pitch	lower	1	1	2	4
	unchanged	2	7	7	16
	higher	0	2	3	5
	total	3	10	12	25

Fig. 1 Effects of wearing an air conduction (AC) receiver on tinnitus matching test. By wearing an AC receiver, loudness of tinnitus became louder in 12 of 25 ears, while pitch remained unchanged in many cases.

4. Loudness of a Sound in the Ear Canal Radiated by Bone Conduction Sound

4.1 Materials and methods

Twenty-two ears of 11 normal volunteers were the subjects of this study. An electret type microphone (Rion AD-02) was placed deep in the ear canal. It was hooked up to a B&K type 2113 amplifier. Test sound was applied via a bone conduction receiver placed on the forehead. The receiver was activated by Rion AA-70 audiometer. Stimulus sound was set to be maximum at each test frequency in order to improve S/N of the emitted sound.

4.2 Results

Fig. 2 shows a sound pressure recorded in the ear canal with and without wearing an AC receiver, when a BC receiver is activated at the maximum output level. Fig. 3 summarizes the changes in sound pressure by wearing an AC receiver. Ear canal sound became larger by wearing an AC receiver by 17.9±4.9dB at 0.8 kHz, although it decreased at 2–4 kHz.

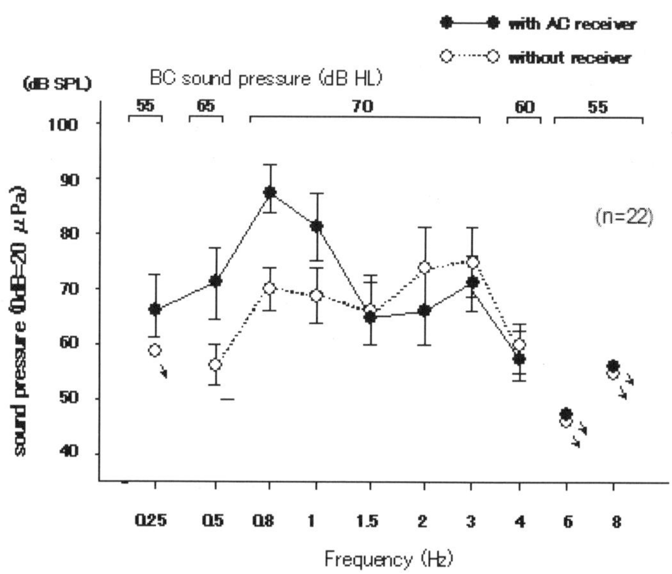

Fig. 2 Sound pressures recorded in the ear canal during bone conduction (BC) test with and without wearing AC receiver. Stimulus sound was set to be maximum at each test frequency in order to improve S/N of the emitted sound. BC sound pressures are shown in brackets.

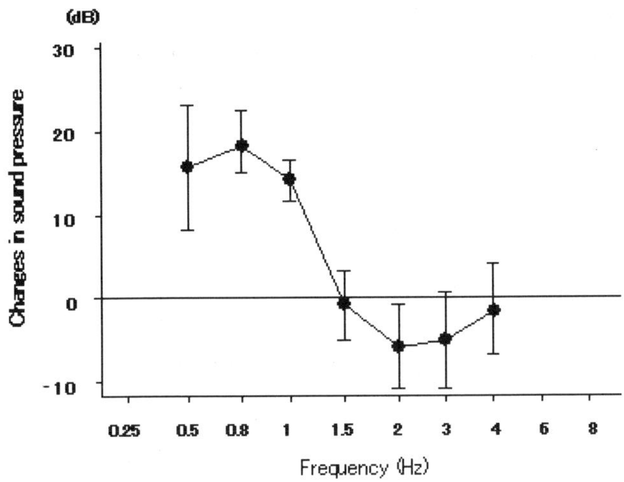

Fig. 3 Increment of the ear canal sound pressure by wearing an AC receiver. The increment was calculated by subtracting the data without the stimuli from those with the stimuli. Ear canal sound became larger by wearing an air-conduction receiver at 0.8 kHz, although it decreased at 2–4 kHz.

5. Discussion

Low tone sound induced by occlusion of the ear canal is supposed to be a mixture of various vital sounds such as vascular pulsation, bruit, respiratory noise, vibration of the mucosal villi, etc. (Fig 4). As shown in the present study, nature of the sound was close to a roaring tinnitus resembling 125 Hz band pass noise. This may indicate that a spontaneous oto-acoustic emission (OAE) does not contribute to this phenomenon, since the pitch of OAE ranges between 1 and 2 kHz [3]. Occlusion-induced sound is rather similar to a tinnitus noticed in a sound-proof room which is normally heard in very quiet circumstances. According to Asakuma et al. [4], such tinnitus is originated from a vital sound in the middle ear, since it is not blocked by intravenous administration of lidocaine that should reduce tinnitus of the inner ear origin.

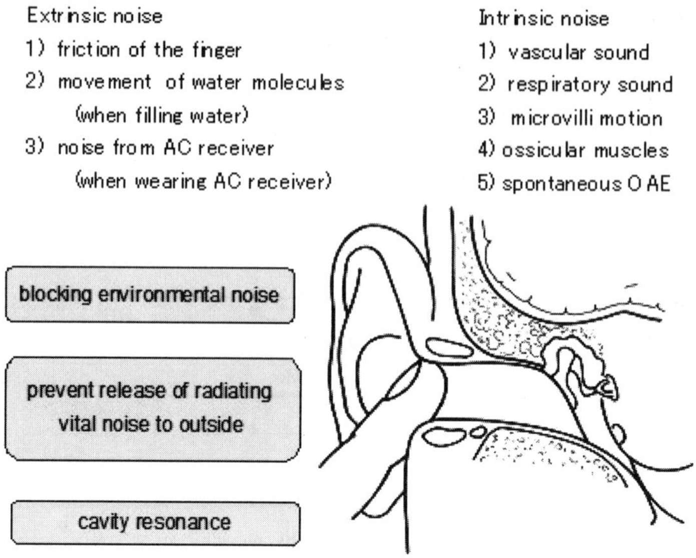

Fig. 4 Origin of a sound induced by occlusion of the ear canal.

Wearing an AC receiver did not induce any sound in all the subjects, probably due to insufficient occlusion of the ear canal. As the sound in the ear canal increased at most 10 dB below 125 Hz by wearing the receiver, we are not aware of such a small change of sound. This phenomenon may modify the results of audiological testing. In the present tinnitus test, loudness was estimated larger by wearing an AC receiver in almost half of the cases. This is probably due to the fact that an AC receiver not only blocked an environmental noise coming into the ear but also enhanced an intrinsic sound by a resonant effect of the ear canal, thus interfering with the loudness of tinnitus.

Occlusion of the ear canal affects variously on audiological testing. Therefore, careful attention should be paid in evaluating the results when measurement is undergone while wearing an AC receiver.

References

1. Gyo K., Nishihara S., Takeda K., Tinnitus induced by closure of the external ear canal. *Practica Otologica* **83** (1990) pp. 1009–1013
2. Gyo K., Hirata Y., Kobayashi T., Effects of wearing air conduction receiver on sound pressure transmitted to external ear canal. *Practica Otologica* **85** (1992) pp. 1545–1549
3. Zurek P.M., Spontaneous narrowband acoustic signals emitted by human ears. *J Acoust Soc Am* **69** (1981) pp. 514–523
4. Asakuma S., Hirashima K., Okada S., The mechanism of tinnitus in the normally hearing person. *Otologia Fukuoka* **31** (1985) pp. 1–6

ESTIMATION OF STAPES PISTON MOTION WITH UNI-DIRECTIONAL MEASUREMENTS IS PRONE TO ERROR

W.F. Decraemer, S.M. Khanna, O. de La Rochefoucauld, W. Dong, J.J.J. Dirckx, E.S. Olson
Univ. of Antwerp, Biomed. Physics, 177 Groenenborgerlaan, B 2020, Antwerp, Belgium; Columbia Univ., Dept. of OTO / HNS, 630 West 168th St., New York, NY 10032, USA

Keywords: stapes, 3-D motion, piston axis component, uniaxial interferometer

In most experiments, access for direct measurement of stapes motion in line with the piston axis is not available and piston motion is estimated from single component interferometric measurements done under observation directions that make angles up to 60° with the piston axis. We measured the vibration velocity of the stapes in human and gerbil from different observation angles and calculated the complete set of 3-D motion components. We expressed the components in an intrinsic reference system and could foretell the motion component to be recorded with a single axis interferometer at an angle with the piston axis. A cosine factor provides a good correction for the axis offset only for low frequencies (f<1.5kHz) in human; at higher frequencies and for gerbil at all frequencies the piston component cannot be accurately estimated from a single off-axis observation and a cosine correction.

1. Introduction

The vibration of the footplate produces the pressure wave in the cochlea that stimulates the sensory cells. We have shown that the vibration of the stapes in human, cat and gerbil exhibits all 3-D components of translation and rotation [1] and that mode changes occur with frequency. It is the piston component – we have good evidence that non-piston components do not contribute to the signal transmission path [2] – that is used in nearly all studies to specify the input to the inner ear.

In most experiments access for measurement of stapes motion in-line with the piston axis is not available, and piston motion is estimated from single component interferometer measurements. These measurements are made with observation angles of up to 60° with respect to the piston axis. A few examples of the observation angle relative to the piston axis and correction method in stapes motion measurements from the recent literature are as follows: gerbil [3], angle maximally 30°, no correction; gerbil [4], angle of incidence between 30° and 45°, cosine correction; gerbil [5], angle ~ 30°, cosine correction; human [6], angle ~ 35° (estimated from their drawing); human [7,8], angle 50°– 60°, cosine correction; human [9], angle 30°–40° (in-vivo!), no angle correction; human [10], angle 5°–20° and 40°– 60°.

We used a heterodyne interferometer/microscope to measure stapes vibration in human and gerbil from different observation angles and calculated the 3-D motion components. The components were transformed into an intrinsic reference system which allowed us to foretell for any point the motion component that will be measured from a given viewing angle with respect to the piston axis. Correcting the amplitude of this component for the cosine of the observation angle does not provide the exact piston component. Phase angle, which as a rule is not corrected, is also flawed.

2. Material and Methods

We use results of experiments on: (i) a fresh human temporal bone of an 83 year old donor (obtained within 24 hours post mortem, kept refrigerated in saline with some antiseptic and first measurements within 4 days) (ii) a Mongolian gerbil directly post mortem. The middle ear cavity was opened to expose the stapes.

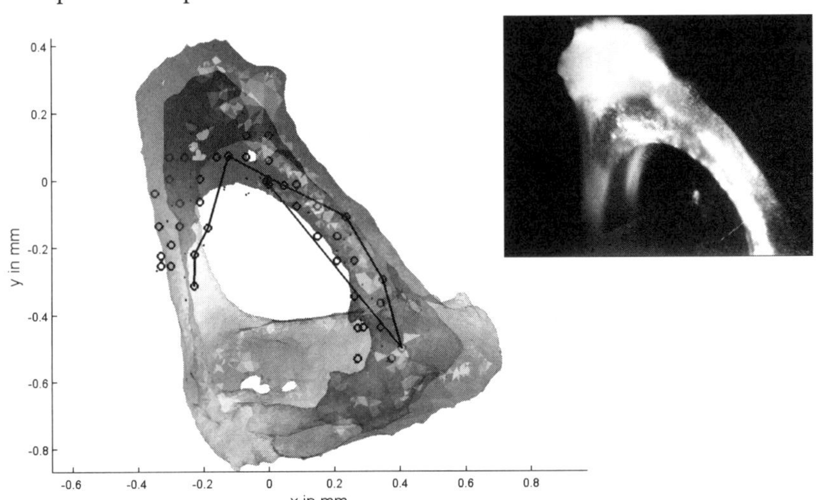

Fig. 1 A 3-D model of the stapes is registered in the position of the stapes during the experiment. Solid dots show points where vibration was recorded. Open dots, extra points on the stapes surface to enhance registration.

We measured the vibration velocity [11,12] of the stapes for pure tone from different observation angles with a heterodyne microscope/interferometer [13] and calculated the 3-D rigid body global translation and rotation for a frequency range covering the entire frequency range of the species under study.

Based on a micro CT scan of the experimental ear, a 3-D model of the stapes was made and registered in its experimental position (Fig. 1).

We determined a coordinate transform to bring the model in an intrinsic frame and used it to express the motion components in the same frame (Fig. 2): piston motion is translation along the y-axis, while tilting about the short and long axis of the footplate are rotation about the x and z axis, respectively.

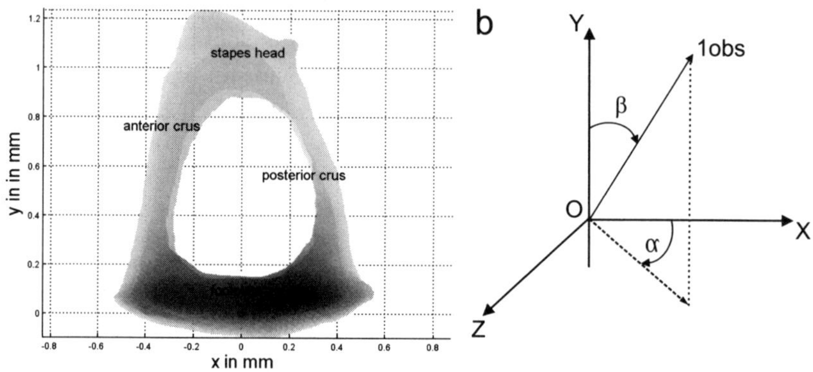

Fig. 2a Model of a gerbil stapes brought in an intrinsic reference system. Piston motion is now along the y-axis.

Fig. 2b Angles specifying the observation direction for a stapes in an intrinsic frame.

The displacement vector of any point can readily be calculated (displacements are so small we may treat them as differentials)

$$\mathbf{ds}_i(t)=\mathbf{ds}_t(t)+\mathbf{d\Theta}(t)\times\mathbf{r}_i \tag{1}$$

$\mathbf{ds}_i(t)$	: displacement of P_i
$\mathbf{ds}_t(t)$	: global translational displacement
$\mathbf{d\Theta}(t)$	: angular displacement about the origin O
$\mathbf{r}_i$	: rest-position vector of point P_i with components x_i, y_i, z_i
$\mathbf{d\Theta}(t)\times\mathbf{r}_i$	: displacement due to the rotation of P_i relative to O_{xyz}

When the motion of the point P_i is observed with a uniaxial measuring system with observation direction along $\mathbf{1}_{obs}$, one records the following component

$$D_i(t) = \mathbf{1}_{obs} \cdot \mathbf{ds}_i(t) \tag{2}$$

We specify the observation direction by angles α (between x-axis and the projection of $\mathbf{1}_{obs}$ in the x,z plane) and β (between the y-axis and $\mathbf{1}_{obs}$) as seen on Fig. 2b.

3. Results with Discussion and Conclusions

3.1 Displacement path for 3 points on the human stapes

For the human temporal bone we determined the 3-D rigid body velocities normalized for ear canal pressure, $\mathbf{ds}_t(t)$ and $\Theta(t)$, and using Eq. (1) we calculated the displacement during a cycle for points on the posterior crus, anterior crus and footplate center for a frequency of 190 Hz. The paths are elliptical and shown, magnified by a factor of 18000, in front, top and sideways views (Fig. 3a). A thick dot marks the displacement at t=0, the smaller dot at t=T/4 which shows sense of the path. All 3 points have a large piston component accompanied by some rocking about the long axis of the footplate.

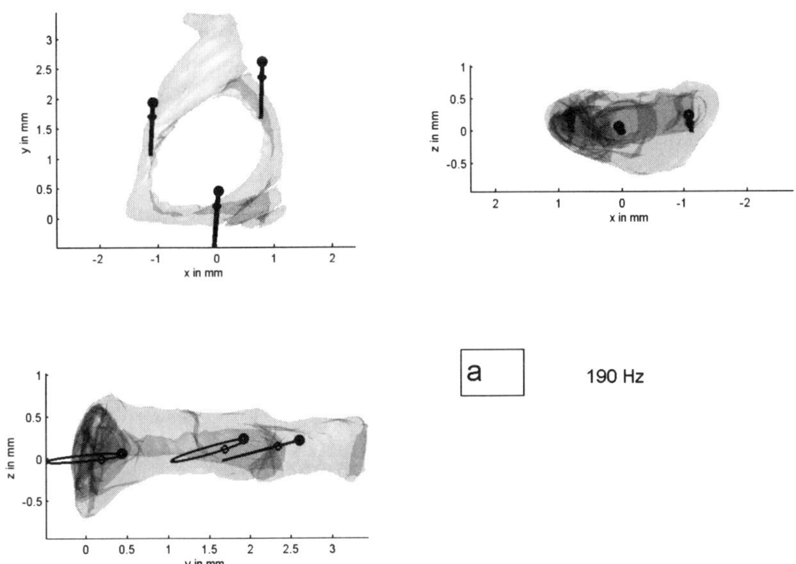

Fig. 3a Three orthogonal views of the displacement at three points of the human temporal bone Y83 at 190 Hz; displacements scaled up by 18000.

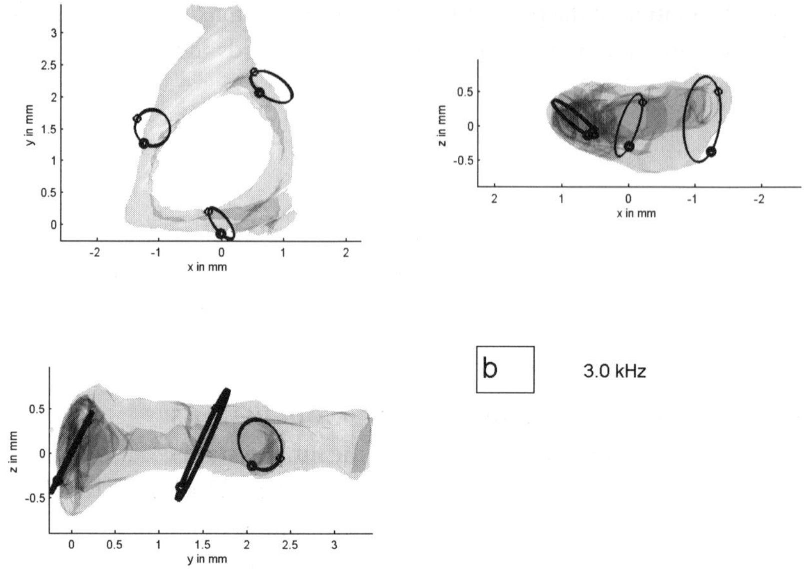

Fig. 3b At 3.0 kHz the displacement path (scaled by 75000) of the 3 points of Y83 is clearly elliptical. Note that the annular ligament is sufficiently soft and wide (~ 14 μm) to allow in-plane footplate displacements (of the order of 10^{-8} m/Pa).

Displacement paths for 3 kHz (magnification 75000, Fig. 3b) are completely different and differ also from point to point. Vibration is no longer dominated by piston motion. If we measured the motion with a unidirectional interferometer and used different observation directions in the x,y-plane we would see no difference in amplitude for the point on the anterior crus (circular path!), while for the 2 other points the amplitude would be large for observation in a direction along the long axis and small along the short axis of the elliptical path.

For elliptical motion paths the phase of the displacement component measured with a uniaxial interferometer will also depend on the observation angle (let us consider an extreme case, and observe a point that follows a circular path in the y-z plane; when we observe along the y direction we will get a motion component that is 90° out of phase with the component observed along the z direction).

3.2 Change in gerbil stapes velocity component with observation angle

Using the experimentally determined rigid body velocities (rel. to ear canal pressure) for a gerbil stapes we calculated with Eq. (1) the 3-D displacement components of a point at the middle of the stapes head (x=0, y=1.0 mm z=0 in Fig. 2). Using Eq. (2) we predicted the velocity amplitude and phase when this point is observed from different viewing angles (values inspired by study [11]: α =10° and β = 0, 20, 40 and 60°).

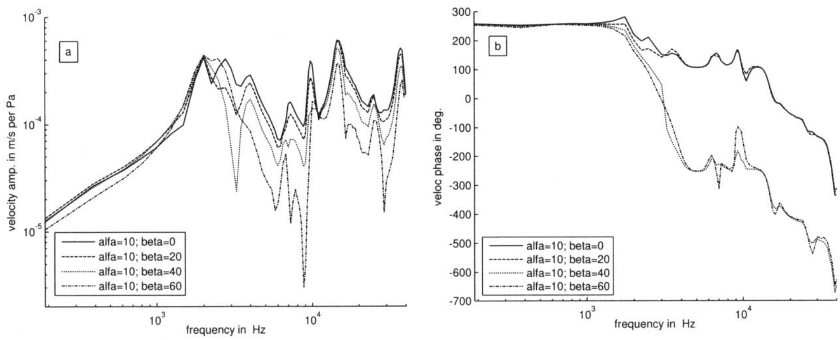

Fig. 4 Predicted amplitude (4a, left panel) and phase (4b, right panel) for the velocity component (in the direction of observation) of a point at the middle front of the gerbil stapes head, when 4 different observation angles, α =10° and β = 0, 20, 40 and 60°, are assumed. Amplitude and phase are relative to ear canal pressure.

The amplitude curves (Fig. 4a) run almost parallel up to 1.5 kHz; at higher frequencies this is no longer true. Top to bottom, curves at most frequencies are in decreasing order of β, but in some frequency bands this order is not respected. Phases (Fig. 4b) are the same for all β for frequencies below 1.0 kHz, at higher frequencies phase differences of 20 to 30° and an extra unwrapping step is seen with increasing β.

In the low frequency region changing β from 0° to 60° the amplitude is reduced less than predicted by the cosine factor (cos60°=0.5). Changing the observation angle introduces contributions from the x and z translation components compensating for the reduction in the y-component.

At high frequencies we found vibration amplitude measured at observation angle β=60° that was even smaller than the 0.1 of the actual piston component and cosine correction will not work.

For the human ear the piston-like motion is quite evident at low frequencies (Fig. 3) and a cosine correction works well below 1.5 kHz.

In general, if stapes motion is measured at an angle β to the piston axis over a wide frequency range and piston motion is estimated using a cosine correction, large errors are introduced due to the presence of multiple modes of vibration.

Acknowledgments

We thank S. Merchant and J.J. Rosowski of Mass. Eye and Ear Infirmary (Boston, USA) for helping with the human temporal bones and M. Ravicz (same institute) for communicating typical α and β angles. Supported by NIH/NIDCD, Capita Fund, FSR (Flanders, Belgium) and RAFO (Univ. Antwerp).

References

1. W. Decraemer, S. Khanna and W. Funnell, "Measurement and modeling of the three-dimensional vibration of the stapes in cat," *Proc. Rec. Developments in Auditory Mechanics, World Scientific,* 36–43 (1999)
2. W. Decraemer, S. Khanna, O. de la Rochefoucauld, W. Dong and E. Olson, "Is the scala vestibuli pressure influenced by non-piston like stapes components? An experimental approach," *Proc. Auditory Mechanisms: Processes and Models, Portland* 491–494 (2005)
3. E. Overstreet, C. Richter, A. Temchin, M. Cheatham and M. Ruggero, "High-frequency sensitivity of the mature gerbil cochlea and its development," *Audiology and Neuro-Otology,* **8**, 19–27 (2003)
4. J. Rosowski, M. Ravicz, S. Teoh and D. Flandermeyer, "Measurement of middle-ear function in the Mongolian gerbil, a specialized mammalian ear," *Audiology and Neuro-Otology,* Vol. **4**, No. 3–4, 129–136 (1999)
5. T. Ren, "Reverse propagation of sound in the gerbil cochlea," Nature Neuroscience, **7** (4), 333–334 (2004) and private communication.
6. K. Heiland, R. Goode, M. Asai and A. Huber, "Human temporal bone study of stapes footplate movement," Am. *Journ. Otology* **20**, 81–86, (1999)
7. N. Hato, S. Stenfelt and R. Goode, "Three-dimensional stapes footplate motion in human temporal bone," *Audiology and Neuro-Otology,* **8**, 140–152 (2003)
8. H. Kurokawa and R. Goode, "Sound pressure gain produced by the human middle ear," *Otolaryngology - Head and Neck Surgery,* 349–365 (1995)

9. A. Huber, T. Linder, M. Ferrazzini, S. Schmid, N. Dillier, S. Stoeckli and U. Fish, "Intraoperative assessment of stapes motion," Ann. Otol. Rhinol' Laryngol. **110**, 31–35, (2001)
10. W. Chien, M. Ravicz, S. Merchant and J. Rosowski, "The effect of methodological differences in the measurement of stapes motion of live and cadaver ears," *Abstract #925 of the 25th Midwinter meeting of the Assoc. Res. in Otolaryngology (ARO),* New Orleans, USA (2005)
11. W. Decraemer, S. Khanna and J. Dirckx, "The integration of detailed 3-dimensional anatomical data for the quantitative description of 3-dimensional vibration of biological structures. An illustration from the middle ear," *Proc. 5th Internat. Conf. on Vibration Measurements by Laser Techniques: Advances and Applications,* SPIE Proc. Series, Vol. **4827**, 148–158 (2002)

12. W. Decraemer and S. Khanna, "Measurement, visualization and quantitative analysis of complete three-dimensional kinematical data sets of human and cat middle ear," *Proc. 3rd Symposium on middle ear mechanics in research and otology,* World Scientific, 3–10, (2004)
13. S. Khanna, C. Koester, JF. Willemin, R. Dändliker and H. Rosskothen, "A non-invasive optical system for the study of the function in the inner ear in living animals", in *Selected papers on Coherence - Domain Methods in Biomedical Optics Valery* Tuchin Ed. SPIE Vol. **2732,** 66–81, (1996)

EXPERIMENTAL INVESTIGATIONS ON THE FUNCTIONAL EFFECT OF OSSICULAR JOINT FIXATION

Ch. Offergeld, M.D.[1,3], **N. Lazurashvili,** M.D.[2,3], **M. Bornitz,** M.Sc.[3], **Th. Beleites,** M.D.[2,3], **Th. Zahnert,** M.D.[2,3]

[1] Dept. of Otorhinolaryngology, Head and Neck Surgery, University of Freiburg, Germany (Chairman: Prof. Dr. Dr. h.c. R. Laszig)

[2] Dept. of Otorhinolaryngology, Head and Neck Surgery, University of Dresden, Germany

[3] Middle Ear Laboratory, Dept. of ORL, HNS, Dresden Medical School, University of Dresden, Germany (Chairman: PD Dr. Dr. h.c. Th. Zahnert)

Corresponding author: Christian Offergeld, M.D., Dept. of Otorhinolaryngology, Head and Neck Surgery, Freiburg Medical School, University of Freiburg, Killianstrasse 5, 79106 Freiburg, Germany
Phone: 49+761+2704212, Fax: 49+761+2704111
Email: offergeld@hno.ukl.uni-freiburg.de

In the normal middle ear, stapes displacement during atmospheric pressure changes is physiologically reduced by the gliding ossicular joints. In fixed ossicular joints, static pressure is assumingly transfered directly towards the inner ear. Therefore unphysiological movements could eventually initiate exceeding displacements and consecutively lead to a risk for inner ear function.

Experimental investigations were performed in order to evaluate the dynamic and quasi-static effect of ossicular joint fixation on the middle ear. Acoustic transfer characteristics and stapes displacement were determined in 12 fresh temporal bone specimens. Stapes vibration amplitude was measured using Laser-Doppler-Vibrometry (LDV) before and after stepwise artificial fixation of the ossicular joints; the same applied to measurements of stapes displacement during standardized pressure changes in the external ear canal.

In comparison to a regular middle ear, fixed ossicular joints demonstrated a minimal decrease of footplate vibration amplitude in the low frequency range whereas an improvement of the transfer characteristics of less than 10 dB was demonstrable in the middle and high frequency region. It furthermore shows that atmospheric pressure changes in the external ear canal lead to an unphysiological footplate displacement.

1. Introduction

In the normal middle ear, a mechanical protection system against exceeding quasi-static and dynamic pressure variations exists [1]. It is the movements of the incudo-malleal joint (IMJ) and incudo-stapedial joint (ISJ) that lead to a certain decoupling of the ossicular chain for protection purposes. Therefore an unimpeded gliding of the ossicular joints is necessary [2]. In cases of ossicular joint fixation (e.g. in tympanosclerosis/ after tympanoplasty) the ossicular chain allows only rigid movements. Assumingly pressure could directly be transfered from the tympanic membrane towards the annular ligament creating exceeding displacements of the footplate into the vestibulum. In consequence, inner ear disorders can be expected.

However, there are only few specific descriptions about the effect of ossicular joint fixation on middle ear transfer characteristics during changes of atmospheric pressure [3,4]. It was the purpose of our experimental study to demonstrate dynamic and quasi-static consequences arising from fixation of the ossicular joints as it helps to understand the function of the reconstructed middle ear (e.g. prosthesis, glueing of ossicular chain).

2. Materials and Methods

We performed experiments in 12 temporal bone specimens without any middle ear pathology.

Fig. 1 demonstrates the experimental setup. A posterior tympanotomy including removal of the facial nerve was performed in order to gain access towards the oval window niche and the footplate. This access was needed for stapes vibration amplitude- and displacement measurements using LDV (Polytec OFV 3001/ OFV 302; Polytec Co., Waldbronn, Germany). The external ear canal was sealed after positioning of a silicone tube connected to a sound source (Praecitronic Co., Dresden, Germany) and a pressure pump which was connected to a tympanometer (Phonak Co., Stuttgart, Germany). Calibration of the sound source was defined for sound excitation of 94 dB at 1000 Hz SPL in the region of the ear drum. The frequency range was defined between 125 Hz and 5 kHz. A probe microphone (Ethymotic Research Inc., Elk Grove Village, IL, USA) was placed through a temporary opening in the external ear canal next to the ear drum for control measurements. Continuous pressure changes were standardized from ± 400 daPa in the external ear canal.

Step 1 included the measurement of the stapes vibration amplitude in regular ossicular joints. Sound excitation was performed using multisinus excitation of 94 dB SPL in the range of 250 Hz until 5000 Hz. LDV-measurements of 3 standardized measuring points (P1–P3) on the footplate were realized. Afterwards we also performed measurements of the stapes displacement during static pressure variations.

Step 2 included the artificial fixation of the ossicular joints using cyanoacrylate glue (Histoacryl®). In 6 specimens, we started fixing the ISJ, in the other 6 cases we initiated with the IMJ. A droplet of Histoacryl® was administered into the joint cleft and distributed properly within.

Step 3 was performed after fixation of the first joint by measurement of the footplate vibration amplitude. Consecutively step 4 included the same procedure after fixation of the second joint. Finally step 5 repeated step 1 after complete fixation of the ossicular chain.

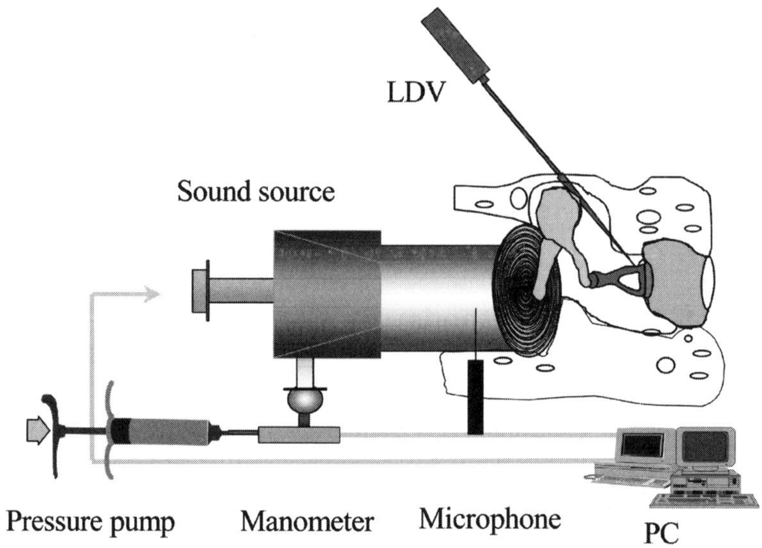

Fig. 1 Schematic view of the experimental setup used for temporal bone investigations.

3. Results

Fig. 2 and 3 show exemplary temporal bone measurements in two specimens concerning footplate vibration amplitude during defined sound excitation in the external ear canal. The differently marked curves indicate measurements of the central footplate region (P2) in normal and prepared temporal bones. Depending on the sequence of fixation, preparation started with either the IMJ or the ISJ before complete fixation of both ossicular joints.

In comparison to normal ossicular joints (Fig. 2, solid curve), fixation of the IMJ leads to an increase of the footplate vibration amplitude in the low and middle frequency region between 1000 Hz and 5 kHz (Fig.

2, dashed curve). This increase, mainly seen in the high frequency range equals less than 10 dB. A comparable improvement was also demonstrable after fixation of both joints including a shift in resonance frequency (Fig. 2, dotted curve). In contrast to the sole fixation of the IMJ it also showed a decrease of transmission of less than 5 dB in the low frequency range.

Very similar results were observed after stepwise fixation of the ISJ (Fig. 3, dashed-dotted curve) and both ossicular joints. While the loss of middle ear transfer function in the low frequency region was almost the same, the increase of vibration amplitude was more emphasized in the high frequencies when both joints were fixed (Fig. 3, dotted curve). In either case of single or combined fixation, a shift of the resonance frequency was demonstrable.

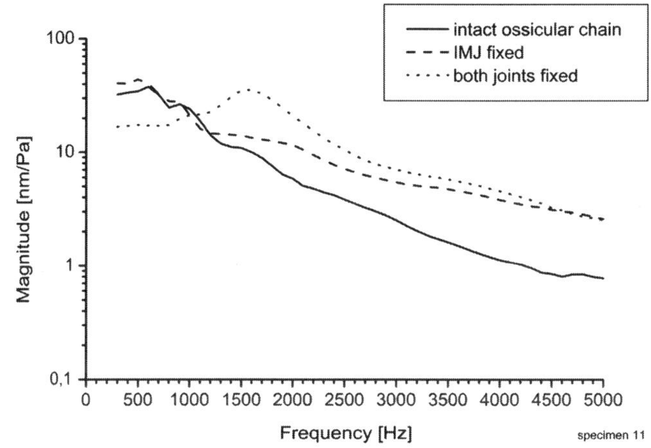

Fig. 2 Diagram demonstrating transfer characteristics of the middle ear in case of intact ossicular chain, fixed IMJ and complete ossicular fixation.

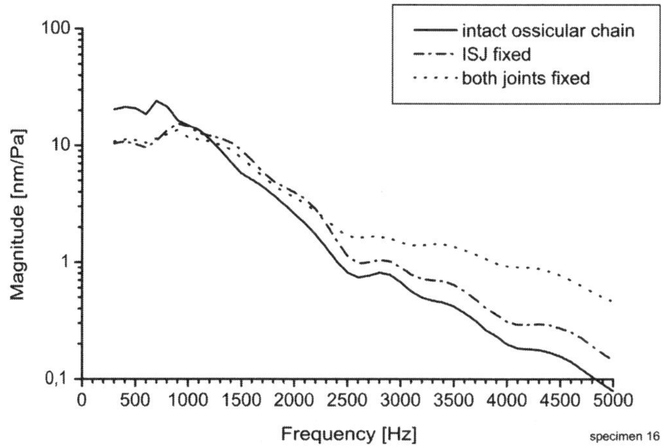

Fig. 3 Diagram evaluating middle ear transfer characteristics in case of intact ossicular chain, fixed ISJ and complete ossicular joint fixation.

Fig. 4 demonstrates the static displacement of the stapes footplate under defined pressure changes before and after stepwise fixation of the ossicular joints. The dashed curve (IMJ-fixation) shows exceeding footplate displacements in comparison to elevated footplate displacements in case of combined joint fixation (dotted curve). The greater displacement for negative pressure can even be more accentuated after fixation of one or both ossicular joints. Fig. 5 demonstrates a dotted curve (both joints fixed) with exceeding footplate displacement, a dashed-dotted curve (ISJ fixed) with decreasing footplate displacement in comparison to the intact ossicular chain (solid curve).

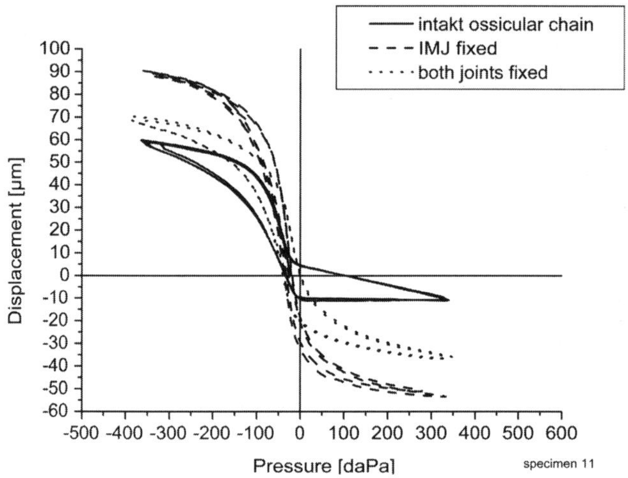

Fig. 4 Stapes footplate displacement after single (IMJ) and combined fixation of ossicular joints.

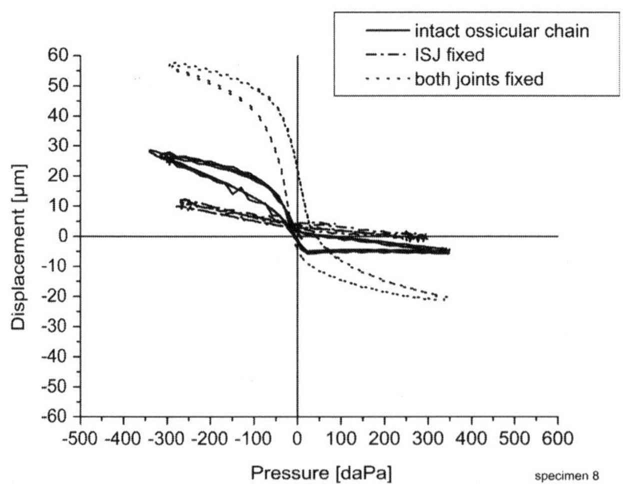

Fig. 5 Footplate displacement after single (ISJ) and combined ossicular joint fixation.

Due to ossicular joint fixation, the footplate displacement is clearly elevated in the majority of cases during application of pressure (± 400 daPa) in the external ear canal. Exceeding footplate displacements of up to 40 μm compared to normal ossicles were observed. Although the increase of the footplate displacement is greater in total for negative pressure, positive pressure application also shows a 3–5fold elevation of the footplate displacement compared to untreated specimen.

4. Discussion

The "buffering" system of the ossicular joints plays an essential role in the function of the normal middle ear determined by its mechanical components [5]. Thus, acoustic and quasi-static functions of the ossicular joints have to be distinguished explicitly from each other [6]. The ossicular joints perform typical gliding movements during changing static pressure or exceeding acoustical pressure loads while being functionally rigid during physiological acoustic sound transmission. It can be assumed that permanent ossicular joint rigidity could endanger the inner ear.

In our experimental results we demonstrated changes of the middle ear sound transfer function after artificial ossicular joint fixation, depending on localization and order of fixation (IMJ/ ISJ/ combined). This experimental study may also explain a possible pathologic pathway of an impaired regulation mechanism of the middle ear ossicular system. After increasing atmospheric pressure in the external ear canal an unphysiological displacement of the footplate was observed. Descriptions in literature evaluated maximum values of 10–30 μm for footplate displacement [4] and served therefore as controls during experimental investigation. Our results definitely exceed the above mentioned values in case of ossicular joint fixation and therefore emphasize descriptions already evaluated by Hüttenbrink [4] for IMJ-fixation. Circumstances like these have been previously rated as dangerous for the inner ear [7].

Atmospheric pressure changes occur very commonly and could therefore mean serious pressure loads for the inner ear according to Moser's description of the crucial role of the malleus-incus articulation [8]. Our results confirm the assumption of an unmitigated transfer of quasi-static pressure loads towards the footplate in case of partially or totally fixed ossicular joints. They furthermore demonstrate the individual significance of the isolated and combined functions of IMJ and ISJ in middle ear transfer function as well as in pressure regulation. The IMJ plays hereby an important role as it seems to be able to partially compensate the quasi-static effects of a fixed ISJ. On the other hand we assume that the gliding motions of the ISJ are able to avoid pre-stress on the annular ligament. These results coincide with descriptions in literature where a multiplefold increase of incus and stapes in- and excursions after artificial fixation of the incudo-malleal joint were described [6]. According to our results alterations in sound transmission depending on IMJ-mobility have also been described previously [9].

Our experimental data demonstrate changes of middle ear function concerning dynamic and quasi-static behaviour after ossicular joint fixation, depending on localization, extent and order of fixation.

References

1. Hüttenbrink, K.B., The middle ear as a pressure receptor. In Hüttenbrink KB (ed.) *Middle ear mechanics in research and otosurgery.* (UniMedia Dresden 1997) pp. 15–20
2. Cancura W., On the statics of malleus and incus and on the function of the malleus-incus joint. *Acta Otolaryngol (Stockh)* **89** (1980) pp. 342–344
3. Murakami S., Gyo K., Goode R.L., Effect of middle ear pressure change on middle ear mechanics. *Acta Otolarygol (Stockh)* **117** (1997) pp. 390–395
4. Hüttenbrink K.B., Ossicle chain mechanics at static air pressures; II: Impaired joint function and reconstructed ossicle chain]. *Laryng Rhinol Otol* **67** (1988) pp. 100–105
5. Marquet J., The incudo-malleal joint. *J Laryngol Otol* **95** (1981) p. 541
6. Eiber A., Kauf A., Computing displacements of middle ear ossicles due to static load. *HNO* **42** (1994) pp. 754–759
7. Pau H.W., Hüttenbrink K.B., Experimental studies in reconstructed middle ears – with special regard to static pressure on the footplate. *Laryngo Rhino Otol* **67** (1988) pp. 331–334
8. Moser M., Fitness of civil aviation passengers to fly after ear surgery. *Aviat Space Environ Med* **61** (1990) pp. 735–737
9. Willi U.B., Ferrazzini M.A., Huber A.M., The incudo-malleolar joint and sound transmission losses. *Hearing Research* **174** (1–2) (2002) pp. 32–44

POSTOPERATIVE TYMPANOGRAM IN TYMPANOPLASTY WITH THIN SECTION CARTILAGE ISLAND

Chin-saeng Cho, MD, **Jae-soo Lee,** MD, **Dong-sik Chang,** MD, **Myung-soo Choi,** MD, **Kyung-you Park,** MD, **Byoung-duk Lim,** Phd*
Department of Otolaryngology-head and Neck Surgery, School of Medicine Eulji University, Dae-jeon, Korea
School of Mechanical Engineering, Yeungnam University, Gyungsan, Korea*

Keywords: Tympanoplasty, Tympanogram, Cartilage
Address: Chinsaeng Cho Dept. of ENT Seo-Gu Dunsan-dong 1306 Eul Ji University Hospital, Daejeon, Korea, Email: chinsaeng@hotmail.com

Background and objectives: The objectives of tympanoplasty are to remove the pathology and to reconstruct an acoustic transfer mechanism. The use of cartilage in the reconstruction of the tympanic membrane has been established especially in cases such as tubal dysfunction and adhesive processes. Cartilage offers the advantage of higher mechanical stability in comparison with membranous transplants. However, it may alter the acoustic transfer characteristics, which may depend on the cartilage thickness. Therefore, the authors have attempted to design a thin section cartilage island with tragal cartilage for grafting material. The purpose of this study is to understand the usefulness of the thin section cartilage island technique by comparing it with conventional temporalis fascia technique using a tympanogram method.

Materials and methods: From March 2002 to August 2005, 101 cases of tympanoplasty type I using thin section cartilage island technique and 50 cases of tympanoplasty type I using temporalis fascia performed by one surgeon had been followed up for 6 months and reviewed. Static compliance, tympanometric width and tympanometric pattern were evaluated after 6 months with an impedance audiometer.

Results: In the thin section cartilage island technique group the percentage of cases with a static compliance within the normal compliance range (0.2~1.6ml) was 72% and 66% in the temporalis fascia group. The tympanometric width in the thin section cartilage island technique group was in 59% of the cases within the normal range (60~150mmH_2O), whereas in the temporalis fascia group 54% of the cases were within this range. In the thin section cartilage island technique group 67% showed a normal tympanometric pattern (A type), whereas in the temporalis fascia group this percentage amounted to 62%.

Conclusion: The results of impedance audiometry show no statistical significance between thin section cartilage island and temporalis fascia. Therefore, it is suggested that the thin section cartilage island technique is suitable for a tympanoplasty.

1. Introduction

The purposes of tympanoplasty are to remove an irreversible pathology and to improve hearing. The middle ear can be protected from harmful environments by this procedure. Since Wullstein and Zollner established the tympanoplasty, temporalis fascia, vein, perichondrium or periosteum have been used as graft materials [1][2]. Recently, most surgeons have widely used temporalis fascia with a success rate up to 90%. Other materials which can be more stable and easier to take at the same operation field have been sought in cases of tubal dysfunction, total perforation or severe mucosal inflammation for achieving uptake rate [3][4]. Cartilage was used for many decades for this reason. It should be also considered because of its acoustic impedance in terms of mass and stiffness effects associated with its thickness. There were some techniques using cartilage for graft material as palisade technique, thin section cartilage plate, and cartilage island technique [5][6][7][8]. Zahnert et al. reported that a cartilage thickness less than 0.5 mm is an acceptable compromise [6]. However, it would not be easy to support the meatal flap with a thin section cartilage plate, and the cartilage island was too thick to transfer the sound. This situation encouraged us to design a thin section cartilage island, which could be satisfactory in terms of size and thickness of the material and be large enough to cover the posterior tympanomeatal flap.

In the present study, we compared the postoperative tympanogram in cases of a thin section cartilage island with temporalis fascia to understand the usefulness of this technique in tympanoplasty.

2. Material and Methods

2.1 Patients

151 ears of 151 patients with chronic otitis media were operated by the same surgeon in Eulji Medical Center between March 2002 and August 2005.

Tympanoplasty type I using Thin Section Cartilage Island Technique had been performed in 101 ears and tympanoplasty with fascia in 50 ears. The median age at operation with Thin Section Cartilage Island Technique and with fascia was 41.1 years and 38.1 years respectively. The number of men and women was 53 and 48 with Thin Section Cartilage Island Technique; and 31 and 19 with fascia.

2.2 Methods

All patients underwent the preoperative Eustachian tube function test. Patients with abnormal Eustachian tubal function, severe mucosal inflammation, or postoperative perforation of the tympanic membrane were excluded from this study. After the perichondrium on one side of the tragal cartilage was elevated, the attached perichondrium was cut partially in C-shape; afterwards it was trimmed to be 0.2–0.3mm and estimated by a micrometer.

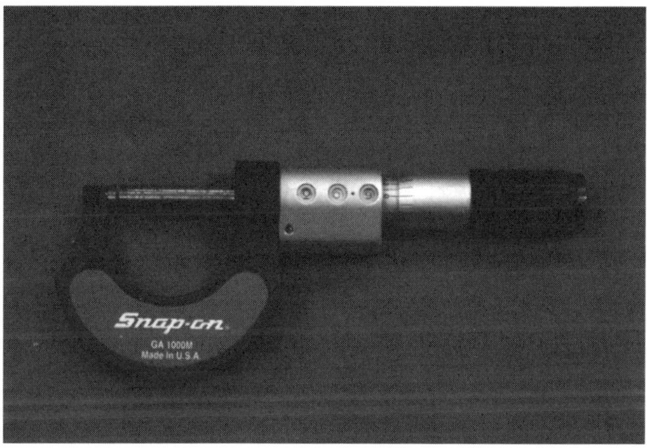

Fig. 1 Micrometer.

The endaural incision was made, and the tympanomeatal flap was elevated to expose the middle ear. The cartilage portion was placed at the perforation site of the tympanic membrane and the perichondrium was placed at the peripheral zone of the tympanic membrane and the tympanomeatal flap.

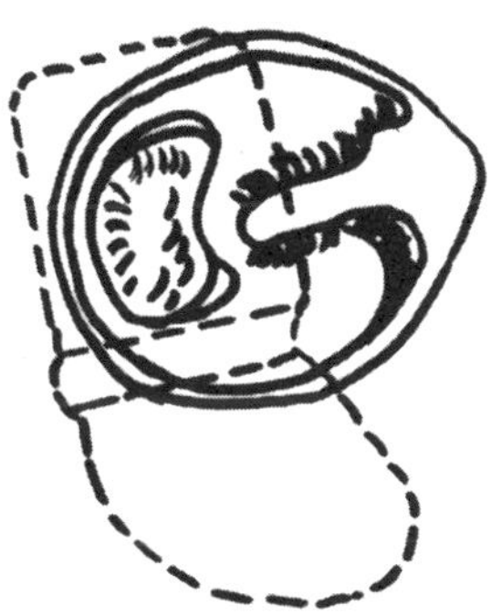

Fig. 2 Underlay graft.

Tympanometric measurements including static compliance, tympanometric width, and tympanometric pattern were done with a Middle-Ear Analyzer (Madsen Electronics ZODIAC 901) after 6 months postoperatively. For the statistical analysis, a χ^2 test was carried out to compare the thin section cartilage island with fascia technique.

3. Results

3.1 Static compliance

The static compliance measurements in the fascia group (n=50) showed that 33 cases (66%) were in the normal range (0.2~1.6ml); 15 cases (30%) showed values of less than 0.2ml and 2 cases (4%) more than 1.6ml. The static compliance of thin section cartilage island graft (n=101) were as follows: 73 cases (72%) within the normal range of 0.2~1.6ml; 22 cases (22%) with less than 0.2ml and 6 cases (6%) with more than 1.6ml. Statistical analysis showed that there was no significant difference between the two groups.

Table 1 Graft material and static compliance.

(P-value > 0.05)

	temporalis fascia graft	thin sliced cartilage island graft
<0.2ml	15(30%)	22(22%)
0.2~1.6ml	33(66%)	73(72%)
1.6ml<	2(4%)	6(6%)
Total	50	101

3.2 Tympanometric width

The tympanometric width indicates the pressure difference between two points on the tympanogram curve where the compliance is half the static compliance.

The results show that the fascia group (n=50) had 7 cases (14%) of normally ranged tympanometric width (60~150mmH_2O); 27 cases of under ranged tympanometric width (< 60 mmH_2O); and 16 cases (32%) of over ranged tympanometric width (> 150 mmH_2O). The tympanometric width of the thin section cartilage island graft group (n=101) were as follows: 60 cases (59%) of 60~150 mmH_2O (normal range); 18 cases (18%) of

< 60 mmH_2O; and 23 cases (23%) of > 150 mmH_2O. There was no significant difference between the two groups.

Table 2 Graft material and tympanometric width.

(P-value > 0.05)

	temporalis fascia graft	thin sliced cartilage island graft
<60mmH_2O	7(14%)	18(18%)
60~150mmH_2O	27(54%)	60(59%)
150mmH_2O<	16(32%)	23(23%)
Total	50	101

3.4 Tympanometric pattern

There were 31 A types (62%), 7 B types (14%), and 12 C types (24%) in the fascia group and 68 A types (67%), 11 B types (11%) and 22 C types (22%) in the Thin Section Cartilage Island Graft group. No significant difference between the two groups was found.

Table 3 Graft material and tympanometric pattern.

(P-value > 0.05)

	temporalis fascia graft	thin sliced cartilage island graft
A type	31(62%)	68(67%)
B type	7(14%)	11(11%)
C type	12(24%)	22(22%)
Total	50	101

4. Discussion

It has been very common to use the perichondrium or fascia in tympanoplasty, in spite of its unacceptable results in cases of tubal dysfunction, adhesive process, tympanic fibrosis, or entire tympanic membrane defect [9]. Several authors preferred to use the cartilage of conchae or tragus in cases of middle ear pressure change [10][11][12]. However, the increased mass and stiffness of thick materials could influence the acoustic transfer properties.

Adkin et al. reported that air conduction threshold depression was 5~10 dB in cartilage grafting. Therefore, they used it only in limited cases. According to other studies there was no significant difference in hearing between graft with fascia and cartilage [8][13][14][15]. We agree that mass and stiffness effect of thick cartilage may lead to high frequency hearing loss. As Zahnert has suggested earlier, thin sections less than 0.5mm could be acceptable as a role of transformer [5].

The fascia has elastic fibers with irregular arrangement and unpredictable and irregular gaps between fibers which are filled with fibrous connective tissue. Therefore it often contracts and is being thickened. Such unstable properties make a surgeon look for other graft material such as tragal or conchal cartilage that is stable and easy to take at the operation field. The cartilage is very useful for its resistance to contraction and absorption in cases of tubal dysfunction, total perforation, or adhesive otitis media [14][16].

Thin section cartilage cannot reach a posterior meatal flap adequately for its limited size and firmness. In order to solve this problem, the authors have developed a thin section cartilage island technique using the section of cartilage attached to the perichondrium. Usually, the cartilage including perichondrium needs to be sectioned into less than 0.3~0.5mm for a proper sound conduction. While the conventional fascia has only fixed thickness, a variable thickness of graft material can be sliced according to the condition of middle ear and Eustachian tube. In this study, graft materials cartilage and fascia were compared by tympanograms which is an indirect method of assessing the sound conduction efficiency. There was no statistical significance between the two techniques observable in static compliance, tympanometric width, and tympanogram type, which are the major parameters of the tympanogram representing the mobility of tympanic membrane. This means that the thin section cartilage island could be similar to fascia in terms of the mobility. However, additional investigations maybe needed to determine whether this applies also to the sound transfer.

5. Conclusion

The authors have compared the conventional fascia technique with the thin section cartilage island by a tympanometric method. Static compliance, tympanometric width and type of tympanogram showed no statistically significant difference between the two techniques. Therefore, this type of surgery could be performed in ordinary cases such as chronic otitis media.

Reference

1. Wullstein H., Theory and practice of tympanoplasty. *Laryngoscope* **66**(1965) pp.1076–1093
2. Zollner F., The principles of plastic surgery of the sound-conducting apparatus. *J Laryngol Otol.* **69**(1955) pp. 637–652
3. Glasscock M.E., House W.F., Homograft reconstruction of the ear. *Laryngoscope* **78**(1968) pp. 1219-1225
4. Sheehy J.L., Glasscock M.E., Tympanic membrane grafting with temporalis fascia. *Arch Otolaryngol.* **86**(1967) pp. 391–402
5. Uzun C., Thomasen P.C., Andersen J., Tos M., A tympanometric comparison of tympanoplasty with cartilage palisades or fascia after surgery for tensa cholesteatoma in children. *Laryngoscope* **113**(2003) pp. 1751–1757
6. Zahnert T., Hüttenbrink K.B., Murbe D., Bornitz M., Experimental investigations of the use of cartilage in tympanic membrane reconstruction. *Am J Otol.* **21**(2000) pp. 322–328
7. Murbe D., Zahnert T., Bornitz M., Hüttenbrink K.B., Acoustic properties of different cartilage reconstruction techniques of the tympanic membrane. *Laryngoscope* **112**(2002) pp. 1769–1776
8. Kirazli T., Bilgen C., Midilli R., Ogut F., Hearing results after primary cartilage tympanoplasty with island technique. *Otolaryngolory-HNS.* **132**(2005) pp. 933–937
9. Palva T., Surgical treatment of chronic middle ear disease. *Acta Otolaryngol.* **104**(1987) pp. 279–284
10. Hüttenbrink K.B., Surgical treatmrnt of chronic otitis media. *HNO.* **42**(1994) pp. 582–593
11. Dornhoffer J.L., Surgical management of the atelectatic ear. *Am J Otol.* **21**(2000) pp. 315–321
12. Heermann J., Heermann H., Kopstein E., Fascia and cartilage palisade tympanoplasty: nine years experience. *Arch Otolaryngol.* **91**(1970) pp. 228–241
13. Adkins W.Y., Composite autograft for tympanoplasty and tympanomastoid surgery. *Laryngoscope.* **100**(1990) pp. 244–247
14. Milewski C., Composite graft tympanoplasty in the treatment of ears with advanced middle ear pathology. *Laryngoscope* **103**(1993) pp. 1352–1356
15. Amadee R.G., Mann W.J., Riechelmann H., Cartilage palisade tympanoplasty. *Am J Otol.* **10**(1989) pp. 447–450
16. Elasfour A.A., Zaghloul H.S., Cartilage tympanoplasty: audiological and otological outcome. *International Congress Series.* **1240**(2003) pp. 73–79

DO NON-PISTON COMPONENTS CONTRIBUTE TO SCALA VESTIBULI PRESSURE BEHIND THE FOOTPLATE IN GERBILS?

W.F. Decraemer[1], O. de La Rochefoucauld[2], W. Dong[2], S.M. Khanna[2], J.J.J. Dirckx[1], E.S. Olson[2]
[1] Univ. of Antwerp, Biomed. Physics, 177 Groenenborgerlaan, B 2020, Antwerp, Belgium
[2] Columbia Univ., Dept. of OTO / HNS, 630 West 168th St., New York, NY 10032, USA

Keywords: 3-D stapes motion, scala vestibuli pressure

In recent papers we have shown that the mode of vibration of the ossicular chain in cat and human temporal bones is more complex than a simple rotation about a fixed axis and that it also changes with frequency. For the stapes e.g. it was shown that rotations of the footplate about its long and short axis are present besides the predominant piston-like velocity component. As the footplate motion gives rise to the pressure wave set up in the cochlea, we investigated whether the non-piston components contribute to the pressure produced in the gerbil cochlea: 3-D vibration velocity of the stapes along with the scala vestibuli pressure were measured in the same animals. We found no correlation between non-piston components and scala vestibuli pressure.

1. Introduction

The motion of the stapes footplate produces the acoustical input into the cochlea. The mode of stapes vibration has been studied mainly in human temporal bones (for an overview: [1,2]) and in a few animal models (anesthetized cat [3], cat temporal bone: [4,5,6]). It is now quite well established that the motion is not purely piston-like but that at higher frequencies rotations about the long and short footplate axis are also present ("rocking", "tilting"). Whether the non-piston motion components are functionally important is still an open question. An argument in favor is the remarkable ability of the middle-ear to produce a gain between the sound pressure in the ear-canal and the acoustic pressure in the perilymph of the scala vestibuli (directly behind the footplate) that is a very smooth function of frequency, while the frequency response of the piston component of the stapes exhibits some maxima and minima. This is especially prominent when we compare gain and motion curves not averaged over experiments of different individual preparations. Could it be that tilting of the footplate of the stapes fills in the gaps in the frequency response of the piston component resulting in a smoother pressure frequency response in the cochlea? Trying to answer this question we have measured in succession scala vestibuli pressure and 3-D vibration velocity of the stapes in the same animals (gerbil) and studied their correlation.

2. Material and Methods

Young adult Mongolian gerbils with healthy ears were used for this study. The animal preparation is described in detail in [7]. The external ear canal (EC) was cut to its bony end and a small plastic tube was cemented in place to hold the sound delivery tube. A probe tube microphone (B&K) measured the sound at about 1 mm from the superior edge of the pars tensa (EC pressure).

Scala vestibuli (SV) pressure directly behind the footplate (distance ~ 0.3mm) was measured with a miniature pressure sensor (Φ = 170 μm, [7,8]) inserted about 0.2 mm deep in a small, hand drilled hole in the cochlea (for a figure with the pressure location, see [9] Fig.1)

The stapes was exposed through a large opening of the bulla and its motion was measured from different viewing angles for single tone stimuli over a wide frequency range (200 Hz–1 kHz, step 200 Hz; 1 kHz–10 kHz, step 250 Hz; 10 kHz–20 kHz, step 500 Hz; 20 kHz–40 kHz, step 500 Hz). SPL for constant input to the driver was between 80 and 90 dB, in the linear range of the middle ear [8]. The procedure and equipment used are described in [10].

The rigid body global translation and rotation about the origin were calculated and transformed in the intrinsic reference system shown in Fig. 1 (z-axis towards reader); piston motion is translation along y and footplate tilt about the long and short axes are rotations about x and z, respectively.

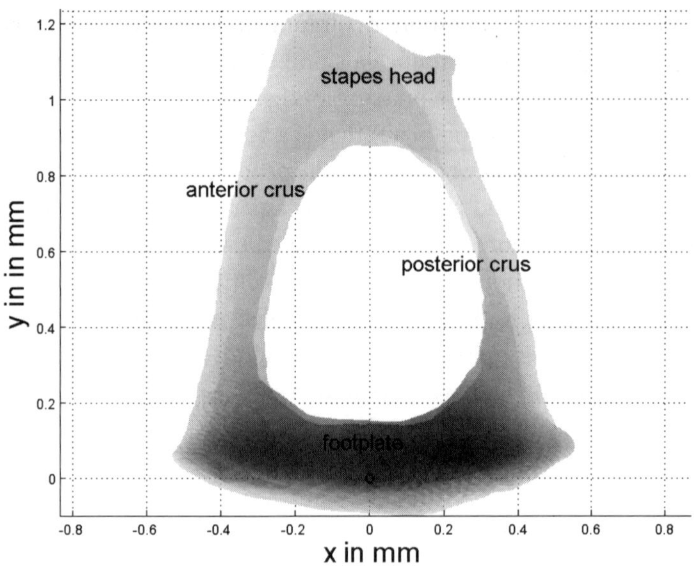

Fig. 1 Model of a gerbil stapes in an intrinsic reference system. (z-axis completing right-handed frame, directed out-of-plane). Piston motion is along the y-axis.

3. Results and Discussion

3.1 Scala vestibuli pressure

Pressure in the scala vestibuli, measured with a calibrated pressure sensor, relative to EC pressure, is shown for 3 animals, 20m4, 25m4 and 27m4, in Fig. 2. The curves represent the pressure gain produced in the middle ear: the gain amplitude (Fig. 2A) was a very smooth function of frequency, fluctuating in a small band around a level of 10 (20.0 dB) with extreme values of 3 (9.5 dB) and 20 (26.0 dB). The low frequency onset for all 3 animals showed a fast increase in gain amplitude towards a small maximum at about 1.5 kHz, then there was a steady decrease to about 6 kHz, where the gain was again somewhat higher in a short frequency interval ending with a small dip at 10 kHz. For animal 25m4 (dashed-dotted line) the gain was remarkably constant all the way up to the highest frequencies. Animals 20m4 and 27m4 had a broad and shallow minimum at 30 kHz, followed by a rise to its overall highest values.

Phase for all 3 animals were very similar (Fig. 2B): the 3 curves started at +0.25 cycle at 190 Hz, rapidly decreased to 0 cycle at about 1.5 kHz (here the amplitude showed a small peak), then decreased further to about 6 kHz where a small peak was formed (here the amplitudes produced a dip). From then on the phases for all animals decreased linearly with frequency and a total phase lag of about −1.5 cycle is built up at 40 kHz.

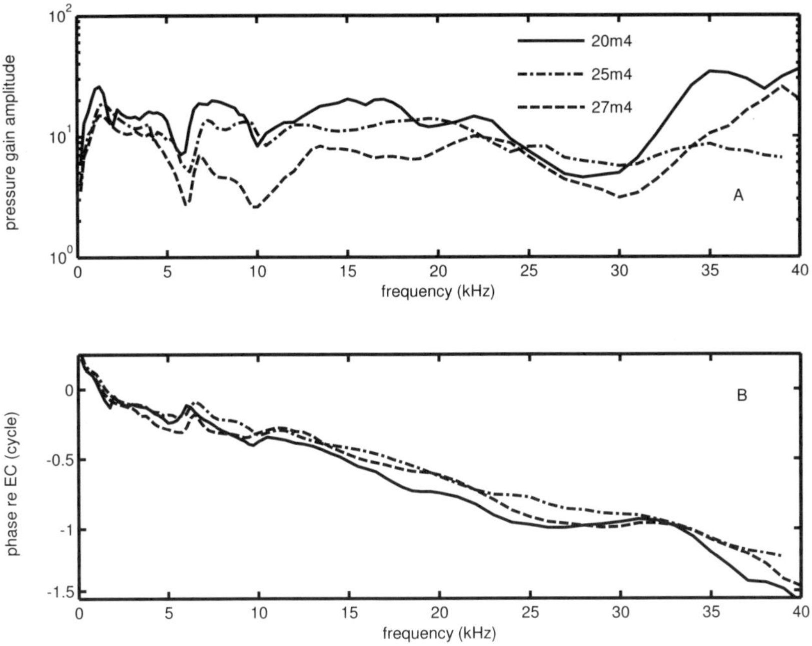

Fig. 2 Middle ear pressure gain is shown for 3 animals. Gain amplitude (panel A) is very smooth with frequency and varies in a small band around a level of ~10 (20.0 dB). Gain phase (panel B) is very similar for all 3 animals and shows a gradual decrease with frequency to a total phase lag of about −1.5 cycle at 40 kHz.

3.2 SV pressure versus piston velocity

In Fig. 3 we compare the stapes piston velocity per EC pressure (thin solid line) with the pressure gain (thick solid line) for animal 27m4, as already shown in Fig. 2. To plot gain and linear velocity on the same axis we multiplied the velocity by a scale factor shown in the figure caption of Fig. 3. The piston velocity component rel. EC pressure is not as smooth a function of frequency as the gain amplitude (Figs. 3A). We show only results for 1 animal but the gross trend of the curves for all 3 animals is fairly comparable. At the very lowest frequencies piston velocity increases more slowly with frequency than the pressure gain; some clear but minor peaks in piston velocity amplitude (total change +/− 6 dB) are not seen in the pressure (27m4: @ 10 and 15 kHz). Some dips in the piston amplitude are accompanied by dips in the pressure (27m4: @ 6 kHz), but sometimes this is not true and a peak in amplitude occurs at dip in pressure (27m4 @10 kHz). Disregarding these small wiggles the piston velocity is quite flat in a wide frequency band from 2.5 to 32.5 kHz (also for 20m4 and 25m4, not shown) and the amplitude stays high up to the highest frequencies measured.

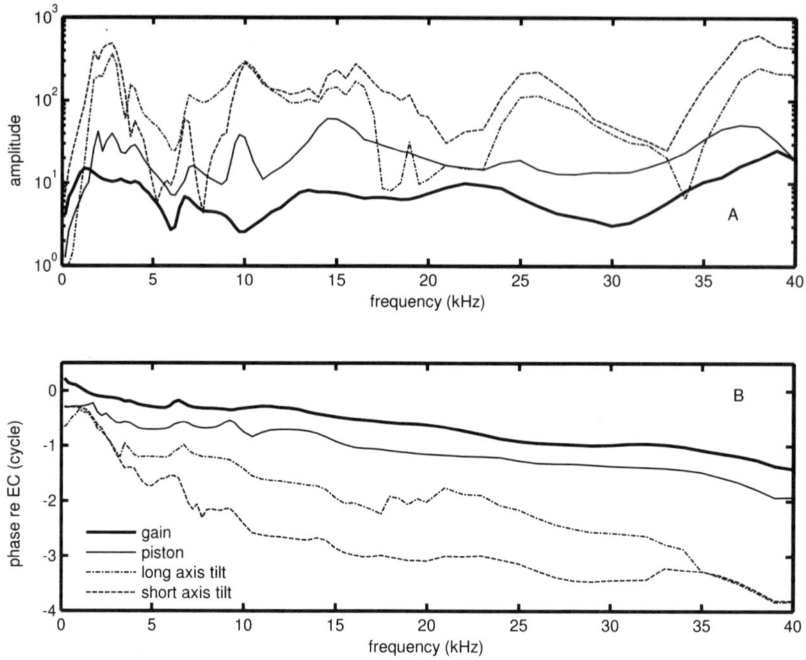

Fig. 3 Amplitude (A) and phase (B) of the pressure gain (SV pressure relative to EC pressure, thick solid line) as a function of frequency for animal 27m4. The piston component velocity (thin solid line) and angular velocities about the long axis (dashed-dotted line) and short axis (dashed line) of the footplate are plotted as well to correlate pressure and velocity. To plot the amplitudes of the velocities on the graph in the scale of the gain, the piston velocity is expressed in units of 10^{-5} (m/s)/Pa, and the angular velocities in 10^{-3} (rad/s)/Pa. (Please refer to the text for further discussion).

3.3 SV pressure versus footplate tilt

Pressure in the inner ear is produced when the footplate compresses the fluid in the cochlea and therefore mainly displacements perpendicular to the footplate will induce pressure. The motion components that give rise to such displacement are the piston component of the translation and the tilt of the footplate about its short and long axes. At first it seems reasonable to exclude the tilting from producing a pressure that can propagate further down the cochlea. Let us nevertheless hypothesize that there might be a mechanism that makes rotations effective in sound transmission. If we allow tilting modes to contribute to the pressure generation and play a role in smoothing of the pressure gain versus frequency curve, we must look for frequency bands where the piston amplitude is small and where this is compensated by high angular amplitude. The effect does not have to be large as there are no frequencies where the piston amplitude goes through a deep minimum. We see (Fig. 3A) that dips in piston amplitude are not systematically accompanied by highs in tilt amplitude. A deep minimum in piston amplitude, not reflected in the pressure would have been a conclusive proof, but it does not occur.

Conversely we see that strong maxima or minima in tilt are not reflected in pressure indicating that tilt can only play a minor role. The same argument is supported by the fact that phase of the tilt motion does not seem to play a role (Fig. 3B). If pressure were generated partly by tilt and partly by piston motion, phase differences between the two kinds of motion should also play a major role in the net pressure production. In frequency regions where the phase difference between the tilt and piston is varying in a different way with frequency (this is in regions where the piston and tilt phase curves are not running parallel to each other), we do not see any systematic effect of this on the pressure curve.

4. Conclusion

We have presented measurements of the 3-D velocity components of the stapes and have correlated these measurements with the SV pressure to verify whether non-piston components of the footplate produce pressure behind the footplate and thus can also eventually give rise to an effective input to the cochlea and can help in realizing the remarkably smooth and flat pressure gain from EC to scala vestibuli as a function of frequency. We found no evidence for this hypothesis: dips in the piston velocity are not systematically filled by peaks in tilt and conversely peaks in tilt are not repeated in the SV pressure. Further we found that SV pressure and piston velocity correlate well overall but differences in trends of the curves are also present.

Acknowledgments

Support by NIH/NIDCD, E. Capita Fund, FSR (Flanders, Belgium) and RAFO (Univ. of Antwerp).

References

1. Heiland K.E., Goode R.L., Masanori A. and Huber A., A human temporal bone study of stapes footplate movement. The Am. Jour. of Otolog. **20**, (1999) 81–86
2. Hato N., Stenfelt S. and Goode R.L., Three-dimensional stapes footplate motion in human temporal bones. Audiol. Neurootolog. **8**, (2003) 140–152
3. Guinan J.J. and Peake W.T., Middle-ear characteristics of anesthetized cats. J. Acoust. Soc. Am. **41**, (1967) 1237–1261

4. Decraemer W.F., Khanna S.M., Funnell W.R.J., Measurement and modelling of the three-dimensional vibrations of the stapes in cat, Proceedings of the Symposium on Recent Developments in Auditory Mechanics, Eds. H. Wada, T. Takasaka, K. Ikeda, K. Ohyama and T. Koike, World Scientific (2000) 36–43
5. Decraemer W.F., Khanna S.M., New insights in the functioning of the middle-ear. The function and mechanics of normal, diseased and reconstructed middle-ears. Ed by J.J. Rosowski and S. Merchant. Kugler Publications, The Hague, The Netherlands, (1999) 23–38
6. Olson E.S. and Cooper N., Stapes motion and scala vestibuli pressure. Abstracts of the 23rd Annual Midwinter Research Meeting, St-Petersburg Beach, Fla, USA, abstract #399, (2000) p 114 (can be read at http://www.aro.org/abstracts/abstracts.html)
7. Olson E.S., "Intracochlear pressure measurements related to cochlear tuning", J. Acoust. Soc. Am. **110** (1), (2001) 349–367
8. Olson E.S., "Observing middle and inner ear mechanics with novel intracochlear pressure sensors", J. Acoust. Soc. Am. **103** (6), (1998) 3445–3463
9. Dong W. and Olson E.S., "Middle ear forward and reverse transmission in gerbil", J. Neurophysiol. **95**, (2006) 2951–2961
10. Decraemer W.F., Khanna S.M., de La Rochefoucauld O., Dong W., Dirckx J.J., Olson E.S., "Estimation of stapes piston motion with uni-directional measurements is prone to error", Memro2006 Proceedings

MECHANICAL EXCITATION OF COMPLEX STAPES MOTION IN GUINEA PIGS

Albrecht Eiber, Christian Breuninger, Institute of Engineering and Computational Mechanics, University of Stuttgart, Pfaffenwaldring 9, 70550 Stuttgart, Germany
Email: eiber.breuninger@itm.uni-stuttgart.de

Damien Sequeira, Alexander Huber, Department of Otorhinolaryngology, Head and Neck Surgery, University Hospital of Zurich, Switzerland
Email: Alex.Huber@usz.ch, Damien.Sequeira@usz.ch

As observed in many studies the natural vibration pattern of the stapes on acoustic stimulation reveals a complex motion pattern dependent on the frequency of excitation. Whereas for low frequencies the motion is predominantly piston-like, significant rocking can be found for higher frequencies. The cochlea fluid is mechanically exited by the piston-like motion and two rotational movements along the short and long axis of the footplate. The rotational components produce no net volume flux of the cochlea fluid and, therefore, their influence on the hearing sensation is still an open question. To investigate the response of the cochlea on complex motion of the stapes footplate, different vibration pattern on the stapes have been mechanically applied in anesthetized guinea pigs.

A test rig was built to position the subject, an actuator and a Laser Doppler Vibrometer adjustable by micro manipulators. A three-axis piezoelectric actuator has been designed and coupled to the stapes head of the surgically prepared guinea pig by a coupling rod. For capturing the effective motion of the stapes three-dimensional laser Doppler vibrometry was applied. The excitation procedure for arbitrary stapes motion consists of both an identification and a measurement phase to determine the transducer behavior and the electrophysiological measurements of the cochlea response on the applied motion. Spatial velocity of stapes and cochlea potentials on repeated transducer activation are captured simultaneously by the data acquisition system for appropriate post-processing.

The task of driving arbitrary motion patterns yields a much higher complexity than classical one-dimensional consideration. The setup enables investigations in electrocochleography with different amounts of piston and rocking-like motions of the stapes.

1. Introduction

As a result of the spatial middle ear structure in normal ears, the vibration modes of the stapes in response to acoustic stimulation shows complex movement patterns [1]. These complex, frequency-dependent vibrations can be expressed as one translational displacement perpendicular to the footplate of stapes and two rotational movements around its long and short axes. In the lower frequency range the motion is predominant piston-like, significant rocking is observed at higher frequencies [2]. Whereas the piston-like motion of the stapes footplate induces a global volume displacement of the perilymph in the scala vestibuli, a pure rotational motion primary results only in local fluid displacements. In the classical hearing theory a hearing sensation is evoked only by piston motion, while for rocking motion no cochlear activity is expected. It is the goal of this study to prove this hypothesis experimentally by electrophysiological measurements in guinea pigs.

An acoustic stimulation applied to the middle ear excites always piston and rocking motions of stapes in combination. Particularly, rocking motion without piston motion can not be achieved in the lower audible frequency range. To drive a stapes in so called elementary motions, i.e. pure piston and pure rocking separately, a mechanical excitation of the isolated stapes structure was realized by coupling a mechanical actuator to the stapes head. The response of the cochlea due to piston and rocking motion is determined by measuring cochlear potentials. The actual elementary motions are measured by a three-dimensional Laser Doppler Vibrometer (3D-LDV) focused on the stapes head.

This paper is concerned with the realization of the mechanical excitation of the stapes motion and its measurement, while the evaluation of the cochlear potentials is discussed in [3].

2. Material and Methods

2.1 General aspects

For statistical evaluation, especially measuring cochlear potentials, a high number of repeated measurement data is needed. To get consistent data sets, it is highly important that the physical condition of subject, the positioning of electrodes and the experimental setup be not changed during measurement. The used multi-axis actuator, capable to stimulate piston and rocking independently, reduces the difficult and time consuming task of positioning the subject with respect to LDV and coupling the actuator to the stapes head without any predeformation.

2.2 Test rig

Since for a spatial, mechanical excitation and measurement of the stapes, a predefined position of stapes, stimulator and velocity sensor is needed, a test rig was built up using commercial aluminium profiles as shown in Figure 1 to align subject, actuator and laser vibrometer. It is installed in a sound-proof, electromagnetic radiation-shielded cabin, while all measurement devices are placed outside. Structural vibrations of the frame are suppressed by damping elements in the profiles and by a vibration-isolated desk.

The guinea pig is placed such that the stapes can be aligned in parallel to the frame of the test rig with respect to an intrinsic coordinate system oriented along the short and long axes of the stapes footplate and perpendicular to it. Actuator and laser are inclined such that the stapes head is accessible by the actuator needle and the three laser beams. By means of micromanipulators (M-332.3MS / M-333.1MS, Physik Instrumente (PI) GmbH & Co. KG, Karlsruhe, Germany) the position of the subject is adjusted to focus all three laser beams on the stapes head. Subsequently, with a micromanipulator (MM-3, Narishige Scientific Instruments Lab., Tokyo, Japan), the actuator needle is attached to the stapes. A firm coupling of actuator needle and stapes head is realized by a thread inside the hollow needle, tighten around the stapes head by a noose.

2.3 Three-axes piezoelectric actuator

A custom-built actuator was designed to fulfill the described requirements of producing motion in any desired direction by using three piezoelectric stacks spaced at 120° intervals to drive the actuator head. The body of the actuator is mounted on the micromanipulator. The stacks are driven by the voltage $\boldsymbol{u}_{\mathrm{Piezo}} = [u_1\ u_2\ u_3]$ supplied by common audio power amplifiers.

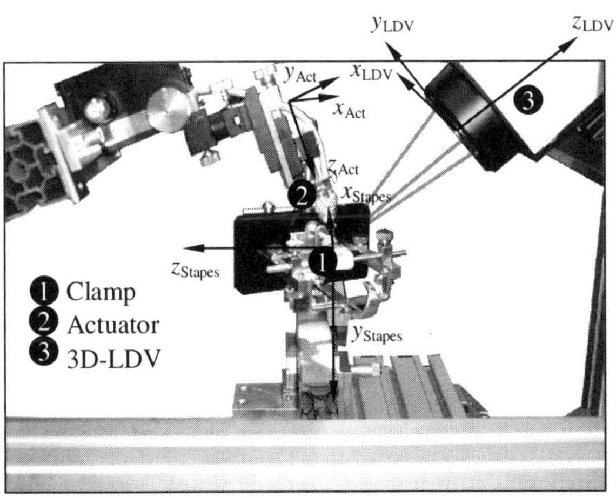

Fig. 1 Clamping support for subject, actuator and 3D-Laser Doppler Vibrometer with its local coordinate systems.

For an ideal actuator in the quasi-static frequency range, the transformation from the elongation of the piezoelectric stacks to needle motion $\boldsymbol{y}_{\mathrm{Act}} = [x_{\mathrm{Act}}\ y_{\mathrm{Act}}\ z_{\mathrm{Act}}]$ in the actuator's coordinate system is a pure geometric property. Due to uncertainties of the setup parameters, e.g. length of the coupling needle and in particular to determine the dynamic behavior up to 10 kHz, an identification of actuator's frequency response function $\boldsymbol{H}(j\omega)$ is carried out. This 3-by-3 matrix yields the relationship $\boldsymbol{y}_{\mathrm{Act}} = \boldsymbol{H}(j\omega)\cdot\boldsymbol{u}_{\mathrm{Piezo}}$ in the frequency domain.

2.4 Three-dimensional Laser Doppler Vibrometry

The 3D-LDV (CLV-3D sensor head, CLV-3000 controller, Polytec GmbH, Waldbronn, Germany) generates three independent laser beams with an incidence angle of 11.6° with respect to the sensor head's longitudinal axis. Hence, the laser beams are crossing at the focal point at a distance of 160 mm from the sensor head's lens defining the measurement point.

The velocity signals along the laser beams are processed in the geometry module of the controller yielding to the velocity components $\boldsymbol{v}_{\mathrm{LDV}}$ in the coordinate system of the sensor head. The velocities in the stapes head coordinate system $\boldsymbol{v}_{\mathrm{Stapes}} = [v_x\ v_y\ v_z]$ are obtained by means of the transformation $\boldsymbol{v}_{\mathrm{Stapes}} = \boldsymbol{S}_{\mathrm{SL}}\cdot \boldsymbol{v}_{\mathrm{LDV}}$ with the rotation matrix $\boldsymbol{S}_{\mathrm{SL}}$ between sensor head and stapes.

2.5 Actuator control

Unlike acoustical stimulus using a loudspeaker, the mechanical excitation of the isolated stapes structure by means of an actuator allows any arbitrary complex motion by superposition of the elementary motions. Nearly pure rocking motion can be applied even in the lower audible frequency range. The actuator control and data acquisition are performed by a real time processor from dSPACE GmbH, Paderborn, Germany, in interaction with the software MATLAB running on a PC.

For a desired motion $\boldsymbol{y}_{\mathrm{Stapes,des}} = [x_{\mathrm{Stapes}}\ y_{\mathrm{Stapes}}\ z_{\mathrm{Stapes}}]$ of the stapes head the actuator needle has to perform the motion $\boldsymbol{y}_{\mathrm{Act}} = \boldsymbol{S}_{\mathrm{AS}} \cdot \boldsymbol{y}_{\mathrm{Stapes,des}}$ according to the rotation matrix $\boldsymbol{S}_{\mathrm{AS}}$ of the actuator orientation with respect to the stapes. By help of the frequency response function of the actuator identified before, the time history $\boldsymbol{u}_{\mathrm{Piezo}}(t)$ of the voltages for driving the three piezoelectric stacks is obtained by the time domain correspondent relation of $\boldsymbol{u}_{\mathrm{Piezo}}(j\omega) = \boldsymbol{H}^{-1}(j\omega) \cdot \boldsymbol{y}_{\mathrm{Act}}(j\omega)$.

2.6 Click design

In case of acoustical stimulation, commonly a sharp click at the loudspeaker is used. Due to a strong low-pass behavior of the dynamic subsystems of loudspeaker, tube to conduct the sound pressure to the ear drum, ear canal and middle ear this click gets strongly low-pass filtered. In mechanical excitation the dynamic chain consists only of stapes and actuator showing a much faster response than in acoustic stimulation. Consequently, an excitation with a higher frequency content can be applied to the cochlea. Even more, by the described control of the actuator, a nearly arbitrary time history of desired motion $y_{\text{Stapes,des}}(t)$ at the stapes head can be applied.

For these investigations, a click for the desired motion of the stapes head was used as shown in Figure 2. This excitation procedure results in a frequency spectrum of excitation similar to an acoustical stimulation with a very short click.

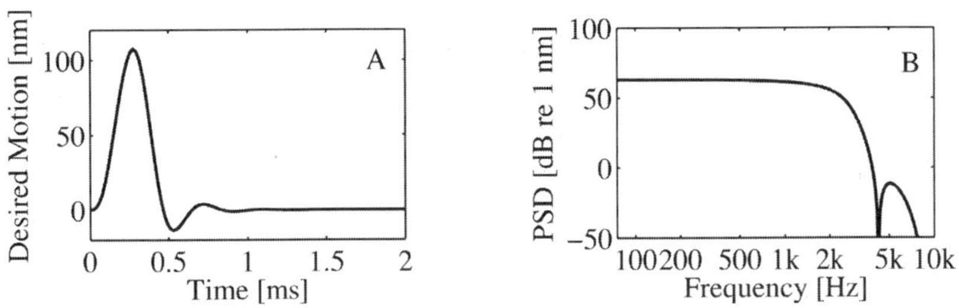

Fig. 2 A: Shape of desired motion of stapes head. B: Spectrum of desired motion.

3. Results and Discussions

The voltage $u_{\text{Piezo}}(t)$ of excitation clicks for piston motion and rocking motion about the long and short axis of the stapes footplate is applied in repetitive cycles of 200 times in intervals of 79 ms. Stapes motion and cochlear response are measured simultaneously and averaged with respect to the cycles to reduce measurement noise. The displacements $y_{\text{Stapes}} = [x_{\text{Stapes}}\ y_{\text{Stapes}}\ z_{\text{Stapes}}]$ of the stapes head are obtained by an integration of the measured stapes velocities.

A typical measurement series is shown in Figure 3. The measured displacements show a predominant motion in the desired direction of excitation. The amplitudes in the other directions are much smaller. The corresponding spectra have a bandwidth up to approximately 3 kHz. Again, the magnitude of the undesired components are about 30 to 40 dB below the desired one.

For these three dominant motions, cochlear potentials with different amplitudes are observed. The greatest potential resulted from translational displacement, but potentials from rocking motions are not negligible.

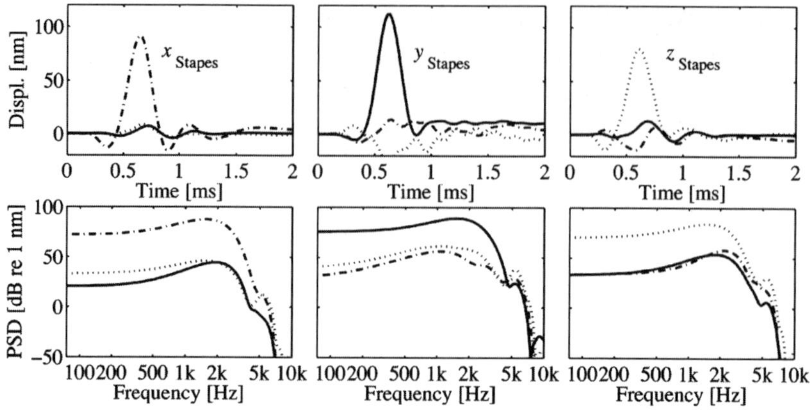

Fig. 3 Time history and spectra of desired elementary motions measured at the stapes head. Piston motion y (solid line), rocking x about short axis (dashed line) and rocking z about long axis (dotted line). Left: Predominant rocking about short axis. Middle: Predominant piston motion. Right: Predominant rocking about long axis.

4. Conclusions

Mechanical excitation of the stapes offers more detailed investigations in electrocochleography compared to classical acoustic stimulation. In particular, the direction of excitation as well as its shape and frequency content can be varied in a wide range. This requires a more complicated experimental setup, a very sensitive and time consuming preparation and a precise positioning of the subject. The developed setup with a three-axes actuator and 3D-LDV sensor is a system to excite and measure predefined motions of the stapes in guinea pigs. Elementary motions, i.e. pure translational piston motion and pure rocking motion, can be defined and nearly achieved in the experiments leading to predominant piston motions and predominant rocking motions of stapes. The subject and actuator can be precisely aligned without giving a statical preload to the stapes. Short clicks with an arbitrary shape can be applied to the prepared guinea pig. Different motion patterns can be imposed by external control while the complete experimental setup remains untouched.

References

1. Decraemer W.F. and Khanna S.M., Measurement, Visualization and Quantitative Analysis of Complete Three-Dimensional Kinematical Data Sets of Human and Cat Middle Ear. In Gyo K. and Wada H. (Eds.) *Proceedings of the 3rd Symposium on Middle Ear Mechanics in Research and Otology.* World Scientific, Singapore, 2004, pp. 3–10
2. Heiland K., Goode R., Asai M. and Huber A., A human temporal bone study of stapes footplate movement. *Am J Otol,* **20** (1999), pp. 81–86
3. Sequeira D., Breuninger C., Eiber A. and Huber A., The effects of complex stapes motion on the response of the cochlea in guinea pigs. In Huber A. and Eib A. (Eds.) *Proceedings of the 4th Symposium on Middle Ear Mechanics in Research and Otology.* World Scientific, Singapore, 2007.

THE EFFECTS OF COMPLEX STAPES MOTION ON THE RESPONSE OF THE COCHLEA IN GUINEA PIGS

Damien Sequeira[1], Christian Breuninger[2], Albrecht Eiber[2], Alexander Huber[1]
[1] Department of Otorhinolaryngology, Head and Neck Surgery,
University Hospital of Zurich, Switzerland
[2] Institute of Engineering and Computational Mechanics, University of Stuttgart,
Germany

Studies into the vibration modes of the stapes in response to acoustic stimulation of the normal ear have revealed a complex movement pattern of its footplate. These complex vibrations can be expressed as one translational displacement and two rotational movements around the long and short axes of the stapes, known as the three elementary motions. According to the classical theory of hearing, the rotational motions induce no volume displacement of cochlear fluid and, therefore, no cochlear activity (i.e. hearing sensation). It is the goal of this study to verify this hypothesis.

A custom-built, three-axis piezoelectric actuator, capable of eliciting any desired vibration mode, was coupled to the surgically prepared stapes superstructure of anesthetized guinea pigs. When producing different movement patterns, electrophysiological measurements of the cochlear potentials were simultaneously recorded.

Mechanical stimulation of the stapes according to the three elementary motions delivered three cochlear potentials of different amplitude. The greatest potential resulted from translational motions.

The results of the present study show a cochlear excitation in all performed movement patterns of the stapes. Hence, the prevailing hypothesis could not be verified.

1. Introduction

Based on recent studies into the vibration modes of the stapes, the normal ear, when responding to acoustical stimulation, exhibits a complex movement pattern of its footplate. Low frequency vibrations exhibit predominantly piston-like motions, which increasingly evolve into rocking-like motions at middle and high frequencies [1, 2]. These complex vibrations can be decomposed into one translational and two rotational movements around the long and short axes of the stapes. Inward translational movements result in an increase of fluid pressure in the scala vestibuli, producing a pressure gradient between the scala vestibuli and the scala tympani, which contains the round window that is a flexible boundary to the ambient middle-ear air pressure. This pressure equalizes by generating a fluid bulk shift that excites the basilar membrane and launches a traveling wave [3].

However, the rotational components of the stapes motion produce no net volume displacement of cochlear fluid at the oval window, since the inward movement of a certain volume on one side of the stapes axis leads to outward movement of an equal volume on the other side. Therefore, no bulk pressure change is induced at a certain distance from the oval window. As the effective stimulus to the cochlea is thought to be the pressure difference between the oval and round windows [4], rotational motion of the stapes represents lost energy that is not transformed into a hearing sensation. However, this hypothesis has never been tested experimentally.

The present study aims to record the electrophysiological activity of the inner ear in response to mechanical excitation of the stapes, as discussed in [5]. This would allow verification of the present hypothesis of sound propagation from the middle ear to the inner ear.

2. Materials and Methods

2.1 Animal preparation

The study was performed in five specific-pathogen-free female guinea pigs showing normal Preyer reflexes, hence disease-free middle ears. A prior two-week acclimatization period to the new environment was implemented. General anesthesia was carried out by means of intramuscular application of Ketamin (35mg/kg) and Xylacin (5mg/kg), as well as additional inhalation narcosis with Sevoflurane (0.4–2%). The guinea pigs were placed within an animal specific head-holder. After prior tracheotomy, the stapes was micro-surgically exposed as shown in Fig. 1. The animals were euthanized at the end of the experiment by an intraperitoneal barbiturate overdose.

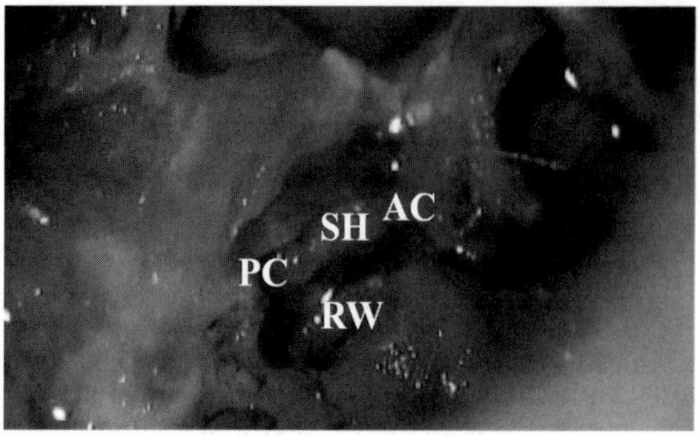

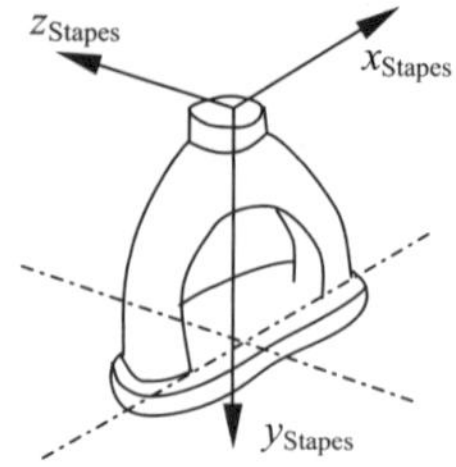

Fig. 1 Left: Intraoperative view of the stapes exposure in a right ear [AC = anterior crus, PC = posterior crus, RW = round window, SH = stapes head]. Right: Stapes with the corresponding coordinate system.

2.2 Mechanical stimulation & 3D-Laser Doppler Vibrometry

A custom-built cylindrical steel actuator with a mounted needle containing a noose was used for exciting the stapes in the three different motion patterns. The actuator, mounted on a micromanipulator, was carefully advanced to the stapes head under direct control of an operation microscope, until firm contact was obtained. The noose enclosed in the needle was then fastened around the stapes head. The stimuli were very short clicks of alternating phase with an interclick-interval of 79ms (Fig. 2, A–C).

A Helium-Neon (HeNe) based CLV-3D compact three-dimensional laser vibrometer (Polytec GmbH, Waldbronn, Germany) was focused on the stapes head. Subsequently, this allowed for both the monitoring and measurement of stapes superstructure displacements in the nanometer range over a wide range of frequencies [5].

2.3 Electrophysiological measurements

In the current experiment the recording of cochlear activity, namely the compound action potentials (i.e. CAP), was executed by means of a custom-made, silver-ball electrode placed in the round window niche of the anesthetized guinea pigs. The measurements were averaged in order to increase the accuracy of these potentials. Additionally, the entire experiment was carried out within a made-to-measure test stand placed on a vibration-free table and in a sound and electromagnetic-proof room.

The actuator stimulation and the recording of the resulting stapes motion and cochlear activity were driven by a computerized and analysis measurement system.

3. Results

The compound action potentials in response to mechanical stimulation, namely rarefaction and condensation clicks, were recorded over displacements ranging up to 200nm. To avoid trauma to the oval window, the maximum displacement level was 200nm.

Being able to generate predominant movement patterns from a single actuator, the stapes footplate vibrations were directly assessed using the three-dimensional laser Doppler vibrometer. The level of accompanying movements in the other two directions occurring while eliciting the desired prevalent vibration pattern was relatively small [5].

By repeating the stimulus for each specific displacement two hundred times, it was possible to obtain a representative cochlear response. The performed experiment showed electrophysiological excitation in all cases of desired movement patterns of the stapes. Thus, the measured compound action potentials were influenced by both translational and rotational vibration patterns as shown in Fig. 2. Occurring with predominantly rotational movements pattern were, nevertheless, small amounts of translational movement. However, the corresponding compound action potential was much greater than the equivalent compound action potential for a predominantly translational movement of equal amplitude. The most

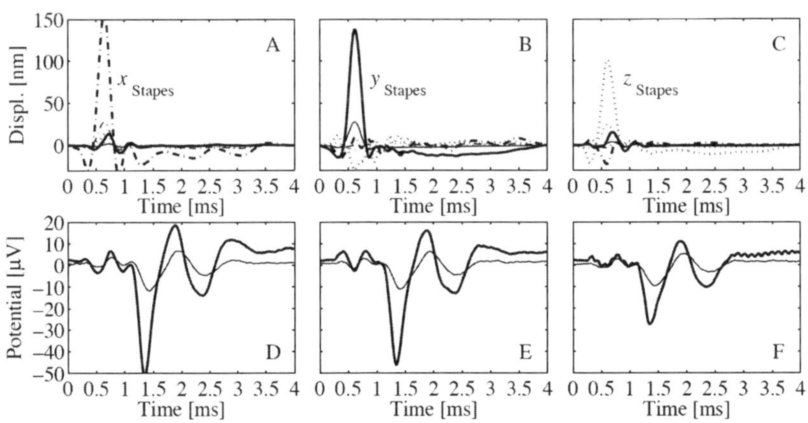

Fig. 2 Compound action potential [CAP] as a function of the displacement of the dominant movement pattern of the stapes. The upper three graphs depict the predominant movement pattern of a click of high and low intensity. A: x-motion inducing rocking-like movement around the short axis. B: y-motion inducing piston-like movement. C: z-motion inducing rocking-like movement around the long axis. The lower graphs represent the corresponding CAP: the thick line in response to a click of high intensity, and the thin line in response to a click of low intensity.

influential vibration mode being the translational movement produced electrical potentials of the highest amplitude. All types of motion induced trends by which increased displacement caused increased compound action potential amplitudes.

A correlation between the translational component of the actual displacement of motion and its corresponding electrophysiological reaction in response to positive clicks was plotted on a logarithmic scale as shown in Figure 3. This correlation depicted the corresponding translational movement patterns with and without the rotational components. Accordingly, the subsequent addition of these rotational motions revealed greater compound action potential amplitudes than for amplitudes in response to translational movement patterns alone. A higher correlation was achieved among rotational motions around the short axis, due to larger volume displacements of cochlear fluid. Hence, a linear relationship between the logarithm of displacement or logarithm of velocity, respectively, and cochlear response amplitudes was found in all three motion types.

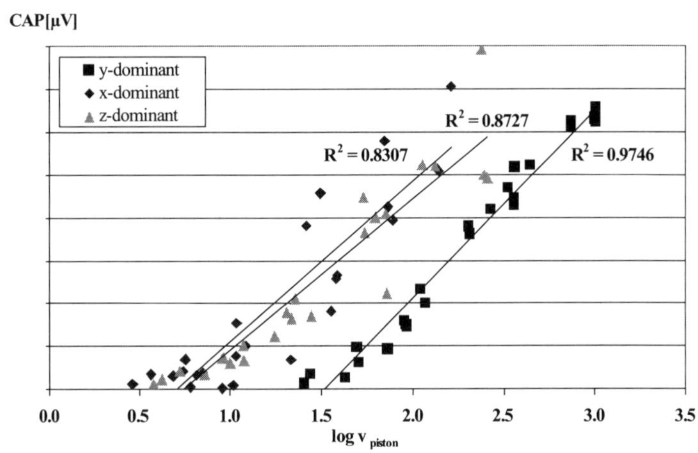

Fig. 3 Correlation between the piston-like velocity components of the actual displacement patterns of motion and its corresponding electrophysiological reaction in response to positive clicks.

4. Discussion

In the present study, it was possible to generate the three desired movement patterns in a preponderant fashion. The main objective was to test whether only translational stapes movements influenced cochlear activity, while rotational movements elicited no reaction.

Having obtained cochlear excitation in all performed movement patterns of the stapes, albeit of different amplitudes, the prevailing hypothesis could, therefore, not be verified. As a result of these findings, it can be concluded that both local pressure differences in the perilymph produced by rotational motions and global pressure differences produced by translational motions give rise to electrophysiological excitation from the stapes to the inner ear.

5. Conclusion

However, since the findings of the present study only represent a limited sampling size, these results need to be verified by a larger animal population size. This would then allow for the formulation of quantitative relations between the three elementary motions and their corresponding cochlear response.

These results have particular clinical relevance in the development of passive and active middle-ear prostheses as well as in the surgical techniques used to position them [6]. Furthermore, basic research into mathematical models of the middle ear and cochlea will need to consider the data presented here, since almost all such models assume that only the translational stimulus mode is effective at exciting the inner ear.

References

1. Decraemer W.F. and Khanna S.M., Three-dimensional vibration of the stapes measured with a heterodyne laser interferometer. In Tomasini E. (ed.) *Vibration Measurements by Laser Techniques: Advances and Applications.* SPIE, **3411** (1998), pp. 592–600
2. Heiland K., Goode R., Asai M. and Huber A., A human temporal bone study of stapes footplate movement. *Am J Otol,* **20** (1999), pp. 81–86
3. Dallos P., Cochlear Neurobiology. In Dallos P., Popper A.H. and Fay P.P. (eds.) *Handbook of auditory research: The Cochlea.* Springer, New York, 1996, pp. 1–43
4. Voss S., Rosowski J. and Peake W., Is the pressure difference between the oval and round windows the effective acoustic stimulus for the cochlea? *J Acoust Soc Am,* **100** (1996), pp. 1602–1616
5. Breuninger C., Sequeira D., Huber A. and Eiber A., Mechanical Excitation of Complex Stapes Motion in Guinea Pigs. In this edition
6. Eiber A., Freitag H.-G., Burkhardt C., Hemmert W., Maassen M., Rodriguez Jorge J. and Zenner H.-P., Dynamics of Middle Ear Prostheses – Simulations and Measurements. *Audiology & Neuro-Otology,* **4** (1999), pp. 178–184

FACTORS AFFECTING MEASUREMENT OF EAR-CANAL PRESSURE TO STAPES VELOCITY TRANSFER FUNCTION

Toshiki Maetani, M.D. [1,2], **Sunil Puria,** Ph.D. [2,3,4], **Richard L. Goode,** M.D. [2,3]

[1] Department of Otolaryngology, Head and Neck Surgery, Ehime University School of Medicine, Shitsukawa, Toon, Ehime, 791-0295, Japan
Email: maeta3@m.ehime-u.ac.jp
[2] Veterans Affairs Palo Alto Health Care System, 3801 Miranda Avenue, Palo Alto, CA
[3] Department of Otolaryngology, Head and Neck Surgery, Stanford University School of Medicine, 801 Welch Road, Stanford, CA
[4] Department of Mechanical Engineering, Stanford University, 496 Lomita Mall, Stanford, CA

Possible factors that affect measurement of the middle ear transfer function were investigated using human cadaveric temporal bones. As done by many others in the past, a laser Doppler vibrometer measured the stapes velocity (V_{st}) and a probe-tube microphone measured pressure (P_{ec}) in the external ear canal (EAC). The ratio of the two variables V_{st}/P_{ec} is the stapes velocity transfer function (SVTF). Three different types of experiments were conducted: (1) artificial vs. natural ear canal, (2) different locations of probe tube microphone relative to the eardrum, and (3) varying levels of humidity. The mean SVTF with artificial EAC (A-EAC) was similar as previously reported data, and the differences between SVTF with the natural EAC and that with A-EAC were less than 5.0 dB in magnitude up to 15 kHz and less than 45 degrees in phase angle. Significant differences between SVTF magnitude slopes with N-EAC and A-EAC were not detectable. The position of the probe-tube microphone (PT mic) significantly changed the SVTF at high frequencies. At 8 kHz 10 mm difference with the PT mic position caused 20 dB elevations in SVTF magnitude. The most influential factor that affects on SVTF at high frequencies was the position of the probe-tube microphone which is well known to be due ear canal acoustics. Dryness due to a decrease in humidity decreased the SVTF mainly at low frequencies.

1. Introduction

Laser Doppler vibrometry has played an important role for more than a decade for basic research of middle ear mechanics using cadaveric temporal bones or animals and for assessment of middle ear of living humans. This instrument is thought to be useful for diagnosis of conductive hearing impairment in some clinical cases with which conventional tympanometry cannot detect the cause of hearing impairment.

Recently stapes velocity (V_{st}) and/or umbo velocity (Vu) data has been reported in living and cadaver ears [1] - [7], [13]. Some measurements suggest that V_u of living humans is quite different from that with human cadaveric temporal bones at frequencies above 2 kHz. [6]. Even in cadaveric temporal bones there appear to be differences in V_{st} at frequencies above 2 kHz arising from possible methodological differences. For example, Aibara et al [8] report a SVTF magnitude slope of –7 dB/octave while O'Connor and Puria [9] report a slope of –2.3 dB/octave at frequencies above 2 kHz. Recently, Chien et al [7] report that some of these differences may be due to differences in the angle of the stapes velocity in relation to the translation axis of the footplate. The purpose of this study is to explore other methodological factors that may affect laboratory measurements of SVTF.

2. Materials and Methods

2.1 Materials

Twelve human cadaveric temporal bones were used that had been extracted from human cadaver within 48 hours after death using a Schuknecht bone saw; mean age was 72, ranging from 60 to 88 years old. These specimens were preserved with a 100 ppm merthiolate in normal saline solution at 5 degrees Celsius. Measurement on individual specimens was performed within 2 to 6 days after death. Abnormal and pathological bones were excluded by inspection using an operating microscope. Two ears were used to develop the procedures. Measurements from the remaining 10 ears are reported.

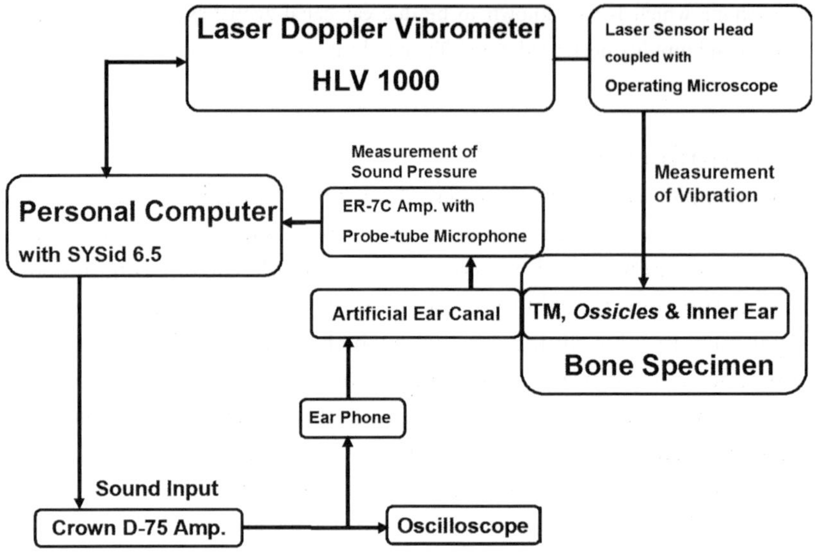

Fig. 1 Schematic representation of the measurement system.

2.2 Measurement system

As shown in Figure 1, all measurements were performed using SYSid 6.5 audio band measurement and analysis system (www.sysid.com, Berkeley, CA, U.S.A.). This software program in conjunction with a DSP-16+ processing board (Granbury, NJ, U.S.A.) produces an output signal used to drive a sound source, and synchronously measures and averages two channel input signals. The magnitude and phase angle at each frequency is obtained through fast Fourier transformation (FFT).

The sound stimuli were stepped tones swept over 200 logarithmically-spaced frequency points from 0.1 to 25 kHz in a manner similar to that described previously [11].

One of the input signals was sound pressure of EAC (P_{ec}) measured by a probe-tube microphone (ER-7C, Etymotic Research, Elk Grove Village, IL, USA) whose tip was placed within 2 mm from the tympanic membrane. In natural EAC experiments this tube was fed through the foam of the eartip into the canal space.

In the experiments with artificial EACs, a small hole was made near the medial end of the plastic tube, which was placed perpendicularly onto the bony tympanic ring as an artificial EAC, and an ER-7C tube was fed through this hole into the canal space, also within 2 mm from the edge of the tympanic membrane.

The second input is peak footplate velocity measured by a laser Doppler vibrometer (LDV) (HLV-1000, Polytec PI, Costa Mesa, CA, U.S.A.).

The LDV was set to the 5 ((mm/s)/V) velocity range, the 30 kHz low pass filter corner frequency, and with the high pass filter turned off.
PT mic and HLV laser calibrations have been previously described [7]. (Figure 2)

2.3 Data analysis

P_{ec} values are RMS values and V_{st} was expressed with the peak values. SVT-Fs were calculated as V_{st}/P_{ec} and its magnitude expressed logarithmically dB units defined as:

$$\text{TF dB} = 20 * \log10((V_{st}/P_{ec}) / 0.1)$$

Here 0 dB is set to 0.1 (mm/s)/Pascal.

Since it is usually hypothesized that the distribution of TF is log-normal, the geometric mean was calculated as the mean SVTF and expressed with units of dB. In other words it is the mean of logarithmic values of SVTFs [12].

2.4 Measurement angle correction

The angles between laser beam and the normal vector of the footplate or piston axis were estimated to be 45 to 60 degrees. V_{st} was calculated by dividing the measured velocity by cosine of 55 degrees at all frequencies so that cosine correction is considered to be within 3 dB as Hato and Stenfelt argued [8]. In this paper a frequency-dependent method was not taken as argued by Chien et al [6].

3. Results

3.1 Signal to noise ratio (SNR)

The noise floor level was measured in all 10 bones. In those ears the SNR of P_{ec} magnitude was more than 60 dB up to 15 kHz and about 60 dB at frequencies from 15 kHz to 25 kHz. The SNR of V_{st} was more than 40 dB up to 8 kHz, 35 dB from 8 kHz to 15 kHz and above 15 kHz the SNR was less than 20 dB.

3.2 Artifact levels

The promontory vibration was measured as the artifact level. It was more than 40 dB from 0.1 to 5 kHz, 20 to 40 dB from 5 to 15 kHz and less than 5 dB above 15 kHz.

3.3 Canal obliquity and SVTF

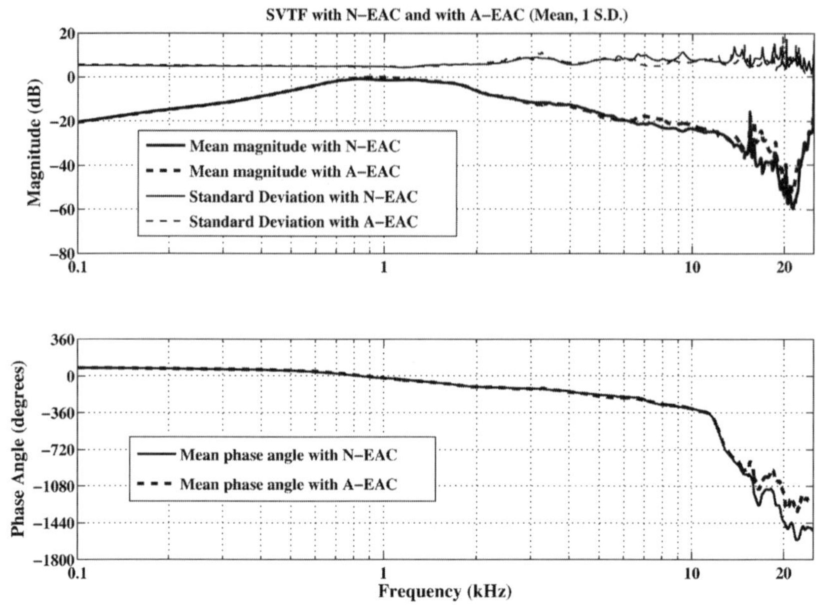

Fig. 2 The mean SVTF with the N-EAC and A-EAC (top figure: magnitude, bottom figure: phase). The magnitude standard deviations are shown above the 0 dB line, which corresponds to the reference of 0.1 mm/s/Pa.

In each of the ten bones, both the SVTF with natural EAC and with artificial EAC were measured within a 24-hour time interval. In experimental procedures, care was taken not to damage the ossicles, especially the footplate.

As shown in Fig. 2, differences in SVTF magnitude with N-EAC and that with A-EAC is within 2.0 dB up to 6 kHz and at 6 to 12 kHz differences were within 5.0 dB. The standard deviation of TF magnitude difference was 4 dB up to 4 kHz and that at 4 to 12 kHz was within 10 dB.

Differences in SVTF phase angle with N-EAC and that with A-EAC was less than 45 degrees below 12 kHz. The standard deviation of TF angle difference was within 45 degrees up to 4 kHz and at frequencies from 4 to 12 kHz within 120 degrees. Mean, SD and range of both SVTF were quite similar and it seemed that the canal obliquity does not affect on the SVTF.

3.4 PT microphone position and SVTF

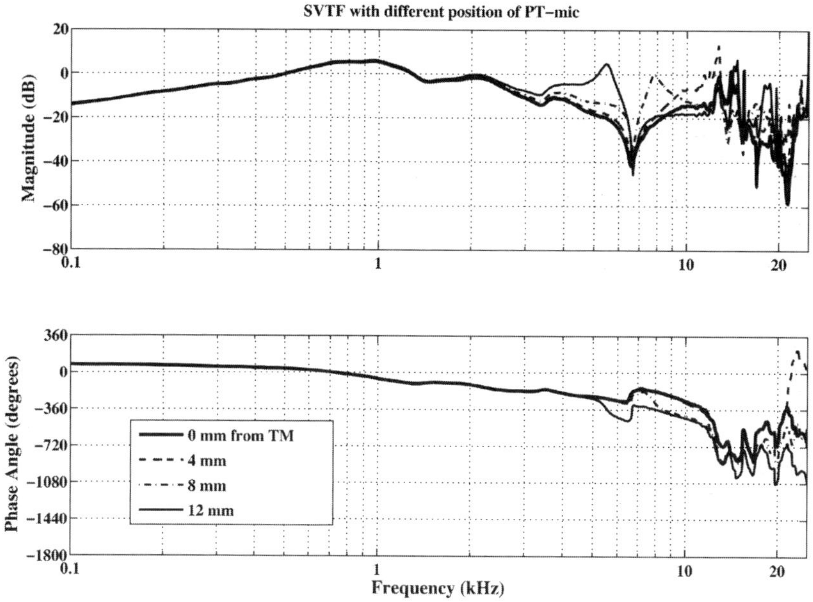

Fig. 3 SVTF (upper figure: magnitude, bottom figure: phase) measured at 4 different positions of the PT microphone tip. The 4 positions are the PT mic position 0 mm from the TM (thick solid), 4 mm the TM (dashed line), 8 mm from the TM (dashed-dot line), and 12 mm from the TM (thin-solid line).

To assess the effect of the position of the PT mic, SVTFs of a single bone with an artificial EAC was measured with different position of the PT mic. The position of the PT mic was set at 0, 2, 4, 6, 8, 10, 12 and 14 mm from the tympanic membrane.

As the PT mic position was moved laterally, P_{ec} magnitude decreased in the 2 to 10 kHz range. Not surprisingly, the PT mic position didn't affect V_{st}. The position of PT mic drastically affected on the measured SVTF values at high frequencies as Khanna and Stinson previously reported [9]. At 8 kHz the difference SVTF magnitude was 20 dB and even at 4 kHz the difference was nearly 10 dB. Since the quarter wavelength at 4 kHz is about 8.5 mm this result is consistent with basic acoustic theory. With this bone V_{st} at 7 kHz was quite low but the reason of this dip remains uncertain.

3.5 Humidity and SVTF

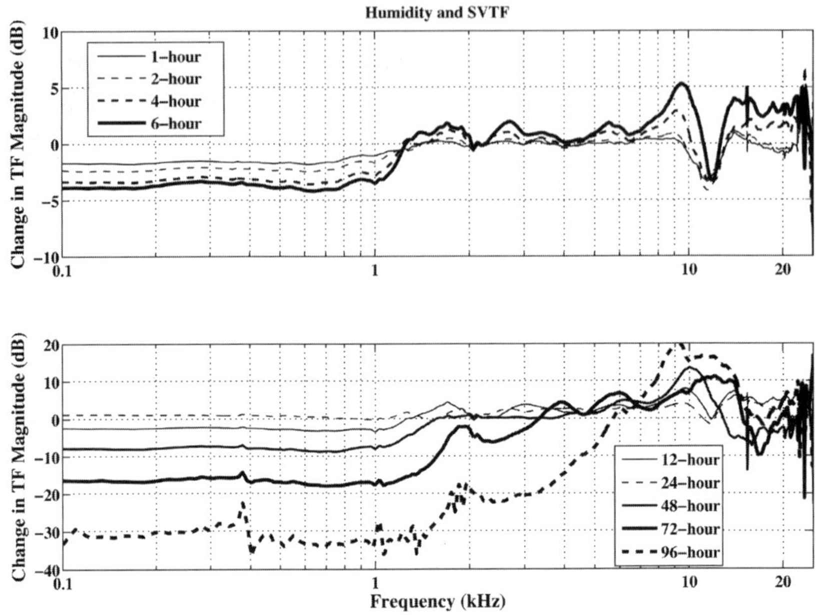

Fig. 4 Change in SVTFs under dry circumstances within 6 hours (top figure: 1, 2, 4, 6 hours; bottom figure: 12, 24, 48, 72, 96 hours). SVTF values were normalized by the initial values (SVTF|T=0). In this period it was sunny and the relative humidity decreased rapidly.

To assess the effect of dryness on SVTF, measurements were repeated for 4 days with a single temporal bone.

This bone had been left in the lab without artificial application of humidity source (i.e., no saline spray or humidifier) throughout the measurement period. The measurements were made at 0, 1, 2, 3, 4, 6 hours (Figure 4, top) and12, 24, 48, 72, 96 hours (Figure 4, bottom) after the initial measurement.

The room temperature was kept constant at approximately 23 degrees Celsius, but the relative humidity varied from 20 to 47 %. Apparently the room humidity was directly influenced by surrounding atmospheric humidity due primarily to changes in the weather. Since the experiment was performed in the rainy season the humidity was comparatively high and it increased when it rained hard (data not shown). Dryness decreased the SVTF by 15 dB at low frequencies by leaving the specimen in a room with 20 to 47 % relative humidity for 3 days. On the contrary, at 8 kHz dryness increased the SVTF by 10 dB for 3 days. These results indicate that in a six hour measurement period, the length of typical laboratory measurements, dryness can affect measurements of SVTF by up to +/– 5 dB if no external humidity is applied.

4. Discussion

Since many factors can affect stapes velocity (V_{st}) and transfer function (V_{st}/P_{ec}), they were classified into two categories. First is the subjective factor which is intrinsic to the bone itself. Pathological bones are excluded but there is certainly some inter-individual variation.

The other factors not intrinsic to the bone are subdivided into storage factors, bone-preparation factors, measurement factors (due to different methodology in experimental settings and instruments), and computation methods. In this paper factors of experimental setting or measurement factors were focused on.

4.1. Canal obliquity

The external ear canal has anatomically complex shape. We hypothesized that due to the oblique position of the eardrum in the ear canal, the medial tapering may amplify the sound energy that enters the EAC at high frequencies. The phase angle of the anterior part of the TM is delayed in terms of that of the posterior part due to the difference in the distance from the sound source. It might cancel or add due to EAC tapering. The results suggest that our hypothesis was incorrect. There does not appear to be an effect due to canal obliquity.

4.2. Position of PT mic

Sound input parameters of auditory system are typically specified in terms of sound pressure level of a single point in the EAC.

When human cadaveric temporal bones are used for the research of auditory system, bony canal is drilled down and a plastic tube as an artificial ear canal is set onto the tympanic annulus perpendicularly and a probe-tube microphone is fixed near the tympanic membrane.

On the other hand in clinical settings it is hard to place the probe-tube microphone near the tympanic membrane. The distance between the annulus and the PT mic is estimated to be 5 to 10 mm since the isthmus of the EAC is located from 7 mm from the annulus. It may cause the difference or error in calculating the middle ear transfer function. In this experiment the effect of the PT mic position was investigated. In this setting, the position of the reflectors (measurement point) and the ear plug, the angle of the laser beam was exactly identical so that the difference in SVTF should be caused only by the difference in the PT mic position.

The PT mic position has an effect on the measured P_{ec} values exclusively which resulted in changes to the calculated SVTF values.

Otolaryngologists should keep in mind that some factors can affect P_{ec} exclusively, the denominator of SVTF, and those values do not always reflect the actual sound energy that enters the EAC at high frequencies. Thus it is also the case with clinical measurements of otoacoustic emissions.

4.3. Humidity

Although some authors [4] mentioned that dryness can affect the SVTF drastically, analytic assessment has not been made. In this paper we measured the effect of humidity but it seems is that this experiment was preliminary and still semi-quantitative. But the tendency that as the relative humidity decreased the SVTF magnitude at low- and mid-frequencies decreased in a manner consistent with an increase in stiffness of the soft tissue (the tympanic membrane and the annular ligament).

5. Summary

Three possible factors that affect the middle ear transfer function were investigated. Significant difference between SVTF with natural EAC and artificial EAC were not measured. As expected the position of the probe-tube microphone and humidity appear to be two important factors.

Acknowledgments

Work supported in part by grant No. DC 05960 from the NIDCD of NIH.

References

1. Goode R. L., Ball G. and Nishihara S., Measurement of umbo vibration in human subjects – methods and possible clinical applications. *Am. J. Otol.* **14** (1993) pp. 247–251
2. Goode R. L., Ball G. and Nishihara S., Laser Doppler vibrometer (LDV) – a new clinical tool for the otologist. *Am. J. Otol.* **17** (1996) pp. 813–822
3. Huber A.M., Schwab C., Linder T., Stoeckli S. J., Ferrazzini M., Dillier N. and Fisch U., Evaluation of eardrum laser Doppler interferometry as diagnostic tool. *Laryngoscope* **111** (2001) pp. 501–507
4. Rosowski J. J., Mehta R. P. and Merchant S. N., Diagnostic utility of laser-Doppler vibrometry in conductive hearing loss with normal tympanic membrane. *Otol. Neurotol.* **24** (2003) pp. 165–175

5. Ruggero M. A. and Temchin A. N., Middle-ear transmission in humans: wide-band not frequency-tuned? *Acoust. Res. Letter Online* **4** (2003) pp. 53–58
6. Whittemore Jr. K. R., Merchant S. N., Poon B. B. and Rosowski J. J., A normative study of tympanic membrane motion in human using a laser Doppler vibrometer (LDV). *Hear. Res.* **187** (2004) pp. 85–104
7. Chien W., Ravicz M. E., Merchant S. N. Rosowski. J. J., The effect of methodological differences in the measurement of stapes motion in live and cadaver ears. *Audiol. Neurootol.* **11** (2006) pp. 183–197
8. Aibara R., Welsh J. T., Puria S. and Goode R. L., Human middle-ear sound transfer function and cochlear input impedance. *Hear. Res.* **152** (2001) pp. 100–109
9. O'Conner K. N. and Puria S., Middle ear cavity and ear canal pressure-driven stapes velocity responses in human cadaveric temporal bones. *J. Acoust. Soc. Am.* **120** (2006) in press, pp. 1517–1528
10. Hato N., Stenfelt S. and Goode R. L., Three-dimensional stapes footplate motion in human temporal bones. *Audiol. Neurootol.* **8** (2003) pp. 140–152
11. Khanna S. M. and Stinson M. R., Specification of the acoustical input to the ear at high frequencies. *J. Acoust. Soc. Am.* **77** (1985) pp. 577–589
12. Puria S., Measurements of human middle ear forward and reverse acoustics: implications for otoacoustic emissions. *J. Acoust. Soc. Am.* **113** (2003) pp. 2773–2789
13. Huber A., Linder T., Ferrazzini M., Intraoperative assessment of stapes movement. *Ann. Otol. Rhinol. Laryngol.* **110** (2001) pp. 31–35

ACUTE TYMPANIC MEMBRANE PERFORATIONS HEAL WITHOUT SIGNIFICANT LOSS OF STRENGTH

M. von Unge, Karolinska University Hospital, Stockholm
Email: magnus.von.unge@ki.se
J.J.J. Dirckx, Bimef, University of Antwerp, Belgium
A Rahman, Karolinska University Hospital, Stockholm, Email: Anisur.Rahman@ki.se
M. Hultcrantz, Karolinska University Hospital, Stockholm
Email: Malou.Hultcrantz@karolinska.se

1. Introduction

The physical and mechanical properties of the tympanic membrane (TM) such as area size, mass, stiffness and 3D-shape defines its vibratory pattern in response to the sound waves and thereby modulates the perception of sound. Changes in some of these parameters will alternate the auditory function of the ear (1, 2). Inflammatory middle ear diseases cause structural aberrations of the TM resulting in changes in its mechanical properties (2–4). There may be changes as well in these parameters after a TM perforation has healed. It has been stated that the healed wound does not recover its complete tensile strength as before although the perforation would heal efficiently (5). There are very few reports on the strength of the TM after perforations have healed.

The aim of the present study was to adjust a moiré interferometry set up for displacement measurements on the Sprague-Dawley rat temporal bone, and to ascertain the degree of the functional and structural restitution of the healed TM following a traumatic fresh perforation.

2. Material and Methods

Ten healthy female Sprague Dawley young adult rats of approx. 300g BW were used. The animals were anesthetized with 100 mg ketamine hydrochloride and 10 mg xylazin hydrochloride intraperitoneally and myringotomy was performed in the right TM using a 0.2 mm KTP laser beam with

0.5 seconds single pulses of 1 Watt. Thereby a calibrated TM perforation was produced. The perforation was made in the upper posterior quadrant. The left TM was left untouched and was used as a normal control. Otomicroscopic inspection was performed thrice a week and the healing pattern was documented. The animals were sacrificed at 2 or 4 weeks (five in each group) after myringotomy. Measurements were made at the University of Antwerp, Belgium.

2.1 Moiré interferometry measurements/moiré principle

Moiré interferometry is an optic, non-contacting technique for shape or deformation measurements. A ruling of straight lines is projected onto the surface of an object and the image of these projected lines is recorded with a video camera. By electronically subtracting images obtained on different object states, interference fringes are obtained. These fringes represent contours of equal object shape or deformation. By subtracting images obtained on an object and on a flat plane, moiré fringes are obtained which correspond to contours of equal object height, and thus display the membrane shape like lines on a topographic map. From these so called "moiré topograms" full field deformation data are obtained. In order to get sufficient moiré fringe image quality white china ink is put behind the eardrum, from the ear canal side.

2.2 Physiological processing

Ten temporal bones were prepared for full-field moiré interferometry measurements of the TM: the tympanic bulla was opened widely, the tensor tympani muscle was cut and part of the medial wall of the tympanic cavity was removed. The incudo-stapedial joint was disarticulated and the stapes was removed. The malleus and incus with their ligaments were kept untouched.

Dehydration of the isolated temporal bone was prevented by performing all the procedures under the air steam of an evaporator according the method of von Unge (6, 7). A plastic tube mimicking the external auditory canal was glued to the bony meatus of the ear canal, through which sequences of static pressures were applied to the ear canal, thereby producing a pressure gradient across the TM. In steps of 50 daPa a first positive sequence was given, starting at 0 daPa increasing up to 350 daPa, and from here back to 0 daPa in descending order. Then a similar sequence but with negative pressures was given. The time interval between each step was 10 seconds (6).

2.3 Morphologic processing

After the interferometry measurements the temporal bones were fixated and decalcified with EDTA according to standard procedures and were studied in light and electron microscope.

3. Results

All perforations were closed, as judged by otomicroscopy, between 9 and 14 days post myringotomy.

3.1 3-D shape

Ten rat and ten mouse ears were recorded. The TM is mounted in the measuring set-up so that the baseline coincides approximately with the plane of the annulus. Thereby the moiré fringes outline the height of the various portions of the TM in relation to the annulus. The peak is located around or at the umbo. The mean peak height for the group was 6.8×10^{-4} m (range, 6–8).

Ten TMs with closed perforations were recorded. There were no significant differences in the patterns of the studied TMs in any of the two groups, as compared with the normal controls. The mean peak height for the group was 7.3×10^{-4} m (range, 7 – 8). There was no statistical difference as compared with the normal controls.

3.2 Displacement

Seven control TMs and eight TMs with closed perforation were successfully recorded in a pressure sequence going up to +350 daPa and down to –350 daPa. As the pressure in the external ear canal is increased a first moiré fringe becomes visible in the center of the posterior portion of the pars tensa followed by a first fringe in the anterior portion. With increasing pressure the fringe expands and its contour moves in centrifugal direction so that it gets closer to the annulus and to the handle of malleus. Meanwhile a second fringe may appear in the same location as the first one did, and so on. The contours of the moiré fringes were compared in the two groups without any notable discrepancy between the two groups.

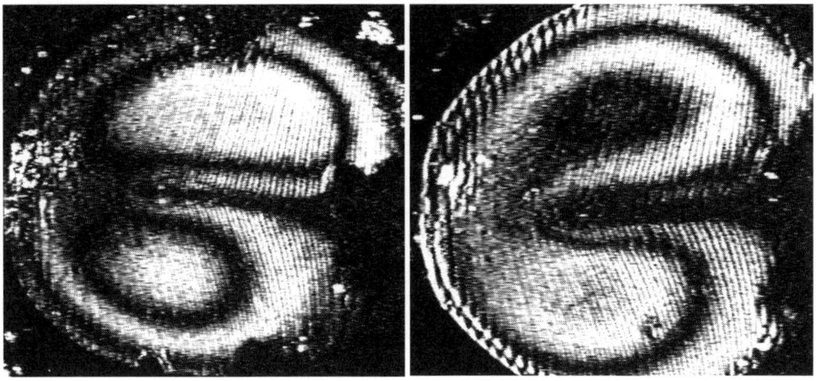

Fig. 1 Displacement interferogram at an ear canal pressure load of 350 daPa of a) normal left TM and b) myringotomized right TM recorded at two weeks after the intervention. Ad a) number two fringe is present in anterior and posterior portion of TM. Ad b) number two fringe is present in posterior portion of TM and hinted in anterior portion.

The peak displacement values were calculated for each ear at each pressure level. Around zero pressure a small pressure alteration induces relatively large displacement, whereas at higher pressures relatively large pressure alterations are needed to induce the same change in displacement. Thereby a displacement versus pressure curve plot displays an "S"-shape (fig. 2). The mean peak displacement at 350 daPa was 2.40×10^{-4} m with a standard deviation of 0.39 for the control group and 2.37×10^{-4} m with a standard deviation of 0.79 for the myringotomized ears. At minus 350 daPa it was 3.20×10^{-4} m with a standard deviation of 0.79 for the controls and 3.14×10^{-4} m with a standard deviation of 0.94 for the studied ears. There seems to be a somewhat larger displacement in the lower pressure range for the studied ears as compared with the controls. The differences are however very small and they are not statistically significant.

In all TM a hysteresis effect was observed, but there were no obvious differences in the hysteresis magnitude between the two groups.

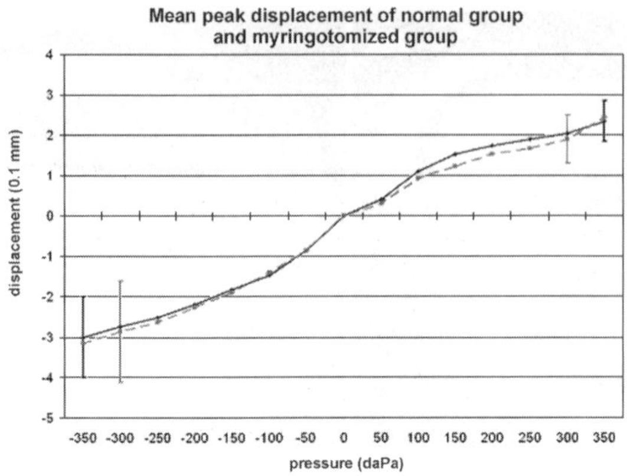

Fig. 2 Mean peak displacement versus pressure in the normal control group and in the myringotomized group. Results obtained during increasing pressurization from zero to 350 daPa and from zero to −350 daPa. Standard deviation indicated with error bars for a few pressure levels. Almost coinciding curve plots.

3.3 Morphology

In light microscopy the pars tensa of the rat TM appears homogenous over its entire surface whereas the site of closed myringotomy appears thicker. The thickness is almost constant in its various portions. In transmission electron microscopy the three layers are readily identified: the dominating lamina propria with its densely packed fibrous bundles and on both sides consisting of thin (outer and inner) epithelial layers (fig. 3). The overall thickness of the pars tensa is approximately 5 μm. In the region of a closed perforation a five-fold thickening is present. The increased thickness consists of invading fibroblasts and large amounts of extra cellular substance. This substance of scar tissue contains fiber-like structures that do not appear densely packed as those in the lamina propria. This tissue does not only cover the site of the myringotomy, but is also spread out around this site and is here located on the medial side of the remaining lamina propria. The epithelial layers appear normal.

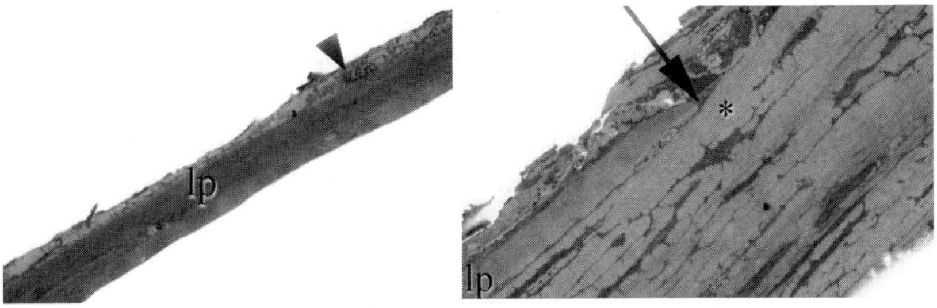

Fig. 3 Transmission electron microscopy, 2.500x, of a) a normal pars tensa, and b) a TM with closed perforation. Note the border of the lamina propria at the perforation site (arrow). Arrowhead in fig. a indicates the outer epithelial layer. The thickness is fivefold increased at the myringotomy site due to invaded fibroblasts and extra cellular matrix (asterisk). lp = lamina propria.

4. Discussion

A purpose of this study was to evaluate the degree of the morphological and functional competence that was restituted in the post-traumatic healing process. As of today chronic TM perforations are most commonly treated with surgical transplants of temporalis fascia, perichondrium or cartilage. Several other substances have been tried out, such as dermal allograft (8), various types of growth factors (9), human type IV collagen, live yeast cell derivatives etc. So far no real alternative to conventional surgical procedures have been presented.

Our aim for a series of investigations is to try out possible remedies for chronic TM perforations as an alternative to open surgery. In order to do so some basic data on the healing of perforations are needed. In the present report we evaluated a set-up for measurements of the strength of the rat TM. The rat was chosen since, among other reasons, there is an established chronic perforation model in rat (10). A moiré interferometry set up was modified in order to perform such measurements on the rat TM.

Our second aim was to establish reference knowledge on the functional outcome of closure and healing of fresh perforations where no infection is at hand and when healing conditions are unimpaired. By using a laser beam for myringotomy the size and location of the perforation thus created was accurately done in a reproducible way. It is the first time data are presented on the strength of the recently closed perforation the TM, with the exception of our previous pilot study on gerbil ears treated with stem cells (11). The most exciting finding in the present report is the almost completely restored static mechanical function, i.e. pressure resistance in the TM already after two weeks. The histology sections reveal a fivefold increase of thickness due to scar tissue formation without an obvious system of orientation. It appears that the lack of fiber orientation is compensated by the large amount of fibers that are produced at the myringotomy sites. The result as tested with moiré interferometry indicates that this action of nature is appropriate in the sense that the strength or resistance to pressures is restored. This healing process, with an "overproduction" of fiber-like structures that do not exhibit an obvious system of orientation, is of utmost clinical importance. Even this recently closed perforated TM has to withstand the challenges of pressure gradients that occur in every day life (sneezing, coughing etc). It may be that over a longer time period the fibers will become reorganized in a more efficient way similar to that of the lamina propria, and thereby the thickness of the TM may be restored. Such an effect may be of importance for hearing. It has been found empirically that "underlay" myringoplasty, where the transplanted tissue is placed medial to the remnant of the TM, is preferable to overlay. The reason has never been proven. This procedure results in a structural situation similar to the repair process as found in the present study.

5. Conclusions

The static stiffness properties of the rat TM can be measured with moiré interferometry. The functional properties as regards pressure resistance are mainly restored already at two weeks after laser myringotomy in the model. The lack of systematic fiber orientation in the closed perforation appears to be compensated by increased amount of tissue.

References

1. von Unge M., Bagger-Sjöbäck D., Tympanic membrane changes in experimental otitis media with effusion. *Am J Otol* 1994; **15**: 663–669
2. von Unge M., Decraemer W.F., Bagger-Sjöbäck D. *et al.*, Tympanic membrane changes in experimental purulent otitis media. *Hear Res* 1997; **106**: 123–136
3. von Unge M., Decraemer W.F., Dirckx J.J. *et al.*, Shape and displacement patterns of the gerbil tympanic membrane in experimental otitis media with effusion. *Hear Res* 1995; **82**: 184–196
4. von Unge M., Decraemer W.F., Dirckx J.J. *et al.*, Tympanic membrane displacement patterns in experimental cholesteatoma. *Hear Res* 1999; **128**: 1–15
5. Cotran R.S., Kumar V., Collins T., Tissue Repair: Cellular growth, fibrosis and wound healing. In: *Pathologic basis of disease. eds: W.B Saunders Co.* 1999: 107–109

6. von Unge M., Decraemer W.F., Bagger-Sjöbäck D. *et al.*, Displacement of the gerbil tympanic membrane under static pressure variation measured with a real-time differential moiré interferometer. *Hear Res* 1993; **70**: 229–242.
7. von Unge M., Bagger-Sjöbäck D., Borg E., Mechanoacoustic properties of the tympanic membrane: a study on isolated Mongolian gerbil temporal bones. *Am J Otol* 1991; **12**: 407–419.
8. Laidlaw D.W., Costantino P.D., Govindaraj S. *et al.*, Tympanic membrane repair with a dermal allograft. *Laryngoscope* 2001; **111**: 702–707.
9. Amolis C.P., Jackler R.K., Lustig L.R., Repair of chronic tympanic membrane perforations using epidermal growth factor. *Otol Head and Neck Surg* 1992; **107**: 669–683.
10. Spandow O., Hellström S., Animal model for persistent tympanic membrane perforations. *Ann Otol Rhinol Laryngol* 1993; **102**: 467–472
11. von Unge M., Dirckx J.J., Olivius N.P., Embryonic stem cells enhance the healing of tympanic membrane perforations. *Int J Ped Oto* 2003; **67**: 215–219

BOOST OF TRANSMISSION AT THE PEDICLE OF THE INCUS IN THE CHINCHILLA MIDDLE EAR

Mario A. Ruggero, Andrei N. Temchin, Yun-Hui Fan, Hongxue Cai
Institute for Neuroscience and Hugh Knowles Center (Dept. of Communication Sciences and Disorders), Northwestern University, Evanston, IL, USA
Email: mruggero@northwestern.edu, a-temchin@northwestern.edu, yhfan@northwestern.edo, h-cai@northwestern.edu

Luis Robles, Dept. of Physiology and Biophysics, Faculty of Medicine, Universidad de Chile, Santiago, Chile, Email: lrobles@med.uchile.cl

We re-examined ossicular vibrations in the widely opened middle ear of the chinchilla, a species with a relatively narrow hearing bandwidth, similar to that of humans. The magnitude of vibration velocity at the head of the stapes is relatively constant (~0.3 mm/s/Pa) up to 24 kHz, thus exceeding the bandwidth of hearing in chinchilla (<20 kHz). Phase lag relative to pressure in the external ear canal increases approximately linearly between 0 and 20 kHz, with a slope equivalent to a pure delay of 76 μs. The present findings support the contention that, in general, the middle ears of amniotic vertebrates do not limit the bandwidth of hearing. The magnitude of vibration of the incus lenticular plate is similar to that of the head of the stapes but substantially larger than the vibration of the incus long process in the range 15–24 kHz. Thus, the flexibility of the incus pedicle seems to boost the bandwidth of middle ear transmission.

1. Introduction

This study was partly motivated by findings that contradicted the commonly held notion that the "tympanic membrane, the ossicles and their supporting ligaments play a large role in band pass limiting the middle-ear function ... determining the band-pass shape of the auditory threshold function" [1]. Those findings led to the conclusion that the velocity magnitudes of middle-ear vibration in several species are relatively uniform over a wide frequency range and thus do not restrict the bandwidth of hearing [2–5].

Seeking further support for that conclusion, we are re-examining ossicular vibrations in the middle ear of the chinchilla, a species with a relatively narrow hearing bandwidth, similar to that of humans. We previously measured middle-ear vibrations in chinchilla [6] but did not report on responses at high frequencies comparable to the upper limits of hearing because of limitations in the vibration-recording methodology (the Mössbauer technique) and in the bandwidth of the acoustic-stimulus system. The present measurements take advantage of an acoustic-stimulus system with wider bandwidth [3] and better vibration-recording apparatus (laser velocimeters) [7]. This study was also motivated by findings in guinea pig and chinchilla suggesting that the magnitudes of stapes vibrations may exceed those of incus vibrations (Figs. 7 of [8] and 6 of [5]).

2. Methods

Middle-ear measurements were carried out in deeply anesthetized chinchillas (*Chinchilla lanigera*). Stimuli were tones produced by a wide-band acoustic-stimulus system [3]. The vibratory responses to tones of the long process of the incus just peripheral to the pedicle, the lenticular plate of the incus, and the head of the stapes were recorded using laser velocimeters (*Dantec* or *Polytec*) coupled to a compound microscope.

3. Results

The magnitude of vibration velocity at the head of the stapes was relatively constant (~ 0.3 mm/s/Pa) up to 24 kHz (Fig. 1A). It decreased at a rate of ~ –20dB/oct at frequencies higher than 30 kHz. Phase lag relative to pressure in the external ear canal (Fig. 1B) increased approximately linearly between 0 and 20 kHz, with a slope equivalent to a pure delay of 76 μs. The phase slope was somewhat steeper at frequencies higher than 20 kHz. Both the large bandwidth and the delay of the middle-ear responses appear to originate principally at the tympanic membrane, since they are present in the vibrations of the incus peripheral to its pedicle. These features, however, are refined by a wide peak in the magnitude of the transfer function across the incus pedicle, i.e., between the long process and the lenticular plate, which is accompanied by a large phase lag. The magnitude peak boosts vibrations by about 16 dB at 25 kHz, further flattening the magnitude middle-ear transfer function. The additional phase lag extends the range of constant delay to about 20 kHz. The vibration of the head of the stapes is similar to that of the incus lenticular plate.

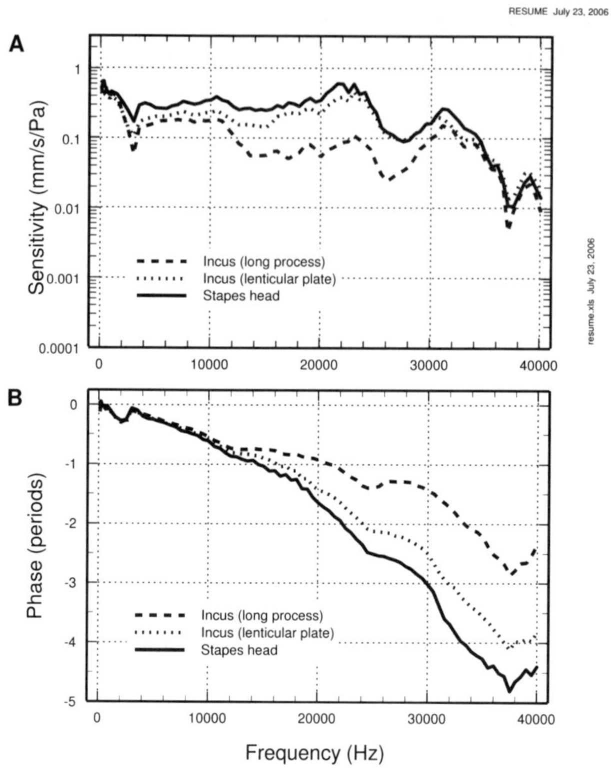

Fig. 1 Average velocity sensitivity (A) and phases (B) of the responses to tones of the long process of the incus at a site peripheral to its pedicle (dashed lines, n=15), the lenticular plate of the incus (dotted lines, n=15) and the head of the stapes (solid lines). The latter were computed by summing the mean response gains (in decibels) or phases of the lenticular plate (dotted lines) and the corresponding gains and phases measured across the incudo-stapedial joint in 5 middle ears.

4. Discussion and Conclusions

The boost of transmission across the pedicle of the incus and the similarity of vibration magnitude at the head of the stapes and at the incus lenticular plate jointly imply that the pedicle of the incus provides more flexibility to the ossicular chain than the incudo-stapedial joint, confirming a recent suggestion [9].

The present results show that the bandwidth of stapes vibration extends to at least 24 kHz and thus exceeds the bandwidth of hearing in chinchilla (< 20 kHz [10]; see also Figs. 1 of [2] and 4 of [5]). Therefore, the present findings support the contention that, in general, the middle ears of tetrapod vertebrates do not limit the bandwidth of hearing. Rather, the bandwidth of hearing is set by the properties of the inner ear [2].

Acknowledgments
We were supported by Grant DC-00419 from the National Institutes of Health (USA).

References
1. Rosowski J.J. and Relkin E.M., Introduction to the analysis of middle ear function. In A.F. Jahn and J. Santos-Sacchi. (eds.) *Physiology of the Ear.* Singular, San Diego, (2001) pp. 161–190
2. Ruggero M.A. and Temchin A.N., The roles of the external, middle, and inner ears in determining the bandwidth of hearing. *Proc Natl Acad Sci USA* **99** (2002) pp. 13206–13210
3. Overstreet E.H. and Ruggero M.A., Development of wide-band middle ear transmission in the Mongolian gerbil. *J Acoust Soc Am* **111** (2002) pp. 261–270
4. Ruggero M.A. and Temchin A.N., Middle-ear transmission in humans: wide-band, not frequency-tuned? *ARLO - Acoustics Research Letters Online* **4** (2003) pp. 53–58
5. Ruggero M.A., Temchin A.N., Robles L. and Overstreet E.H., A new and improved middle ear. In K. Gyo, H. Wada, N. Hato and T. Koike. (eds.) *Middle Ear Mechanics in Research and Otology.* World Scientific, Singapore, (2004) pp. 134–141
6. Ruggero M.A., Rich N.C., Robles L. and Shivapuja B.G., Middle-ear response in the chinchilla and its relationship to mechanics at the base of the cochlea. *J Acoust Soc Am* **87** (1990) pp. 1612–1629
7. Ruggero M.A. and Rich N.C., Application of a commercially-manufactured Doppler-shift laser velocimeter to the measurement of basilar-membrane vibration. *Hear Res* **51** (1991) pp. 215–230
8. Cooper N.P. and Rhode W.S., Basilar membrane mechanics in the hook region of cat and guinea-pig cochleae: sharp tuning and nonlinearity in the absence of baseline position shifts. *Hear Res* **63** (1992) pp. 163–190
9. Funnell W.R., Heng S.T., McKee M.D., Daniel S.J. and Decraemer W.F., On the coupling between the incus and the stapes in the cat. *J Assoc Res Otolaryngol* **6** (2005) pp. 9–18
10. Heffner R.S. and Heffner H.E., Behavioral hearing range of the chinchilla. *Hear Res* **52** (1991) pp. 13–16

FROM IMAGING OF THE MASTOID TO MECHATRONIC SURGERY: THE ROBIN-PROJECT

Marcus M. Maassen[1], Florian Damman[3], Jesus Rodriguez Jorge[1], Dirk Malthan[2], Armin Schäfer[2], Erwin Schwaderer[3], Raphael Ciuman[1], Jan Stallkamp[2], Stefan Wössner[2], Dirk Bartz[5], Zein Salah[4], Hans P. Zenner[1]

[1] Laboratory for Medical Robotics, Department of Otolaryngology, University Hospital of Tuebingen, Germany
[2] Fraunhofer-Institute for Manufacturing Engineering and Automation (IPA), Stuttgart, Germany
[3] Department of Radiology, University Hospital of Tuebingen, Germany
[4] WSI/GRIS – VCM, University of Tuebingen, Germany
[5] ICCAS / VCM, University of Leipzig, Germany

For the past years, surgeons performing lateral skull base surgery have been paying more attention to the development and advancement of mechatronically aided surgical procedures. Especially the interconnection between electronic hearing implants (i.e. MET Otologics Transducer) and the ossicular chain requires an accurate milling of skull cavities to ensure a proper angle of coupling and a long term stable fixation. We developed a PC-based computer and robot assisted system (CAS / RAS) for the precise and efficient planning and execution of surgical processes at the lateral skull. Employing multimodal sensory feedback, the geometry of the surgical area can be analyzed with a resolution of several μm.

1. Introduction

In otosurgery, one of the most challenging surgical procedures is the implantation of electronic hearing devices, requiring a highly reproducible and accurate fixation technique. Here, the interconnection between the amplifier's vibratory actor and the ossicular chain, and the fixation of so-called mountain brackets, requires an accurate milling of the required skull cavities [1]. In order to avoid a distortion of the transmitted acoustical signals, the implantation angle has to be defined very carefully. In addition, milling of the implant bed for the electronic module is usually time-consuming. Mechatronical devices may have the potential to perform this milling in a very short time with high precision. Computer assisted surgical systems are expected to provide an essential improvement of both efficiency and precision for interventions at the lateral skull base in the nearer future [2,3].

2. Planning- and Control System

We developed a software system for the precise planning and carrying-out of computer and robot assisted interventions at the lateral skull base. The development efforts are based upon a PC-based platform, utilizing the available libraries "Visualization Toolkit" (VTK) [4], "Insight Segmentation and Registration Toolkit" (ITK) [5] and "Apache XML-Parser" (Xerces) [6].

In order to realize a both flexible and dependable CAS/RAS- system, a modular and distributed control and communication architecture was realized. It consists of several modules, being classified into the so-called hardware, control and interaction-layer. All modules are physically independent executable software programs. Thus, they all have the ability to supervise the correct function of the other modules and are not affected by eventually occurring malfunctions of associated software components. This way, a redundant software system is built, as described also in other critical application scenarios [7].

The communication between the modules is based upon "Industrial Ethernet", a real-time variant of the well-known TCP/IP-protocol. The command sequences are transmitted utilizing the XML ("eXtended Markup Language") standard, being a flexible and expandable method of message transfer. Furthermore, employing XML, the transferred message syntax can be checked automatically in order to avoid transfer errors. The interconnection of the robot system is realized in a bi-directional way. Whereas control sequences and parameter messages are transferred to the hardware-layer, throughout feedback of the robot position and the status of the hardware components takes place. Additionally, sensory information like the force impacts on the tool tip and the information of the optical sensor systems are looped back to the higher level algorithms. These algorithms make comparisons between actual measured values and expected target values. The computed differences are visualised and the robot's trajectory and speed are modified accordingly.

3. Hardware Set-up

In order to evaluate the developed planning and control system for computer and robot-assisted interventions at the lateral skull base, a laboratory test scenario was realized. The central element of the hardware set-up is built by a modified industrial robot system "Adept Six-300" (Adept Technology GmbH, Dortmund, Germany). The employed robot system distinguishes six degrees of freedom (6-DOF) of its articulated kinematics allowing for flexible preparation angles. It is equipped with a 6-DOF force and momentum sensor system "Adept Force" (Adept Technology GmbH, Dortmund, Germany) so that any impact on the robot's tool tip can be recorded and supervised.

In addition to the mechanical sensor systems, two different optical sensor systems have been utilized. A laser-based triangulation distance sensor "LT 100" (ElcoTec GmbH, Dortmund, Germany) has been integrated for the precise identification of the in-situ geometry. It consists of a laser source being reflected by the patient's surface and a CCD-camera recording the reflection angle. This way, in combination with the robot's kinematics, a laser scanner has been realized, allowing a determination of the patient's topology with a precision better than 10 μm in every direction. For the differentiation of tissues, an auto fluorescence sensor system "S2000", (OceanOptics Europe B.V., Duiven, The Netherlands) has been integrated. The tissue region to be analysed is radiated with ultra-violet light, the resulting auto fluorescence spectra are recorded and automatically interpreted. The milling of the skull cavities is done by a conventional bone drilling system "Elan EC" (Aesculap AG & Co KG, Tuttlingen). This way, the results of the robot-assisted intervention are comparable to the manual preparation of the required skull cavities.

4. Closed-loop Robot Control

The integration of sensory systems feeding back in-situ information allows for an employment of the robot system in a so-called closed loop control architecture. Here, actual and nominal values are compared continuously, so that e.g. planned milling paths can be adjusted to intra-operative changes. This results in an increased precision and safety of the milling procedure.

The surveillance of the affecting forces assures non-pathologic force impacts on the patient. The measured forces are recorded and transmitted to the control system. For the estimation of forces within a surgical step, algorithms were implemented, that allow a simulation of the force impacts. In case of unacceptable errors, the robot-assisted surgical process is interrupted. Current research efforts show that the analysis of recorded forces may help identifying anatomical structures e.g. dura mater [8]. These results may supplement the developed sensory system in the nearer future.

5. Topology Comparison and Registration

In particular the transition of the computer-assisted planning of a surgical procedure to its execution is regarded as a critical step. For this step a transformation of the planning coordinate system into that of the patient is necessary: the patient has to be registered. Within the developed system, the comparison of the nominal geometry against the actual surface geometry using a laser scanner builds the basis for an intra-operative and continuous registration step.

In contrast to existing surface-based registration techniques like ICP- (Iterative Closest-Points) algorithms, the developed algorithms do not match the whole surface to realize a registration. Rather, significant associated anatomical landmarks in the actual and nominal data set are identified and assigned to one another. The technique is based upon a procedure called "spin-images" [9], was however modified in important pre and post processing steps. The advantages include the robustness against malformed surface reconstructions, resulting e.g. from blood and rinsing liquids.

The precision of the surface-based registration was evaluated by the measuring of artificial landmarks in form of registration metal beads. After the performed surface-based automatic registration, the position of the registration beads was identified by the robot system. For the determination of the robustness of the procedure a test series with 50 experiments was performed (Fig. 1), whereby the head model was deformed using polygon reduction and smoothing, and the addition of error noises [10]. The registration was accomplished in 48 of the 50 cases with an absolute error smaller than +/–0.7 mm (Fig. 2). In two cases the registration was, however, not accomplished correctly.

Furthermore, within the milling process the planned and simulated surface topology of the skull cavity can be compared with the performed milling process. Prior to the shift of the milling head, the in-situ geometry is evaluated in real-time. Only in case of negligible error values, the milling process is continued. In other cases, a re-registration of the patient is performed automatically.

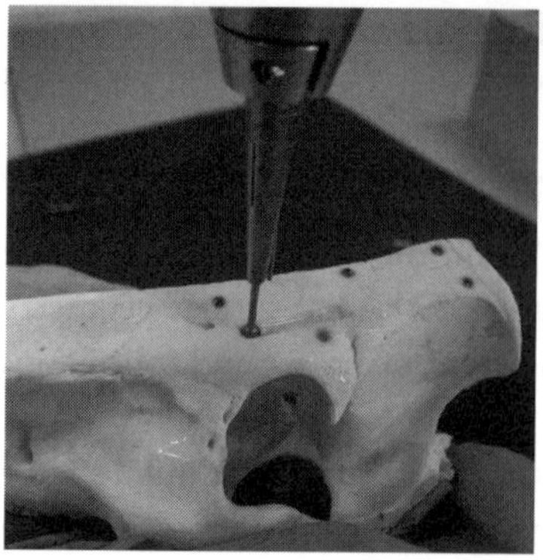

Fig. 1 Laboratory setup for milling tests on animal samples.

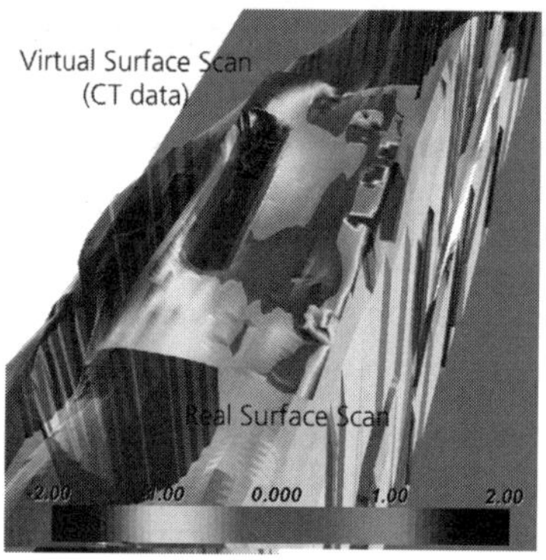

Fig. 2 Visualization of milling error by comparison of simulated and actual surface.

6. Conclusion

A computer and robot assisted system for microsurgical high-precision interventions at the lateral skull base has been developed. The system employs different sensor systems, like force sensors and laser triangulation sensors for precision measurements, in order to realize quality assurance and documentation steps. Employing multimodal sensory feedback, the geometry of the surgical area can be analyzed with a resolution of several μm. Using this enhanced data, a robust surface based registration procedure could be implemented. Its evaluation showed a success rate of 96% with an absolute error smaller than +/–0.7 mm. It could be shown that the feedback of sensory information using spin image technology improves the safety and the precision of mechatronical-assisted surgical procedures [11].

This work was supported by grant No. MA 1458/2 of the German Research Foundation (DFG).

References

1. Maassen M.M., Dammann F., Malthan D., Stallkamp J., Schwaderer E., Zenner H.P.: Development of a robot prototype with sensory feedback. 3rd Symposium of Middle Ear Mechanics in Research and Otology. Matsuyama, Ehime, Japan, 9th–12th July, 2003
2. Dammann F., Schwaderer E., Seemann M.: Einsatz von Methoden der 3D-Visualisierung im Kopf-Hals-Bereich. Fortschr Röntgenstr 2003; **175**: 86.
3. Plinkert P.K., Plinkert B., Hiller A., Stallkamp J.: Einsatz eines Roboters an der lateralen Schädelbasis. Evaluation einer robotergesteuerten Mastoidektomie am anatomischen Präparat. *HNO*. 2001 Jul; **49** (7): 514–522
4. http://www.vtk.org, 27.02.2004
5. http://www.itk.org, 27.02.2004
6. http://xml.apache.org/xerces-c/index.html, 27.02.2004
7. Bowen, J., Stavridou V.: Safety-critical systems, formal methods and standards. Oxford University Technical Report PRG-TR-5-92, *Software Engineering Journal*, 178–183
8. Federspil P.A., Geisthoff U.W., Henrich D., Plinkert P.K.: Development of the First Force-Controlled Robot for Otoneurosurgery. *Laryngoscope* 2003 Mar; **113** (3): 465–471
9. Johnson, A.E.: *Spin-Images: A Representation for 3-D Surface Matching*. Carnegie Mellon University, Pittsbugh, Pennsylvania, August 1998
10. Malthan D., Stallkamp J., Wössner S., Dammann F., Zenner H.P., Maassen M.M.: *Lasertriangulationsgesteuerte Sensorik und miniaturisierte Roboterkinematik können Implantationen an der lateralen Schädelbasis verbessern*, 5. Oktober 2002, Leipzig, II Jahrestagung der Sektion Neuroendoskopie, Neuronavigation und intraoperative Bildgebung der Deutschen Gesellschaft für Neurochirurgie.
11. Malthan D., Ehrlich G., Stallkamp J., Dammann F., Schwaderer E., Maassen M.M.: Automated registration of partially defective surfaces by local landmark identification. *Comput Aided Surg*. 2003; **8** (6): 300–309

OSSICULAR RECONSTRUCTION USING STORED INCUS IN PLANNED TWO-STAGE TYMPANOPLASTY

Kiyofumi Gyo, Toshiki Maetani, Naoto Hato, Masamitsu Hyodo
Address: Kiyofumi Gyo, MD, Department of Otolaryngology, Ehime University
Shizukawa, Toon, Ehime 791-0295, Japan, Email: kiyofumi@m.ehime-u.ac.jp

Keywords: ossicular chain, mastoid bowl, cholesteatoma, staged tympanoplasty,

The incus once removed at the first stage can be used in ossicular reconstruction at the second stage, when it is preserved appropriately. The present study was conducted to investigate if the mastoid bowl is a suitable site for storage. The study group included 24 ears of 23 patients who underwent staged tympanoplasty for the treatment of middle ear cholesteatoma. The average interval between the two stages was 8.3 months (range 6–12 months). The incus was identified in all cases at the second stage: ten incudes were found to be covered with a thin mucosa layer, 12 were buried in fibrous or granulation tissue, and two were joined to the surrounding bone. In 19 cases, the incus was available as a short columella for ossicular reconstruction. The remaining five cases were reconstructed using a hydroxyapatite ossicle as a long columella, since the stapes superstructure was missing at the second stage. Preservation of the incus in the mastoid bowl is an effective option in staged tympanoplasty, when the incus is considered useful for ossicular reconstruction at the second stage.

1. Introduction

According to Sheehy and Crabtree [1], planned two-stage tympanoplasty is indicated when the middle ear is severely affected by diseases such as middle ear cholesteatoma. At the first stage, the incudostapedial joint is disarticulated and the incus is removed for safe, complete exenteration of the disease. When the incus is deemed useful as a columella in ossiculoplasty, it is often stored outside the body until use at the second stage. We previously kept the incus in a tiny cell filled with pure alcohol and stored it in a refrigerator. This procedure is convenient for eradicating possible residual squamous epithelium attached to the incus. However, it also includes risks, such as accidental loss during storage, mistaken use as someone else's ossicle, viral or bacterial contamination, and death of the living osteocytes, which may induce atrophy of the incus after repositioning.

To prevent these problems, we recently stored the incus in the eradicated mastoid bowl after stripping the diseased surface, when the incus seemed useful for ossicular reconstruction. This paper describes the results of stored incus at the second stage and the hearing outcomes of ossiculoplasty by use of it.

2. Methods

Subjects were 24 ears of 23 patients who underwent staged tympanoplasty for treating extensive middle ear cholesteatoma. The patients were 12 males and 11 females, and their ages ranged from 4 to 62 years, with an average of 25.6 years. The patients were chosen for this study because the incus remained in good shape and was considered suitable as a columella in ossicular reconstruction at the second stage. Surgery was conducted using the intact canal wall technique.

Results of ossiculoplasty were evaluated using the criteria proposed by the Otological Society of Japan in 2000. Audiometric data were obtained by calculating the pure-tone averages of 500, 1000, and 2000 Hz before the first stage, and at least 6 months after the second stage. The surgery was considered successful when at least one of the following three criteria was achieved: a postoperative air-bone gap within 15 dB, a hearing gain of more than 15 dB, or a threshold of postoperative air conduction hearing within 30dB.

3. Results

At the second stage, the incus was identified at the original sites of storage in all cases; 10 incudes were found to be covered with a thin layer of mucosa (Fig. 1), 12 were buried in fibrous or granulation tissue (Fig. 2), and 2 had adhered to the surrounding bone via bony adhesions (Fig. 3). These results were closely related to the preoperative condition of the mastoid cavity; when the mastoid disease was mild and the mucosa was preserved, the incus tended to be covered with a thin layer of mucosa. When the mastoid cavity was severely diseased, necessitating extensive mastoidectomy, the incus tended to be buried in fibrous or granulation tissue. Age and gender did not influence the outcomes of the incus.

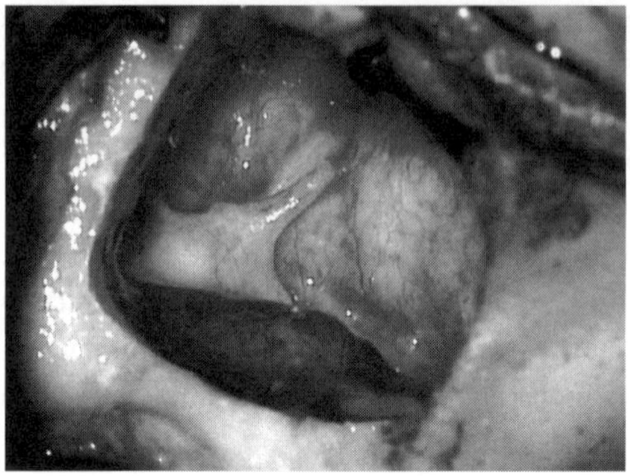

Fig. 1 The incus covered with a thin layer of mucosa. Findings at the second stage. The operation was conducted 9 months after the first stage. The patient was a 9-year-old girl suffering from sinus cholesteatoma.

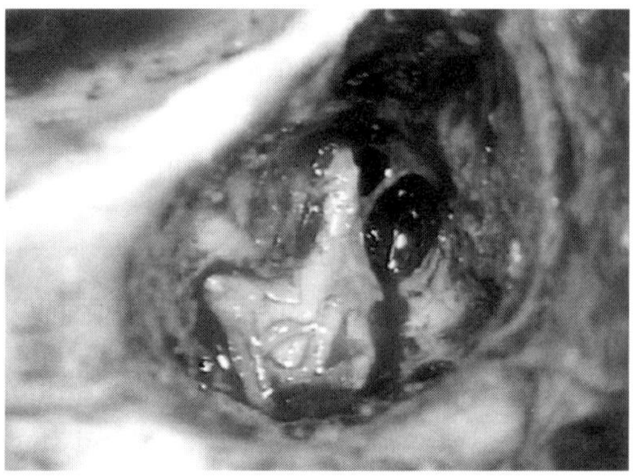

Fig. 2 The incus burried in granulation. The operation was conducted 11 months after the first stage. The patient was a 55-year-old woman suffering from totally adhesive type of cholesteatoma.

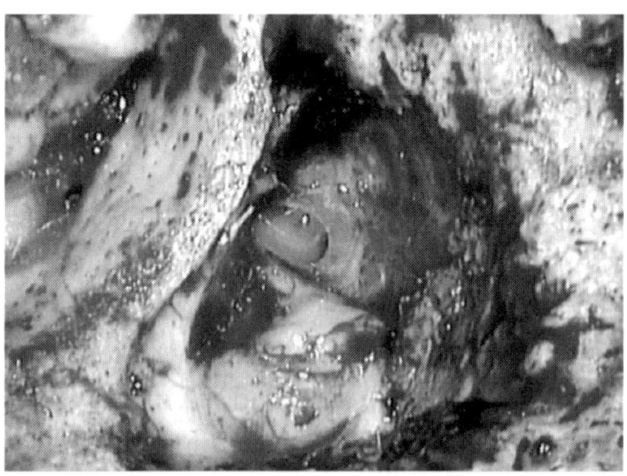

Fig. 3 The incus subjected to bony adhesion to the surrounding. The operation was conducted 7 months after the first stage. The patient was a 55-year-old woman suffering from sinus cholesteatoma.

Residual cholesteatoma was discovered as a pearly mass in 6 ears, either at the attic (3 ears) or the tympanic sinus (3 ears). These cholesteatomas were localized and easily removed. No residual disease was ever observed in the mastoid bowl where the incus had been stored.

In 19 of 24 cases, the ossicular chain was reconstructed using the incus as a short columella. In the remaining 5 cases, the stapes superstructures that had been identified at the first stage disappeared between stages. These 5 cases were reconstructed using a hydroxyapatite ossicular prosthesis as a long columella.

Postoperative hearing was assessed in 17 of the 19 patients who had undergone ossicular reconstruction with a stored incus; 2 cases were lost for follow-up. When the latest audiometric results were analyzed, the ossiculoplasty was judged success in 11 out of 17 cases (65%); there was closure of the air-bone gap within 15 dB in 11 cases (65%), a hearing gain of more than 15 dB in 5 cases (18%), and postoperative air conduction hearing within 30 dB in 9 cases (53%).

4. Discussion

Although ossiculoplasty is performed using a variety of materials, autologous ossicles are considered best as columellae because of their easy availability, low cost of preparation, and good biocompatibility. They also resulted in good postoperative hearing in a long-term follow-up study. At present, however, use of incus in the cholesteatomatous ear remains controversial because of the possibility of recurrent cholesteatoma and progressive bone absorption. Steinbach et al. [2] studied 203 incudes taken from patients with cholesteatoma. Their histological examination revealed the frequent existence of tiny deposits of squamous tissue on the incudes that appeared free of cholesteatoma under an operating microscope. Dornhoffer et al.[3] also stated that gross examination of the incus with an operating microscope was not accurate in assessing cholesteatoma involvement. To reduce the risk of cholesteatoma recurrence, Muller-Hermann [4] advocated that the incus be autoclaved during surgery to kill the squamous epithelium adhering to it, although the procedure simultaneously destroys the living osteocytes.

In the case of staged tympanoplasty, we can avoid the problems related to reuse of the incus. The simplest procedure is to store the incus in a cell filled with alcohol until it is used at the second stage. This procedure is sufficient to kill any squamous epithelium anchored to the incus, although it was somewhat cumbersome and risky. Storage of the incus in the mastoid bowl during staging can overcome most of the disadvantages of external storage. It is accomplished without the risk of loss during storage, avoids accidental contamination by viruses or bacteria, and provides favorable conditions for culturing the living tissue.

At the second stage, we found no residual cholesteatoma in the mastoid bowl where the incus had been stored. This suggests that the incus is now free of cholesteatoma and is safe for use in ossiculoplasty, although the period of storage might be too short to conclude that the incus is disease-free. If residual cholesteatoma is found around the incus at the second stage, we should use another material as a columella for ossiculoplasty. Progressive bone absorption is another risk when using the autologous incus for ossiculoplasty, and is one of the major causes of late conductive hearing loss after initial good postoperative hearing. This problem may be avoided to some extent by staging the procedures, since we can check the status of the stored incus at the second stage. In our cases, prominent atrophy of the incus occurred in 1 of 24 ears. In this case, the incus underwent necrotic demineralization, probably due to progressive osteitis. Note that the stapes superstructures were also absent in 5 of 24 ears at the second stage, although they had appeared normal or almost normal at the first stage. According to the surgical records, the stapes was surrounded by cholesteatoma or granulation tissue at the first stage, suggesting that the bone was resorbed as a consequence of progressive osteitis. When the stapes superstructures were missing at the second stage, we used a hydroxyapatite ossicle as a long columella.

References

1. Sheehy J.L., Crabtree J.A., Tympanoplasty: staging the operation. *Laryngoscope* 1973; **83**: 1594–1621
2. Steinbach E., Hildmann H., Re-use of incus in cholesteatoma and it chronic mucosal disease. *Z Laryngol Rhinol* 1972; **51**: 659–664
3. Dornhoffer J.L., Colvin G.B., North P., Evidence of residual disease in ossicles of patients undergoing cholesteatoma removal. Acta Otolaryngol 1999; **119**: 89–92
4. Muller-Hermann E., The autogenous autoclaved incus. *Laryngol Rhinol Otol* 1983; **62**: 369–370

INCUS INTERPOSITION: SURGICAL HIGHLIGHTS AND AUDIOLOGICAL RESULTS

Ch. Röösli, A. de Ataide, Ch. Schlegel-Wagner, T. E. Linder
Department of Otorhinolaryngology, Head and Neck Surgery, Kantonsspital Lucerne, Switzerland

Address for Correspondence: Christof Röösli, HNO-Klinik Kantonsspital Luzern, Spitalstrasse 100, 6000 Luzern, Phone: 0041 41 205 13 56, Fax: 0041 41 205 49 60
Email: christof.roeoesli@ksl.ch

Introduction: A wide variety of pathologies cause diminished sound transmission efficiency of the middle ear. If the malleus handle and the stapes suprastructure are intact, incus ossiculoplasty is the treatment of choice. We describe the technique used for incus interposition and report the 1-year postoperative functional results.

Methods: Sixty consecutive patients with an intact malleus handle and stapes suprastructure underwent incus interposition between October 2001 and January 2004 using either the patient's own ossicle or a Titanium prosthesis. The surgeries were either primary interventions, revision surgeries or planned staged ossiculoplasties in closed or open cavities.

Pre- and postoperative air and bone-conduction thresholds and air-bone gaps for pure-tone averages of three and four frequencies and for single frequencies were analyzed.

Results: Ossiculoplasties were performed using autografts (34 patients) and titanium prosthesis (26 patients). The mean postoperative air-bone-gap improved from 26dB to 15dB for the frequencies of 0.5kHz to 2kHz and from 25dB to 17dB for the frequencies of 0.5kHz to 4kHz. The largest improvement could be reached in the lower and middle frequencies, whereas smallest improvements were achieved at 4kHz. A favorable postoperative air-bone-gap of 20dB or less was achieved in 91% of patients using autograft and in 65% of patients using a titanium prosthesis. These differences were statistically not significant.

Conclusions: Sculpted autologous incus interposition provided the maximum hearing threshold improvement. However the audiologic results of the new titanium prosthesis did not differ significantly ($p = 0.11$).

Further studies may verify why the closure of the air-bone-gap at 4kHz was less successful than in lower frequencies.

1. Introduction

A wide variety of pathologies may affect the sound transmission of the middle ear. A precondition for successful reconstruction of acoustical middle ear function is a reliable transduction of sound energy through a reconstructed ossicular chain besides an intact and vibrating tympanic membrane in a well ventilated middle ear.

If the handle of the malleus and the suprastructure of the stapes are preserved (Fisch group I [1] or Austin-Kartush group A [2, 3]), the incus interposition is the preferred choice to reconstruct the ossicular chain. The position of the malleus towards the capitulum of the stapes is crucial for optimal placement of the ossicle. If the patient's incus is destroyed by the middle ear pathology or not available at staged surgeries, several prostheses made of many different materials are commercially available.

We report our experience of interposing the patient's own incus or a new Titanium incus prosthesis with a postoperative follow-up of at least one year using the American Academy of Otolaryngology-Head and Neck Surgery guidelines.

2. Materials and Methods

2.1 Patients

Sixty-seven consecutive patients underwent incus interposition between October 2001 and January 2004 at the ENT-Department of Kantonsspital Lucerne, Switzerland. Sixty patients (89.5%) with a mean age of 38 years (range 5–77 years) were available for clinical and audiometric follow-up. Mean follow-up time was 1.5 years (range 1–2.75 years). The pathologies leading to the discontinuity of the ossicular chain are presented in Table 1.

Table 1 Pathologies responsible for the discontinuity of ossicular chain (n=60).

Diagnosis	**n**	**%**
Cholesteatoma	27	45
Chronic otitis media (central perforation)	19	32
Trauma	5	8.5
Atelectasis	4	6.5
Malformation	2	3.2
Previous ear inflammations	2	3.2
Tympanosclerosis	1	1.6
Total	**60**	**100**

2.2 Type of surgery

The patient's own incus was the preferred option for reconstruction using the principle outlined by U. Fisch [1, 4]: The incus was removed, the long process eliminated with a diamond drill and a groove for the malleus handle drilled at the previous incudomalleal joint area. The indentation for the stapes head was made opposite to the malleus groove within the posterior process of the incus using 1.0 and 0.8mm diamond drills. The proper length of the incus interposition was determined using the 2.5mm micro-raspatory as a guide and by repeatedly placing the incus in its perfect position. All autologous incus interpositions were performed as first stage surgeries, since the incus was not preserved for a staged reconstruction.

In patients with a medialized malleus or fixation of the anterior malleal ligament, the malleus head was removed in order to lateralize the malleus handle perpendicular to the stapes capitulum. In contrast to others [5] the tensor tympani tendon was never sacrificed.

If the patient's own incus was not available, the Fisch Titanium Incus (Karl Storz GmbH Tuttlingen, Germany) was used. Its shape that resembles the modified patient's own incus can be modified using conventional diamond drills [1]. The contact surfaces were always roughened with a drill, even if the custom made length was ideal. A too smooth surface may allow sliding of the prosthesis away from the ossicles during wound healing.

2.3 Evaluation of the hearing results and statistical analysis

Pure tone averages and air-bone gaps for three frequencies (500Hz, 1000Hz and 2000Hz) as well as for four frequencies (500Hz, 1000Hz, 2000Hz and 4000Hz) were compared using pre and postoperative measurements.

Cross-tabulation statistics were performed with Chi-square test to analyze differences in air-bone-gaps. Values of $p \leq 0.05$ were considered significant.

3. Results

The patient's own incus could be used in 34 patients (57%). In the remaining 26 patients (43%) it had to be replaced using the titanium incus prosthesis. The malleus head was resected in 35 patients (58%). A closed cavity was present in 54 (90%), an open cavity in 6 (10%) of the 60 patients. Eight cases (15%) were planned staged interventions.

The mean pre and postoperative air-conduction thresholds in all 60 patients are shown in Table 2.

Table 2 Mean pre and postoperative air-conduction threshold and mean pre and postoperative ABG.

Frequencies (kHz)	0.5-2	0.5-4
Mean preoperative air conduction threshold (dB)	40.3	41.6
Mean postoperative air conduction threshold (dB)	26.9	33.7
Mean preoperative air bone gap (dB)	26.3	25.1
Mean postoperative air bone gap (dB)	14.9	17.1

The distribution of the postoperative air bone gap for the three and four frequencies as well as for single frequencies is presented in Figure 1. The strongest improvement was achieved in the lower and middle frequencies. The smallest improvement was seen at 4kHz, where a closure of the ABG within 20dB was achieved in only 46%. The range encompassed a decline of 50dB to an improvement 60dB.

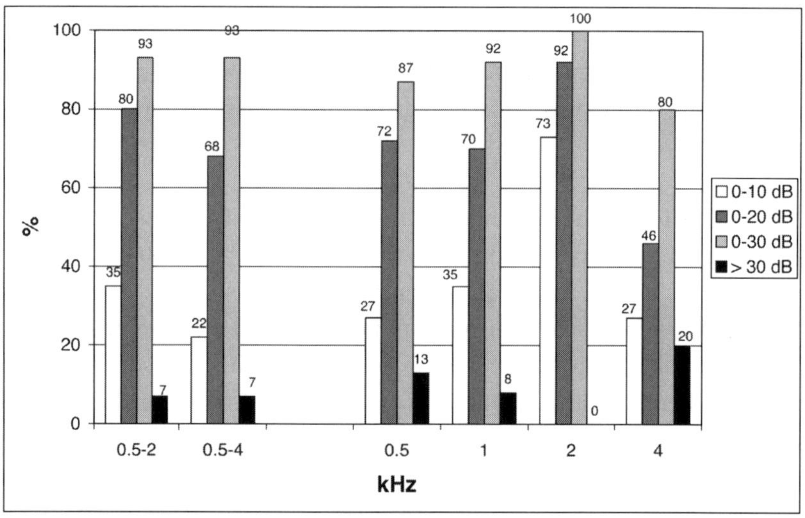

Fig. 1

A closure of the air-bone gap within 20dB could be achieved in 91% (0.5kHz to 2kHz) and in 76.5% (0.5kHz to 4kHz) using the patient's own incus. The same goal was accomplished in 61% (0.5kHz to 2kHz) and in 58% (0.5kHz to 4kHz) using a titanium prosthesis (Table 3). These differences were statistically not significant (p = 0.11). Failures (ABG > 30dB) occurred in 3 patients after dislocation of the prosthesis and in one patient with tympanosclerosis and partial stapes fixation.

Table 3 Postoperative air-bone-gap in correlation to the type of prosthesis used and the frequencies evaluated.

0.5kHz - 2kHz					**0.5kHz - 4kHz**				
air-bone-gap	**material**				**air-bone-gap**	**material**			
	autologous incus		Titanium			autologous incus		Titanium	
dB	n	%	N	%	dB	n	%	n	%
0-10	13	38	7	27	0-10	7	21	6	23
0-20	31	91	17	65	0-20	26	77	15	58
0-30	33	97	23	89	0-30	33	97	23	89
> 30	1	3	3	11	> 30	1	3	3	11
Total	34	100	26	100	Total	34	100	26	100

The resection of the malleus head did not lead to a significant change of the postoperative ABG ($p = 0.65$). On the contrary, it was crucial to be able to perform incus interposition in 35 patients (58%). The nature of disease ($p = 0.17$), the type of the surgical cavity ($p = 0.78$), revision surgeries ($p = 0.79$) or staging of the intervention ($p = 0.19$) did not significantly influence the outcome.

No partial or total extrusion of the prosthesis or total deafness was observed in any of the 60 patients.

4. Discussion

Chronic middle ear disease and middle ear atelectasis most often lead to damage of the ossicular chain and an incus interposition may become necessary. Once the patient's own incus is extensively involved with the underlying disease autograft materials or allograft prosthesis may be used.

An autograft can be shaped in different ways [6]. The goal is to obtain a slim, direct graft without touching the bony sulcus or the promontory. Our preferred method is to remove the long process of the incus and the posterior part of the incus body using diamond burrs as described by U. Fisch [1, 4]. Lately, titanium has become a frequently used material for ossicular prostheses [7] due to its excellent biocompatibility [8], low weight and ease of shaping using standard diamond drills.

Among the studies comparable to our series (including more than 20 patients and a follow-up lasting at least one year), the postoperative air-bone gap was calculated for the frequencies of 0.5kHz to 2kHz (three frequencies) in 8 studies [5, 9–15] and for the frequencies of 0.5kHz to 4kHz (four frequencies) in 4 studies [16–19]. Our results using an autograft are in the higher range compared to the literature and the results achieved using the Fisch titanium prosthesis are well comparable to materials used by others [5, 9–19]. A direct comparison of the optimal material is not possible due to many factors (operation technique, technique for reconstruction of the tympanic membrane, aeration of the middle ear) influencing the results.

In our series, all investigated factors that may affect the audiological outcome (original disease, type of cavity, revisions surgery, staging, type of prosthesis) turned out not to be significant as described by others [20].

The guidelines of the Committee on Hearing and Equilibrium of the American Academy of Otolaryngology-Head and Neck Surgery for the evaluation of treatments for conductive hearing loss suggest calculating a four tone pure tone average for air and bone conduction using the thresholds at 0.5, 1, 2 and 3kHz. In most European centers the 3kHz tone is not measured, however the 4kHz tone is included in the calculation. Analyzing our own results and reviewing the literature, the calculation of 0.5–2kHz offers the best outcome, whereas the inclusion of the 4kHz tone drops the success rate. Therefore measuring only up to 2kHz seem to bias the results. This bias might be related to the variability of stapes movement at different frequencies (predominantly piston-like at lower frequencies, rocking motion at higher frequencies) [21]. Whether after incus interposition only the piston-like movements are transmitted needs to be proven.

5. Conclusions

This long-term evaluation after incus interposition demonstrates that excellent hearing results with an air-bone gap of 20dB or less can be achieved in 91% of the patients using an autograft and in 65.5% using a titanium prosthesis. Optimization of all factors that may influence the audiological results as well as technically perfect incus interposition is necessary to further improve the audiometric results and achieve reproducible excellent postoperative audiometric results.

Further investigations must answer the question why the closure of the air-bone gap at 4kHz is less successful compared to lower frequencies.

References

1. U. Fisch and J. May, Tympanoplasty, mastoidectomy and stapes surgery. In U. Fisch and J. May (eds.). Thieme, Stuttgart, New York 1994, p. 47
2. D. F. Austin, Ossicular reconstruction. *Otolaryngol Clin North Am* **5** (1972) pp. 145–160
3. J. M. Kartush, Ossicular chain reconstruction. Capitulum to malleus. *Otolaryngol Clin North Am* **27** (1994) pp. 689–715
4. U. Fisch and T. E. Linder, Temporal bone dissection, the Zurich guidelines, Tuttlingen 2005) 20–1
5. P. W. Slater, 2nd, Practical use of total and partial ossicular replacement prosthesis in ossiculoplasty. *Laryngoscope* **110** (2000) pp. 176–177
6. M. Tos, Manual of Middle Ear Surgery: Approaches, Myringoplasty, Ossiculoplasty and Tympanoplasty (Eds.). Thieme, New York (1997) p. 305
7. C. V. Dalchow, D. Grun and H. F. Stupp, Reconstruction of the ossicular chain with titanium implants. *Otolaryngol Head Neck Surg* **125** (2001) pp. 628–630
8. P. Dost, Animal experiments and cell culture studies on stapes reconstruction with diverse biomaterials. *Laryngorhinootologie* **79** (2000) p. 193
9. J. A. Romualdez, E. Stauffer, R. Hasler and M. A. Hotz, A new ossicle homograft inactivation/preservation procedure: clinical results. *ORL J Otorhinolaryngol Relat Spec* **67** (2005) pp. 34–38
10. H. P. Zenner, A. Stegmaier, R. Lehner, I. Baumann and R. Zimmermann, Open Tubingen titanium prostheses for ossiculoplasty: a prospective clinical trial. *Otol Neurotol* **22** (2001) pp. 582–589
11. J. D. Macias, M. E. Glasscock, 3rd, M. H. Widick, D. G. Schall, D. S. Haynes and A. F. Josey, Ossiculoplasty using the black hydroxylapatite hybrid ossicular replacement prostheses. *Am J Otol* **16** (1995) pp. 718–721
12. H. Silverstein, A. B. McDaniel and R. Lichtenstein, A comparison of PORP, TORP, and incus homograft for ossicular reconstruction in chronic ear surgery. *Laryngoscope* **96** (1986) pp. 159–165
13. C. G. Jackson, M. E. Glasscock, 3rd, M. K. Schwaber, A. J. Nissen, S. G. Christiansen and P. G. Smith, Ossicular chain reconstruction: the TORP and PORP in chronic ear disease. *Laryngoscope* **93** (1983) pp. 981–988
14. K. R. Rust, G. T. Singleton, J. Wilson and P. J. Antonelli, Bioglass middle ear prosthesis: long-term results. *Am J Otol* **17** (1996) pp. 371–374
15. V. D. Janzen, Ossiculoplasty using a hemi-incus interposition. *J Otolaryngol* **13** (1984) pp. 211–212
16. R. L. Daniels, F. M. Rizer, A. G. Schuring and W. L. Lippy, Partial ossicular reconstruction in children: a review of 62 operations. *Laryngoscope* **108** (1998) pp. 1674–1681
17. L. M. Menendez-Colino, M. Bernal-Sprekelsen, I. Alobid and J. Traserra-Coderch, Preliminary functional results of tympanoplasty with titanium protheses. *Otolaryngol Head Neck Surg* **131** (2004) pp. 747–749

18. A. Nikolaou, Z. Bourikas, V. Maltas and A. Aidonis, Ossiculoplasty with the use of autografts and synthetic prosthetic materials: a comparison of results in 165 cases. *J Laryngol Otol* **106** (1992) pp. 692–694
19. C. H. Stupp, H. F. Stupp and D. Grun, Replacement of ear ossicles with titanium prostheses. *Laryngorhinootologie* **75** (1996) pp. 335–337
20. R. C. O'Reilly, S. P. Cass, B. E. Hirsch, D. B. Kamerer, R. A. Bernat and S. P. Pozanovic, Ossiculoplasty using incus interposition: Hearing results and analysis of the middle ear risk index. *Otol Neurotol* **26** (2005) pp. 853–858
21. A. Huber, T. Linder, M. Ferrazzini, S. Schmid, N. Dillier, S. Stoeckli and U. Fisch, Intraoperative assessment of stapes movement. *Ann Otol Rhinol Laryngol* **110** (2001) pp. 31–35

PREVENTION AND TREATMENT OF TYMPANIC MEMBRANE BLUNTING

Thomas L. Eby, M.D., Division of Otolaryngology Head and Neck Surgery
University of Alabama Birmingham, BDB 563, 1530 3rd Ave. S, Birmingham
AL 35294-0012 USA, Email: eby@uab.edu

Anterior tympanic membrane blunting results in persistent conductive hearing loss and patient dissatisfaction despite successful closure of a perforation. Tympanic membrane compliance and efficiency in sound transmission are impaired. In extreme cases the entire tympanic membrane may lateralize giving a false fundus with maximal conductive loss. The causes of blunting may be both surgical technique and poor wound healing. We describe our techniques for prevention of blunting which include adequate support and anchoring of the fascia graft in an underlay technique and the use of thin split thickness skin grafts. Post operative follow up in clinic to monitor healing is important. Examples of the techniques and results are presented.

1. Introduction

The normal function of the tympanic membrane depends on its shape, integrity, compliance and orientation with the external canal and ossicular chain. When the tympanic membrane heals with a more obtuse angle of the anterior sulcus or a thickening near the anterior annulus, some degree of conductive hearing loss invariably occurs. A maximal conductive hearing loss can occur if the tympanic membrane heals lateral to the malleus. The cause of tympanic membrane blunting or lateralization is most often the unfavorable result of tympanoplasty surgery. The patient is understandably disappointed with the result even though the tympanic membrane perforation has been closed. In some cases the same pathology is the end result of an indolent inflammatory condition of the tympanic membrane and adjacent canal skin. Patients who have tympanic membrane blunting most often complain of fullness, tinnitus and hearing loss in the affected ear.

Tympanic membrane blunting may include a spectrum of pathology ranging from an abnormal contour limited to the anterior sulcus to lateralization of the entire tympanic membrane giving rise to a false fundus. Some authors also consider complete external canal stenosis as a severe form of blunting. Tympanic membrane blunting can be recognized clinically by the following features: the absence of the normal acute angle at the anterior sulcus, or rounding along the anterior or inferior margin of the tympanic membrane. In more severe cases normal landmarks such as the malleus profile are lost and the tympanic membrane may be smaller than normal, have a convex contour or a blind sac appearance. There is always a conductive hearing loss.

The prevention and treatment of tympanic membrane blunting requires adherence to several important principles of reconstruction. The fascia graft must be anchored or secured in several locations including both anterior and posterior annulus as well as the malleus. Methods to encourage early epithelialization of the graft and bony canal must be used to prevent graft thickening or migration. The technique presented here is a reliable procedure to address the problem of tympanic membrane blunting.

2. Methods

In order to correct a blunted anterior annulus or lateralized tympanic membrane, the area of abnormal tissue must be completely excised. If there is any doubt about the condition of the remaining tympanic tissue it is removed. Efforts to preserve the epithelium and excise the underlying fibrosis are usually unproductive. After excision, there is an area of absent skin in the bony canal adjacent to the tympanic defect. This can be a large part of the bony canal when the entire tympanic membrane is lateralized.

The keys to successful correction of the blunting are to anchor the fascia graft and to re-epithelialize the denuded bony canal and graft. The two main anchors to secure the temporalis fascia graft are the anterior bony annulus and the malleus handle. The fascia graft must be large enough to reach underneath the tympanic perforation and far anterior under the anterior annulus to reach the Eustachian tube opening. The superior edge of fascia is positioned medial to the malleus handle. The fascia is supported by gelfoam placed in the middle ear.

Thin split thickness skin grafts are best to re-epithelialize the exposed areas. These are obtained by a free hand technique from the upper arm near the axilla. A straight razor blade is used to obtain thin skin grafts approximately 2cm by 4cm in size. One or more of these grafts may be obtained as needed. The skin in this area is thin with few hairs, easy to access, and leaves a hidden and cosmetically acceptable scar. A dermatome is not necessary and usually results in a graft that is too thick. The thin skin is placed on a backing of rayon cloth with a thin layer of antibiotic ointment. This serves as a support for the placement and initial healing of the skin graft. The rayon must be removed postoperatively in the clinic within two weeks or a foreign body reaction may occur.

Placement of the split thickness skin graft with its backing is important. The most critical placement is at the anterior sulcus, where a strip of skin is tucked tightly into the anterior angle, covering both the anterior bony wall and the fascia tympanic graft. Other strips of split thickness skin graft with their rayon backing are placed around the circumference of the canal to cover all areas without epithelium. The strips are cut so that the skin covers all of the rayon and there are no gaps in coverage. Slight overlap of the skin strips is acceptable because the overlapping skin will slough. If any areas are not covered, or covered only with the rayon backing, there is a risk of granulation development with the end result of recurrent fibrosis.

In order to hold the grafts in place, gelfoam soaked with antibiotic solution is placed on top of the rayon backing for the skin grafts near the reconstructed tympanic membrane. The remainder of the external canal is packed with a ribbon of ¼ inch gauze with antibiotic ointment. All of the packing including the gauze and rayon skin graft backing is removed between postoperative day 10 and 14. After packing removal antibiotic drops are given for ten days. Follow up visits one month and two months after surgery insure that healing is progressing properly. If the skin graft does not take in some areas, excess granulation tissue is controlled with silver nitrate cautery.

3. Results

Six patients with tympanic membrane blunting as their primary pathology were treated from 2000–2006. Patients with congenital aural atresia, acquired stenosis of the external canal due to trauma or infection, cholesteatoma of the middle ear or external canal or those with active chronic otitis media were excluded from this study.

Five of the six patients gave a history of previous tympanoplasty surgery. The technique used for their surgeries whether overlay, underlay or other, was not known. In two of these patients the previous surgery was several years before their initial visit and hearing seemed to worsen after a period of otorrhea. The sixth patient had a history of chronic myringitis for more than four years treated intermittently with oral and topical medications. At presentation all patients had no tympanic perforation or otorrhea.

The preoperative and postoperative audiograms from all the patients were reviewed. Hearing results are reported according to the American Academy of Otolaryngology Head and Neck Surgery committee on hearing and equilibrium guidelines[1]. The pure tone averages for air and bone conduction at 0.5,1,2,3 kHz for each audiogram determined the air bone gap. Preoperative hearing results showed conductive hearing loss in all patients. The postoperative audiograms were at least six weeks after surgery and showed varying degrees of improvement. Three patients had closure of the A–B gap to 10dB or less, one to 15 dB and two to less than 30 dB. All the results are shown in Table 1.

Table 1 Prev Surg= previous surgery, Hx Otorrhea= history of otorrhea, PreOP A–B gap, PostOp A–B gap= preoperative and postoperative air bone gap in dB.

Patient	Age	Gender	Prev Surg	Hx Otorrhea	PreOp A-B gap	PostOp A-B gap
1	49	F	+	+	25	10
2	60	F	-	+	22	0
3	57	M	+	-	36	15
4	49	M	+	+	40	24
5	59	M	+	-	20	9
6	29	F	+	-	45	25

The postoperative position of the tympanic membrane was normal in all patients with recreation of the anterior sulcus. In patient 4, the reconstructed tympanic membrane appeared thicker than normal and the malleus profile was not distinct. It is suspected that tympanosclerosis affecting the ossicular chain as well as the tympanic membrane resulted in limited improvement in the air bone gap. Patient 6 had a history of cholesteatoma and underwent re-exploration of the middle ear. No recurrence was found and no explanation for her residual conductive loss was found.

4. Discussion

Causes of blunting or lateralization of the tympanic membrane have been described previously. In his review of 48 cases, Plester[2] found blunting to be a complication of the onlay technique of tympanoplasty. He found anterior angle fibrosis but also deep penetration of a fold of epithelium into subepithelial tissue and even cholesteatoma in some cases. He concluded that blunting was a nearly unavoidable problem with the onlay method. Blunting was also found to be a complication of lateral onlay tympanoplasty by Segal et.al [3] in their seven cases. The incidence of iatrogenic tympanic membrane blunting may be decreasing with the increase in use of the underlay technique and cartilage grafting methods[4]. In their series of fourteen cases, Sperling[5] found that nine occurred after previous tympanoplasty and four after atresia surgery all in children. The only adult case of lateralization occurred without previous surgery. They also note the overlap of pathology with other conditions such as external canal stenosis and external canal as well as middle ear cholesteatoma. The cases in this study follow this pattern with five of six having previous tymanoplasty surgery, although it is not known whether the overlay technique was used. Cases of aural atresia, external canal stenosis and external canal or middle ear cholesteatoma were excluded in this study. In many of these cases the same operative techniques for reconstruction can be applied with success, but outcomes vary depending on the pathology.

Blunting can be the end result of a chronic inflammatory condition of the tympanic membrane and adjacent skin of the bony canal. These patients have a moist thin layer of granulation tissue replacing the epithelium which is refractory to most topical treatments and persists for years with gradual distortion of the anterior annulus and development of conductive hearing loss. This has been called chronic myringitis or chronic external otitis, but is clearly an unusual complication of these conditions and may represent a different pathologic process. The one patient in our study who did not have previous surgery falls into this category. It is also interesting to note that infection or inflammation may have played a role in the tympanic blunting of at least two of the patients with previous tympanoplasty. Both went several years with stable hearing but developed a noticeable drop in hearing after a period of otorrhea.

The techniques for treating tympanic membrane blunting vary. The underlay technique with various ways to anchor the fascia have been described[5,6,7]. This is almost always followed by skin grafting of denuded bone and fascia, usually using split thickness grafts. The abnormal skin and underlying fibrosis is usually excised and discarded, but Sperling[5] describes a technique of skin preservation with thinning to remove fibrosis using a laser. He also augments this with fascia covered in split thickness skin. The fascia is split so that a tongue of the graft is placed along the anterior bony canal while the remainder lies under the anterior annulus. A method using a cartilage-perichondrium composite graft from the tragus has also been suggested instead of temporalis fascia. This technique uses a full thickness skin graft and silastic sheeting to cover exposed canal bone[4].

5. Conclusion

Tympanic membrane blunting is an uncommon but frustrating complication of tympanoplasty surgery. It can also occur spontaneously as the end result of a chronic inflammation of the tympanic membrane. The technique presented here utilizing a well anchored underlay fascia graft with properly placed split thickness skin grafts can reliably correct this problem.

References

1. No author, Committee on Hearing and Equilibrium guidelines for the evaluation of results of treatment of conductive hearing loss. *Otolaryngol Head Neck Surg* **113(3)** (1995) pp. 186–187
2. Plester D., Pusalker A., The anterior tympanic angle: the aetiology, surgery and avoidance of blunting and annular cholesteatoma. *Clin Otolaryngol Allied Sci* **6(5)** (1981) pp. 323–328
3. Segal S., Winerman I., Man A., Surgical correction of the lateralized eardrum. *J Larngol Otol* **95** (1981) pp. 675–678
4. Boone R., Dornhoffer J., Surgical Correction of the Lateralized Tympanic Membrane. *Laryngoscope* **112(8)** (2002) pp. 1509–1511
5. Sperling N., Kay D., Diagnosis and Management of the Lateralized Tympanic Membrane. *Laryngoscope* **110(12)** (2000) pp. 1987–1993
6. Farrior J.B., The anterior tympanomeatal angle in tympanoplasty: surgical techniques for the prevention of blunting. *Laryngoscope* **93(8)** (1983) pp. 992–997
7. Gyo K., Hato N., Shinomori Y., Hakuba N., Lateralization of the tympanic membrane as a complication of canal wall down tympanoplasty: a report of four cases. *Otol Neurotol* **24(2)** (2003) pp. 145–148

THE INTACT OSSICULAR CHAIN IN CHOLESTEATOMA SURGERY

John Hamilton, FRCS, Gloucestershire Hospitals Trust

John Hamilton, Dept of Otolaryngology, Gloucestershire Hospitals NHS Foundation Trust, Great Western Road, Gloucester, GL1 3EE, United Kingdom,
Phone: + 44 8454 226207, Email: john.hamilton@dial.pipex.com

A prospective parallel group study was performed of hearing outcomes in ears undergoing primary cholesteatoma surgery using a laser-assisted intact canal wall technique.

Group A had a continuous ossicular chain. Group B had a disrupted chain with an intact stapes superstructure onto which an ossiculoplasty had been performed.

The four frequency air-bone gap was calculated for each operated ear.

The Belfast Rules of Thumb were also used to calculate a dichotomous measure of whether the operated ear would provide useful hearing.

61 patients underwent surgery resulting in an intact chain. The median air-bone gap in this group was 15dB HL. 82% satisfied the requirements of the Belfast Rules.

84 patients underwent surgery requiring an ossiculoplasty onto an intact stapes. The median air-bone gap in this group was 20 dB HL. 50% satisfied the Belfast Rules.

The two groups are statistically discernible by both outcome measures ($P < 0.001$, Mann-Whitney ; $P < 0.0002$, χ^2, $\nu = 1$ respectively).

Preservation of the ossicular chain provides better hearing than any reconstructed chain after cholesteatoma surgery. Moreover, the requirements of hearing preservation influence the entire surgical technique for the treatment of cholesteatoma.

1. Introduction

At the second MEMRO conference in Boston in 1999, an analysis of the long term audiological results of ossiculoplasty in cholesteatoma surgery by Hamilton and Robinson showed that, although there was a small deterioration in results for all ossiculoplasties in the first five years after surgery, the long term results remained stable. The most important determinant of both the long term and immediate outcome of ossiculoplasty was the state of the ossicular chain after removal of cholesteatoma.

Preservation of the intact ossicular chain was shown to provide markedly better results than any reconstruction of the chain, whether onto the capitulum or stapes footplate[1].

In view of this finding, it was determined to preserve the ossicular chain in all patients undergoing cholesteatoma surgery who presented with the chain intact.

There are three difficulties with this stratagem.

The most testing problem arises because cholesteatoma can be firmly adherent to the ossicles. Under this circumstance, the use of conventional steel instruments to remove disease is liable to cause movement of the ossicles, with the potential transfer of damaging energy into the cochlea. To minimize the risk of permanent sensorineural hearing loss and yet remove the cholesteatoma, the ossicles hitherto have been sacrificed along with the adherent disease.

The fibre-guided, visible light laser has provided the means for preservation of the ossicular chain despite adherent cholesteatoma. This instrument uses a glass optical fibre to deliver light energy to the disease. The light energy vaporizes the cholesteatoma without causing any movement of the ossicles.

A second problem is that cholesteatoma can grow medial to the ossicular chain so that it can be difficult to identify. The fibre-guide laser solves this difficulty as well, as the optical fibre provides the means to conduct the vaporising energy around corners. In difficult cases the action of the laser can be monitored with the use of a small otological mirror. In extreme cases the laser light can be reflected off the mirror onto the disease on the far side of the ossicle.

The third problem is the tendency of the disease to recur *de novo* by retraction. This problem does not directly affect hearing results but may necessitate further surgery in the event that cholesteatoma should recur. If the ossicular chain is preserved intact and draped by epithelium, as in an "open" mastoid cavity, there is a high risk of keratinizing epithelium retracting behind the epitympanic region of the chain. To minimise this risk, it is prudent to shield the epitympanic part of the chain by preservation of the ear canal wall. This study is therefore restricted to patients in whom the ear canal has been preserved.

2. Method

2.1 Inclusion criteria

Ears undergoing primary cholesteatoma surgery using a laser-assisted intact canal wall technique from 1999 to 2005. Patients were separated into two groups on the basis of the state of the ossicular chain at the end of surgery. Group A had a continuous ossicular chain. Group B had a disrupted chain with an intact stapes superstructure onto which an ossiculoplasty had been performed.

2.2 Exclusion criteria

Ears that did not have an intact stapes superstructure at the end of surgery were excluded.

Also excluded were ears which had an intact stapes superstructure at the end of surgery but which did not undergo any form of reconstruction of the ossicular chain. This usually occurred because of prior documentation of significant sensorineural hearing loss in the operated ear.

2.3 Outcome

Outcome was assessed in the second year following surgery.

The air-bone gap was calculated for each operated ear. The air-bone gap was defined as the mean of the difference between the air conduction threshold and the bone conduction threshold at four frequencies (500Hz, 1kHz, 2kHz and 4kHz).

The Belfast Rules of Thumb were also used to calculate a dichotomous measure of whether the ear would provide useful hearing.

The air bone gap provides a measure of the function of the operated middle ear, whereas the Belfast score provides a measure of the benefit to the patient[2].

2.4 Analysis

The null hypothesis was that the distributions of the hearing results of the two groups should be the same.

The distributions of the hearing results, as measured by the air-bone gap, were assessed by the Mann-Whitney *U*-test.

The distributions of the hearing results as measured by the Belfast rules were assessed by the Chi Square test with Yates correction.

3. Results

61 patients underwent cholesteatoma surgery resulting in an intact canal wall and an intact chain. The median air-bone gap in this group was 15dB HL with a range of 2.5–30 dB HL.

84 patients underwent cholesteatoma surgery resulting in an ossiculoplasty in the presence of an intact canal wall. The median air-bone gap in this group was 20 dB HL with a range of 7–55 dB HL.

The raw data are shown in figure 1. The cumulative distribution of each group is shown so that the two groups can be clearly distinguished.

The two groups are statistically discernible ($z = 5.57$ $P< 0.001$, Mann-Whitney)

Patient benefit as assessed by the Belfast Rules of Thumb is a more stringent test of audiometric outcome. Fifty of the intact chain group (82%) satisfied the requirements of this test. Forty of the ossiculoplasty group (50%) satisfied this test (see figure 2). The two groups are also statistically different when measured by this outcome ($\chi^2 = 14.22$, $\nu = 1$, $P < 0.0002$)

4. Conclusions

This investigation has confirmed the hypothesis, suggested by the study presented at the Second Middle Ear Mechanics meeting in Boston in 1999, that preservation of the ossicular chain provides better hearing than any reconstructed chain after cholesteatoma surgery.

Comparison of the median outcomes may suggest that the improvement in middle ear function with chain preservation is "small". This evaluation ignores the stringent constraints required of a reconstructed middle ear to be part of a functionally useful ear. To benefit the patient the ear must have good cochlear and middle ear function and any loss of cochlear function stiffens the demands on middle ear reconstruction. In this context, any procedure which improves middle ear function, even if only by a "small" amount, is important: a 12 dB cochlear loss combined with a 20dB conductive loss may result in an air conduction threshold which does not provide the patient with any benefit. The same cochlear loss with a 15dB conductive loss would be regarded as useful to the patient. In this study the 5 dB improvement in conductive hearing is sufficient to increase the rate of useful hearing from 50% to 82%.

The desire to consistently preserve the ossicular chain in cholesteatoma surgery results in an obligation to adopt a very particular surgical technique, in which both the use of a fibre-guided laser and the preservation of the ear canal wall are necessary.

This perspective is entirely new in cholesteatoma surgery: instead of being a mere afterthought at the end of the surgical procedure, the requirements of hearing preservation now influence the entire surgical technique for the treatment of cholesteatoma.

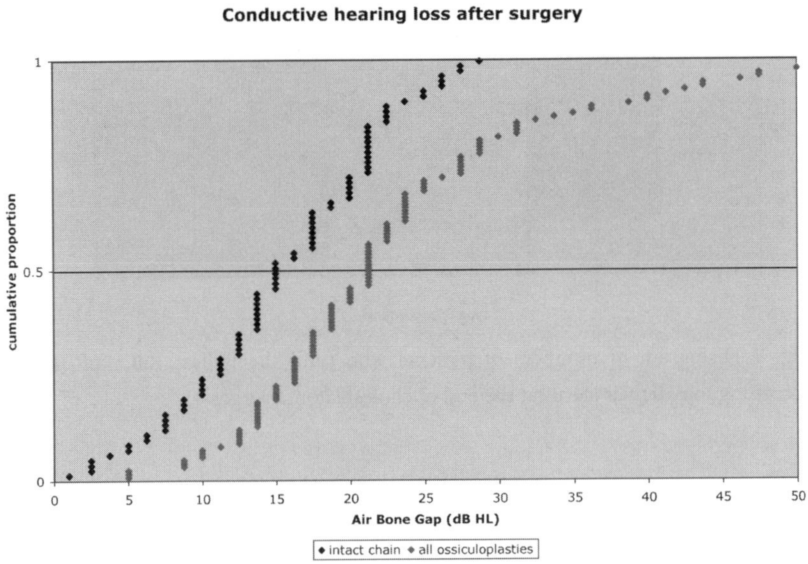

Fig. 1 Cumulative distribution of audiological assessment of middle ear function (air-bone gap) for ears with intact chain and ears with ossiculoplasty onto intact stapes at the end of cholesteatoma resection with intact canal wall.

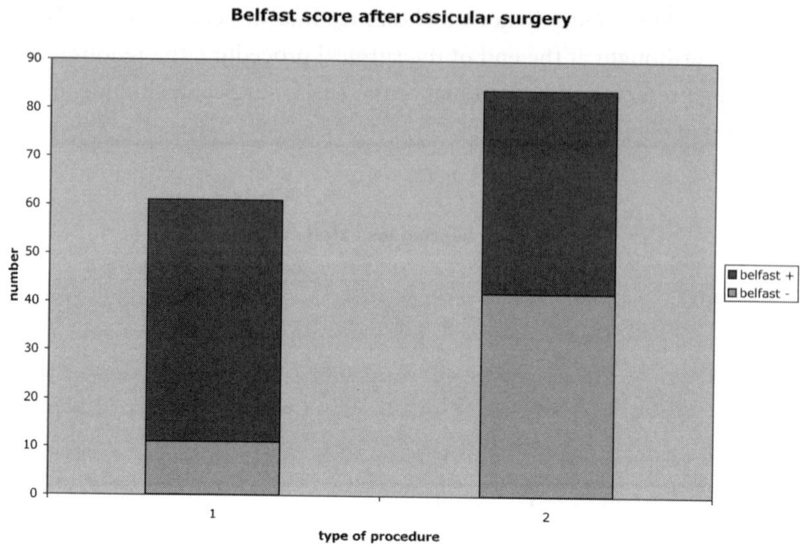

Fig. 2 Histogram of numbers of patients who fulfil the Belfast Rules of Thumb according to ossicular status at the end of cholesteatoma surgery.

References

1. Hamilton J., Robinson J., Short and long-term hearing results after middle ear surgery. *In The function and mechanics of normal, diseased and reconstructed middle ears. Eds* Rosowski JJ, Merchant SN. Kugler Publications, The Hague. 2000; 205–214
2. Smyth G.D.L., Results of middle ear reconstruction: Do patients and surgeons agree? *Am J Otol* 1985; **6**: 276–279

THE EFFICACY OF ONE-STAGE TYMPANOPLASTY WITH MASTOID OBLITERATION AND TYMPANOPLASTY BY TRANSCANAL APPROACH

Ken Hayashi, Atsushi Shinkawa, Department of Otolaryngology, Shinkawa Clinic, 1-2-3, Minamiyana, Hadano, Kanagawa, 257-0003, Japan.

Corresponding author: Ken Hayashi,
Phone: +81-463-76-3341, Fax: +81-463-76-3342,
Email: ken.hayashi@jcom.home.ne.jp, john.hamilton@dial.pipex.com

Purpose: To confirm the effect of one-staged tympanoplasty with mastoid obliteration and tympanoplasty by transcanal approach using ceramic prosthesis.

Materials and Methods: A retrospective chart review was performed on 516 patients undergoing ossicular chain reconstruction between June 2001 and December 2005. We use one-stage tympanoplasty with mastoid obliteration, a modified canal wall down procedure for chronic otitis media with aeration trouble in mastoid. On the other hand, we use a tympanoplasty by transcanal approach for chronic otitis media without aeration trouble in mastoid.

Results: In modified canal wall down, mean ABG for partial ossicular replacement prostheses was 29.5 Db postoperatively. Mean ABG for total ossicular replacement prostheses was 38.1 Db. Mean hearing gain in the P-type ceramic group was 10.3 dB. Mean hearing gain for patients following placement of T-type ceramic group was 9.3 dB. On the contrary, in tympanoplasty by transcanal approach, postoperative mean ABG for partial ossicular replacement prostheses was 40.4 dB. Mean ABG for total ossicular replacement prostheses was 42.7 dB. Mean hearing gain in the P-type ceramic was 7.8 dB. Mean hearing gain for patients following placement of T-type ceramic was 6.2 dB. A modified canal wall down group using ceramic P-type and ceramic a T-type group had 33.3% and 67% success rates. A tympanoplasty by transcanal approach using ceramic P-type and ceramic T-type had 10% and 20% success rates.

Discussion: We confirmed that the total ossicular reconstruction using ceramic T-type was satisfactory for one-stage tympanoplasty with mastoid obliteration. However, the patients requiring tympanolasty by transcanal approach had significantly worse results than those with one-stage tympanoplasty with mastoid obliteration. In this study, we considered that patients undergoing a tympanoplasty by transcanal approach had more severe disease including tympanosclerosis than those requiring one-stage tympanoplasty with mastoid obliteration. In addition, our results showed that hearing results tended to be worse in unplanned revision surgery.
Conclusion: We hope that a variety of material for reconstruction of the ossicular chain will be used in the near future in Japan as well.

1. Introduction

Various operative procedures have been developed for the surgical treatment of chronic otitis media with or without cholesteatoma. The principal objective in chronic otitis media with cholesteatoma surgery is the complete eradication of the disease to produce a safe ear and the improvement of hearing. Over the past years, one goal of the complete eradication of the disease has been consistently achieved using the canal wall down procedure [1]. However, this technique has several problems, such as difficulty with fitting a hearing aid and a higher rate of infection. For this reason, the canal wall up procedure is more commonly used [2, 3]. In reality, the incidence of cholesteatoma recurrence is higher with canal wall up procedure than canal wall down procedure. Therefore, staged operation is in heavy usage, and then patients with cholesteatoma must go through operations a number of times [4, 5].

Consequently, we use one-stage tympanoplasty with mastoid obliteration, a modified canal down procedure, for the treatment of otitis media with aeration trouble in mastoid, while we use a tympanoplasty by a transcanal approach for chronic otitis media without aeration trouble in mastoid. In addition, all these operations were performed as day surgery.
On the contrary, otologic surgeons have used a variety of material for reconstruction of the ossicular chain [6–8]. In Japan, autograft replacement is still the most commonly used materials, and it is very rare that biocompatible synthetic materials are used. However, we have used ceramic prosthesis (Type P and Type T) and reported excellent results including good hearing improvement and low extrusion rates [9].

This time, we describe the effect of one staged tympanoplasty with mastoid obliteration and tympanoplasty by transcanal approach using ceramic prosthesis.

2. Materials and Methods

A retrospective chart review was performed on 516 patients undergoing ossicular chain reconstruction between June 2001 and December 2005. The procedure included one stage tympanoplasty with mastoid obliteration and tympanoplasty by transcanal approach. Demographic information about these patients is summarized in Table 1.

Air-bone gap (ABG) data were obtained by comparing the most recent bone and air-conduction results. Air-bone gap was calculated by the use of four-frequency pure tone averages (500, 1000, 2000, and 3000 Hz) of air and bone conduction from the same test intervals. "Successful" reconstruction was defined as a postoperative PTA-ABG less than or equal to 20 dB.

3. Surgical Procedure 1

We use one-stage tympanoplasty with mastoid obliteration, a modified canal wall down procedure for chronic otitis media with aeration trouble in mastoid [9]. In this procedure, mastoid cavity is opened by resecting bone of the posterior and superior walls of external ear canal, and then antrum and epitympanum are opened. However, the intact canal skin is maintained. After cleaning of the lesions, changes in the ossicular chain, particularly at the long process of the incus and the superstructure of the stapes, are carefully observed. If cholesteatoma included whole incus, incus is removed by separating from the lesions around the stapes. The tendon of the tensor tympani muscle is also cut. After the opening of Eustachian tube to the tympanic cavity is confirmed, the eardrum is reconstructed by closing the perforation underlying it with the fascia.

The ossicular chain was reconstructed using the ceramic ossicular prosthesis (P-type and T-type). The ceramic ossicular prosthesis is used with trimming the shaft to the appropriate size. We performed a partial ossicular chain reconstruction using the P-type ceramic when the superstructure of the stapes could be utilized, while we performed a total chain reconstruction using the T-type ceramic when the superstructure of the stapes could not be used.

After reconstruction of the ossicular chain, the reconstruction of posterior and superior walls of the external ear canal and the obliteration of mastoid cavity was performed with the bone plate from mastoid cortical bone (Figure 1). Through this surgery, we consider that it is most important to preserve the skin of the external canal and keep the position of tympanic membrane intact except for the perforation area of the tympanic membrane.

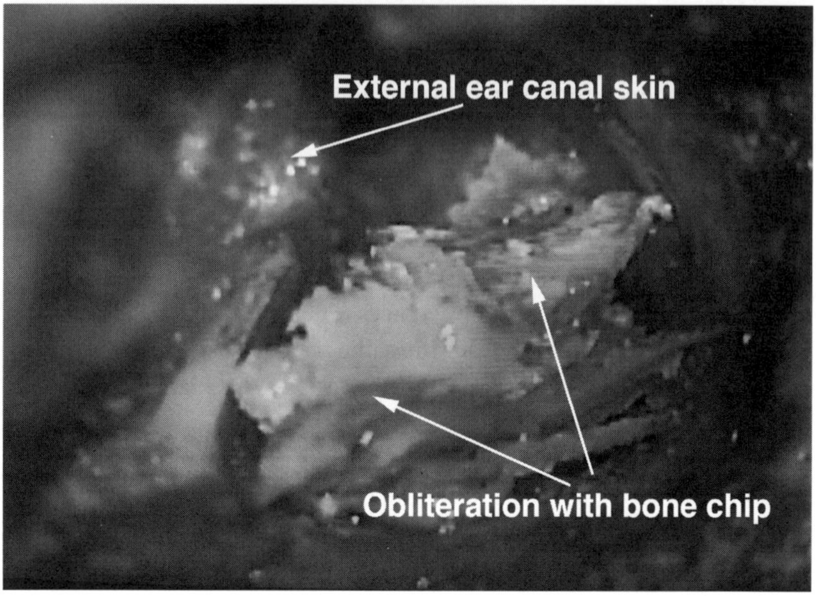

Fig. 1 After reconstruction of the ossicular chain, the reconstruction of posterior and superior walls of the external ear canal and the obliteration of mastoid cavity was performed with the bone plate from mastoid cortical bone.

4. Surgical Procedure 2

On the other hand, we use a tympanoplasty by transcanal approach for chronic otitis media without aeration trouble in mastoid. An incision is made with a lancet at 12 and 7 o'clock, and the meatal skin is elevated to the level of the fibrous annulus. The bone edge of the posterior canal wall is removed little by little with chisel until the pyramidal eminence and the stapes tendon are clearly visible. After the annulus is raised, the middle ear is entered. We performed a partial ossicular chain reconstruction using the P-type ceramic when the superstructure of the stapes could be utilized, while we performed a total chain reconstruction using the T-type ceramic when the superstructure of the stapes could not be used.

5. Results

Ninety-three of 100 cases (93%) represented primary surgery in modified canal wall down, while three hundred nineteen of 416 cases (77%) were performed as an unplanned revision surgery in tympanoplasty by transcanal approach (Table 2).

In modified canal wall down, mean ABG for partial ossicular replacement prostheses was 29.5 dB (SD±15.3) postoperatively. Mean ABG for total ossicular replacement prostheses was 38.1 dB (SD±12.8). Mean hearing gain in the P-type ceramic group was 10.3 dB (SD±7.41). Mean hearing gain for patients following placement of T-type ceramic group was 9.3 dB (SD±6.83). No patient had a significant acute worsening of bone conduction postoperatively. On the contrary, in tympanoplasty by transcanal approach, postoperative mean ABG for partial ossicular replacement prostheses was 40.4 dB (SD±11.9). Mean ABG for total ossicular replacement prostheses was 42.7 dB (SD±10.2). Mean hearing gain in the P-type ceramic was 7.8 dB (SD±12.8). Mean hearing gain for patients following placement of T-type ceramic was 6.2 dB (SD±9.54). No patient had a significant acute worsening of bone conduction postoperatively.

In modified canal wall down group using ceramic P-type group, 8.3% patients had a postoperative ABG of less than 10 dB. 25% patients had a postoperative ABG between 11–20 dB, on the other hand, in tympanoplasty by transcanal approach using ceramic P-type, no patient had a postoperative ABG of less than 10 dB. 10% patients had a postoperative ABG between 11–20 dB. In modified canal wall down group using ceramic T-type, 17% patients had a postoperative ABG of less than 10 dB, 50% patients had a postoperative ABG between 11–20 dB, In tympanoplasty by transcanal approach, no patients had a postoperative ABG of less than 10 dB, 20% patients had a postoperative ABG of 11–20 dB. We defined success as postoperative air-bone gap of 20 dB or less. A modified canal wall down group using ceraic P-type and ceramic T-type group had a 33.3% and 67% success rate (Figure 2). A tympanoplasty by transcanal approach using ceramic P-type and ceramic T-type had a 10% and 20% success rate.

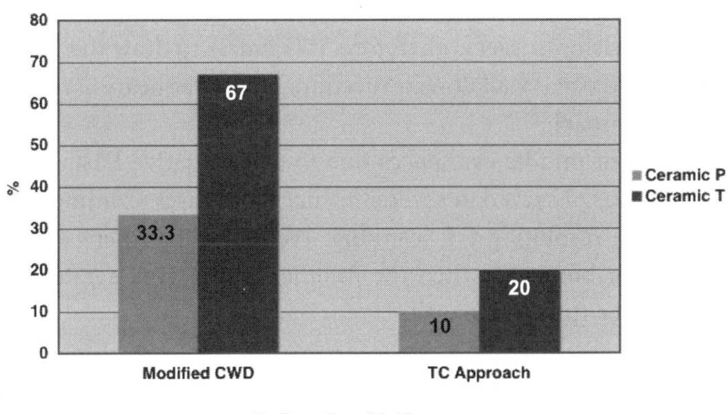

Fig. 2 A modified canal wall down group using ceramic P and ceramic T group had a 33.3% and 67% success rate. A tympanoplasty by transcanal approach using ceramic P and ceramic T had a 10% and 20% success rate.

6. Discussion

We have used one-stage tympanoplasty with mastoid obliteration as a modified canal wall down procedure for chronic otitis media with aeration trouble in mastoid [9]. The major advantage of the canal wall down procedure is that surgical area is visible through a microscope. On the contrary, we maintain the external canal skin intact and fill the cavity formed by the removal of the bone of the external ear canal with the patient's own bone fragments obtained from the temporal bone, even though we remove the external ear canal bones and the mastoid cavity. After that, our procedure makes it easy to remove cholesteatoma and granulation, reduces the risk of infection, and prevents perforation of the tympanic membrane. Our results show that air-bone gaps could be reduced to 20 dB or less in 33.3% of patients with ceramic P-type ceramic and 67% of patients with T-type ceramic. In this study, we confirmed that the total ossicular reconstruction using ceramic T-type was satisfactory for one-stage tympanoplasty with mastoid obliteration. In fact, we broke down the disadvantage of the canal wall down procedure.

On the other hand, tympanoplasty by transcanal approach for chronic otitis media without aeration trouble in mastoid was performed. However, we reported the success rate of 10% for ceramic P-type and 20% for ceramic T-type with tympanoplasty by transcanal approach. In fact, the patients requiring tympanolasty by transcanal approach had significantly worse results than those with one-stage tympanoplasty with mastoid obliteration. In this study, we considered that patients undergoing a tympanoplasty by transcanal approach had more severe disease including tympanosclerosis than those requiring one-stage tympanoplasty with mastoid obliteration. In addition, our results showed that hearing results tended to be worse in unplanned revision surgery. Therefore, it is unfair to draw the conclusion that a modified canal wall down procedure has better hearing results than transcanal approach.

Insufficient middle ear spaces due to postoperative Eustachian tube dysfunction was observed in several unsuccessful cases examined by postoperative high resolution CT scanning. We found that there was a trend for a better air-bone gap when the middle ear was well aerated and the Eustachian tube functioned well.

7. Conclusion

In conclusion, our observation is that unsuccessful cases may not have a secure attachment to the stapes footplate because of not allowing tissue integrations. Therefore, we hope that a variety of material for reconstruction of the ossicular chain will be used in the near future in Japan as well.

Table 1 Demographic information.

	Modified CWD	TC approach
Patients	100	416
Mean age±SD	44.3±15.3	55.5±14.5
Sex (M:F)	42:58	187:229
Affected side (R:L)	54:46	203:213

CWD; Canal Wall Down, TC; Transcanal

Table 2 Primary Surgery versus Revision Surgery.

	Modified CWD		TC approach	
	Ceramic P	Ceramic T	Ceramic P	Ceramic T
Primary Surgery	68	25	89	8
Revision Surgery	4	3	208	111
Total	72	28	297	119

CWD; Canal Wall Down, TC; Transcanal

References

1. Sheehy J., Cholesteatoma surgery: canal wall down procedures. *An Otol Rhinol Laryngol,* **97** (1988) pp. 30–35
2. Smyth G.D., Canal wall for cholesteatoma: up or down? Long-term results. *Am J Otol,* **6** (1988) pp. 1–2
3. Palmgren O., Long-term results of open cavity and tympanomastoid surgery of the chronic ear. *Acta Otolaryngol* **88** (1979) pp. 343–349
4. Smyth G.D. and Kerr A.G., Staged tympanoplasty. *J Laryngol Otol* **84** (1970) pp. 757–764
5. Hinohira Y., Yanagihara N. and Gyo K., Surgical treatment of retraction pocket with bone plate: scutum plasty for cholesteatoma. *Otolaryngol Head Neck Surg* **133** (2005) pp. 625–628
6. Emmett J.R., Biocompatible implants in tympanoplasty. *Am J Otol.* **184** (1989) pp. 215–219
7. House J.W. and Teufert K.B., Extrusion rates and hearing results in ossicular reconstruction. *Otolaryngol Head Neck Surg* **125** (2001) pp. 135–141
8. Fisch U., May J., Linder T., Naumann IC., A new L-shaped titanium prosthesis for total reconstruction of the ossicular chain. *Otol Neurotol.* **25** (2004) pp. 891–902
9. Shinkawa A., Sakai M., Tamura Y., Takahashi H. and Ishida K., Canal-down tympanoplasty; one-stage tympanoplasty with mastoid obliteration, for non-cholesteatomatous chronic otitis media associated with osteitis. *Tokai J Exp Clin Med* **23** (1998) pp. 19–23

"CONCEPTUAL DESIGN" OF THE HUMAN MIDDLE EAR

Herbert Hudde, Institute of Communication Acoustics, Ruhr University Bochum, D 44780 Bochum, Germany, Email: herbert.hudde@rub.de

If the functionality of the middle ear is considered, mostly the ability of effectively transmitting sound energy from the air in the ear canal to the fluids in the inner ear is examined. However, to assess the "quality" of the middle ear it is necessary to consider also other aspects such as the reaction to external forces and to general changes in the mechanic system. The human middle ear turns out to provide a larger auditory frequency range, lower general parameter sensitivity and better protection of the inner ear than a columella ear found in birds and reptiles.

The favourable properties are best understood by regarding the vibrations of the ossicular chain under normal and impaired conditions and for different kinds of excitation. Vibrations were computed by means of a generalised circuit model. All the resulting patterns of vibration taken together reveal a remarkable conceptual design of the human middle ear: The incudomalleal joint acts as an element protecting the inner ear against external forces. Such a robust overload protector necessarily introduces a rather heavy mass centre which tends to worsen the transmission at high frequencies. It turns out that the design of the human middle ear does not only circumvent a decrease in transmission at too low frequencies, but even takes advantage from the mass centre. The surprising features are achieved by the position of the mass centre outside the direct path of transmission in combination with a favourable design of the elastic elements involved.

1. Introduction

In the middle ears of reptiles and birds the connection between the sound collecting tympanic membrane and the input window of the inner ear is simply shaped as a kind of rod called "columella". Thus the question arises why mammals including humans have a rather sophisticated connection which is usually referred to as "ossicular chain" (Fig. 1). In spite of natural discrepancies between different species one observes that the two middle ear systems are about as sensitive as any other. However, ossicular chains are usually able to work at higher frequencies than columella middle ear can do [1].

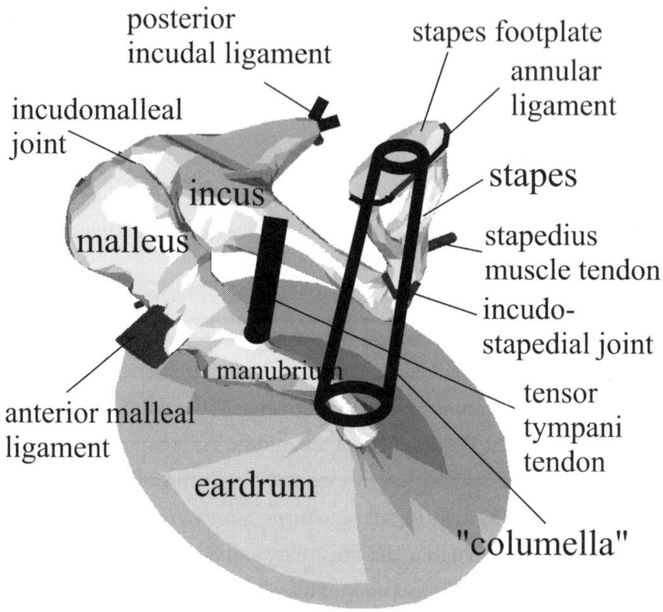

Fig. 1 Human ossicular chain and a schematically drawn "columella".

Looking at Fig. 1 this fact is all the more surprising as the ossicular chain obviously contains more mass which should worsen the transmission of high frequencies because of inertial forces. The main mass is concentrated on both sides of the incudomalleal joint. One can assume that the comparably large masses of the malleus head and the incus body are necessary to implement a particularly robust joint in between. It is known that the incudomalleal joint serves as an overload protector which reduces the effect of external forces and static pressure on the inner ear. The role of the mass centre formed by the malleus head and the incus body has to be elucidated in the following.

The similar sensitivity of both systems in spite of different masses is explained by different kinds of vibration. At low frequencies the malleus and incus jointly rotate about the so called "main axis" which lies near the centre of gravity of both ossicles. This reduces the effective mass. In contrast, the columella mainly vibrates translationally along the rod axis. On the other hand, at *low* frequencies inertial forces are small in any case. Thus a rotational vibration of the ossicles should be particularly expected at high frequencies.

2. Ossicular Vibrations for Acoustic Excitation

The vibrations of the ossicular chain were investigated using a "generalised circuit model" [2]. The model is based on a great variety of transfer functions measured by means of laser vibrometry. Simulations using a mathematical model have an invaluable advantage compared with experiments: conditions can be altered very easily and exactly to study the effect of changes. In this short paper mostly normal conditions are considered.

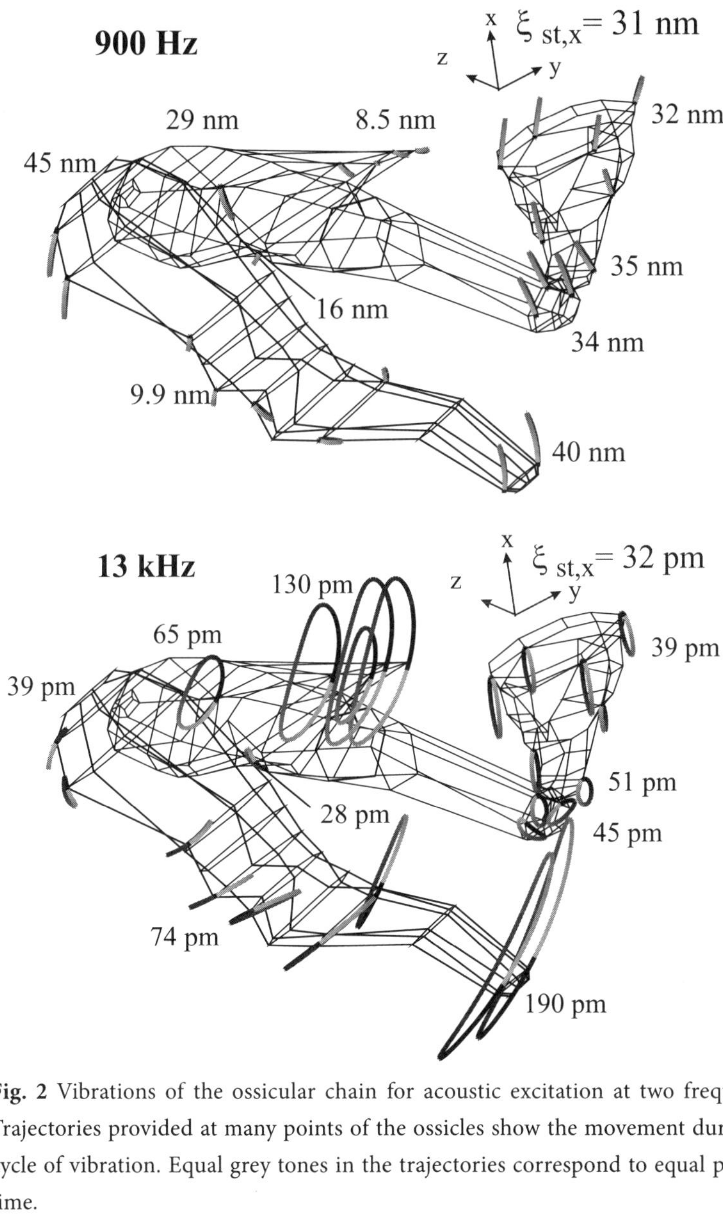

Fig. 2 Vibrations of the ossicular chain for acoustic excitation at two frequencies. Trajectories provided at many points of the ossicles show the movement during one cycle of vibration. Equal grey tones in the trajectories correspond to equal points in time.

The patterns of vibration at different frequencies are best seen in animations, but also the representations in Fig. 2 can give an impression. At low frequencies the already mentioned rotation about the main axis is confirmed (not shown). At medium frequencies above 700–800 Hz we observe rocking motions. At high frequencies above 3–4 kHz particularly the manubrium vibrates very vigorously. At very high frequencies above 10 kHz even the short process of the incus begins to vibrate strongly (Fig. 2). In this way instead of an axis of rotation more and more a centre of rotation occurs in the middle of the incudomalleal joint. In summary, surprisingly different patterns of vibration appear if the frequency varies in the audio frequency range form 20 Hz to 20 kHz. The chain is astonishingly flexible. The incudostapedial joint, fairly compliant ligaments and bending of ossicles contribute to flexibility.

Looking at the stapes one observes strong lateral vibrations of the stapes head. However, only the motion perpendicular to the oval window essentially contributes to the pressure generated in the vestibule. Thus at the stapes and also elsewhere strong vibration components arise which could be regarded as unnecessary and therefore ineffective. Certainly an engineer would avoid unnecessary vibrations and prefer a simple mode of vibration which does not change as a function of frequency. In fact, unnecessary motions would worsen the transmission if strong damping was present in the ossicular chain. However, this is not the case. Actually the flexibility of the chain leads to generally large vibration components, and therefore also to large vibration in the desired direction.

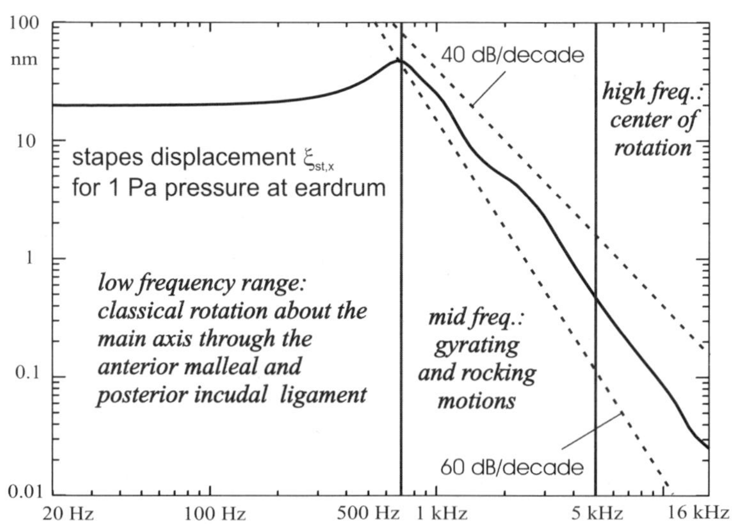

Fig. 3 Frequency response of the middle ear for acoustic excitation. The stapes displacement perpendicular to the footplate is given for a constant pressure of 1 Pa at the eardrum.

The positive effect of the lateral vibrations is proven by the frequency response of the middle ear. In Fig. 3 the stapes displacement in the direction perpendicular to the oval window is used as indicator. The frequency response resembles that of a simple mass-spring vibrator which has a decrease of 40 dB per decade beyond the resonant frequency. The actual drop is somewhat steeper. However, this does not indicate inefficiency of the ossicular chain, but is the result of the effective size of the eardrum area which decreases at higher frequencies.

The irregularity of vibrations means that not only a single mode of vibration – as would be aimed at by an engineer – occurs in the middle ear. The system of suspended ossicles has several modes of vibration in the frequency range of audio signals. The actual pattern of vibration is mainly governed by the eigenfrequencies which are close to the frequency of the excitation. The kind of vibration is flexibly adapted to the frequency and the kind of excitation. In this way the kinetic energy of the ossicles is kept low. For instance, at high frequencies the mass centre encasing the incudomalleal joint does not significantly worsen the transmission because not the bulk of the masses, but only the manubrium and the two incudal processes vibrate around the mass centre.

Changing patterns of vibration seem to be part of the conceptual design we are looking for. The irregular motions found are not unfavourable. On the contrary, a fixed pattern enforced by bearings and guideways would tend to fail if the ossicles were slightly misaligned. Further investigations which cannot be reported here in detail show that the ossicular chain is fairly insensitive to changing relative positions of the ossicles and to artificial stiffenings of ligaments and joints. A partial reduction of flexibility does not produce a break-down of transmission. Only a combination of two or more stiffenings can severely degrade the transmission. The decisive flexible element is the incudostapedial joint which is only stiff in the direction of main transmission (proc. lenticularis to stapes head). Therefore stiffening this joint provokes particularly strong degradations.

3. Ossicular Vibrations for Mechanic Excitation

Another advantage of the mass centre is revealed when also mechanic excitation of the middle ear is considered. In this case the ossicular chain is not driven by a pressure at the eardrum, but by motions of the bony walls of the tympanic cavity. Vibrations of the cavity walls are transmitted via ligaments, muscles and the tympanic membrane to the ossicles. This effect is part of the bone conduction path to the inner ear.

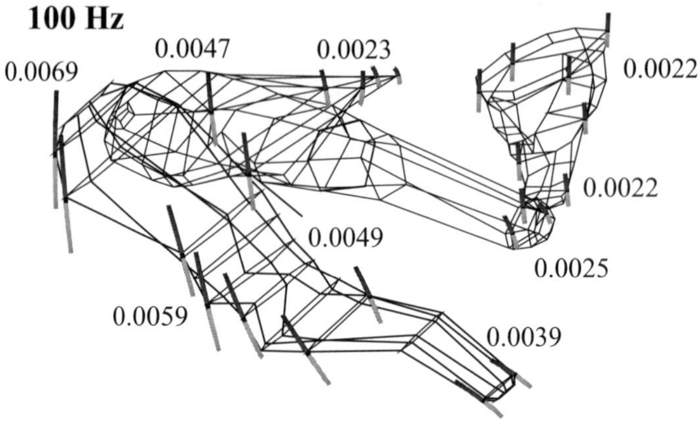

Fig. 4 Vibrations of the ossicular chain for mechanic excitation at 100 Hz. The tympanic cavity wall is shaken in the direction perpendicular to the stapes footplate. The trajectories represent the relative motions of the ossicles referred to the stimulating vibration of the cavity wall. The numbers denote relative vibration amplitudes (spatial effective values).

Fig. 4 shows the vibrations arising at a low frequency (100 Hz) for excitation in the most sensitive direction perpendicular to the stapes footplate. The maximum vibrations occur at the mass centre. This is caused by inertial forces which are mostly effective at the mass centre, not at the stapes. Thus, due to the position of the mass centre outside the direct transmission path from the umbo to the stapes head (see Fig. 5), the transmission of wall vibrations to the inner ear is successfully reduced. External forces are deflected by the mass centre avoiding direct impact onto the stapes head.

With increasing frequency the insulation against bone conduction explained above unavoidably decreases. At high frequencies beyond the cut-off frequency of the system, which is about 2 kHz, the ossicles are almost at rest. Thus the relative vibration approaches the vibration of the tympanic cavity wall. Hence the bone conduction transmission of the middle ear is that of a high-pass filter. The laterally displaced mass centre outside the direct transmission path of the ossicular chain has the advantage to shift the cut-off frequency to higher frequencies.

4. Summary and Conclusions

In addition to the often mentioned transformer principle based on the area ratio of the tympanic membrane and the stapes footplate, three further principles of the "conceptual design" are pointed out in this paper (Fig. 5):

— Implementation of a robust (incudomalleal) joint protecting the inner ear.

— Placement of a comparably heavy mass centre (malleus head and incus body) outside the main transmission path of the ossicular chain.
— High flexibility of the ossicular chain. This is implemented by rather compliant suspensions, non-rigid ossicular processes and particularly by the very elastic incudostapedial joint. The joint is only stiff in the direction of main transmission from the processus lenticularis to the stapes head.

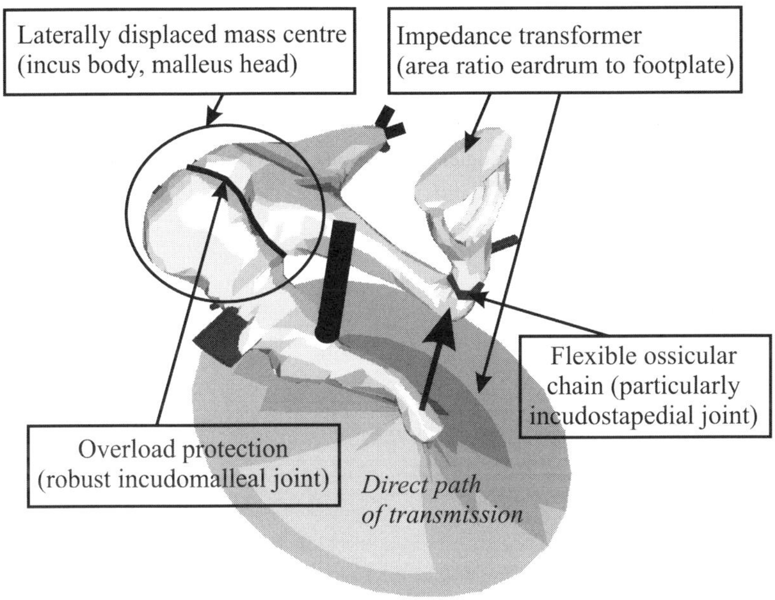

Fig. 5 "Conceptual design" of the middle ear.

This yields the following properties:
— Broad-band air conduction is maintained also under unfavourable conditions: In this respect the human ossicular chain is clearly superior to a columella. The combination of high flexibility and a laterally displaced mass avoids blocking effects (for this aim a real columella possesses an additional elastic element, the "extracolumella", which causes the lower cut-off frequencies found in birds and reptiles).
— Generally low parameter sensitivity: Due to the high flexibility the ossicular chain "finds" favourable patterns of vibration at each frequency in the audio range. Neither the interindividual variability of the exact shape of the ossicles nor temporary intraindividual changes (e. g., due to variations of static pressure) can substantially alter the middle ear transmission.

— Improved insulation from mechanic shock: Inertial forces due to external impact on the head are deflected by the laterally displaced mass, even if they are applied in the sensitive direction perpendicular to the footplate. This increases the cut-off frequency of the bone conduction high-pass filter.

References

1. Manley, G. A., *Peripheral hearing mechanisms in reptiles and birds;* Springer, Berlin 1990
2. Hudde, H. and Weistenhöfer, C., Circuit models of middle ear function. In: J. Rosowski and S. Merchant (eds.) *The function and mechanics of normal, diseased and reconstructed middle ear.* Kugler Publications, The Hague, Netherlands (2000), pp. 39–58

ACOUSTIC-STRUCTURAL COUPLED FINITE ELEMENT ANALYSIS FOR SOUND TRANSMISSION IN HUMAN EAR – MIDDLE EAR TRANSFER FUNCTION

Rong Z. Gan[1], Tao Cheng[1], Mark W. Wood[2]
[1] School of Aerospace and Mechanical Engineering and Bioengineering Center, University of Oklahoma, Norman
[2] Hough Ear Institute, Oklahoma City, Oklahoma, USA, Email: rgan@ou.edu

A 3-D finite element (FE) model of human ear with accurate geometry of the ear canal and middle ear has been recently published by our group. In this paper, the acoustic-structure-acoustic coupled FE analysis was conducted to the model for normal and pathological ears such as the tympanic membrane (TM) perforations. Two laser vibrometers were used to measure simultaneously the TM and stapes footplate vibrations. The transfer function of the middle ear under normal and perforation conditions from the model show frequency-dependent behavior similar to that measured from temporal bones. The FE model provides good prediction on effect of perforation location and size on middle ear transfer function.

1. Introduction

The transfer function of the middle ear for sound transmission cannot be measured readily in living humans and different theoretical models have been developed to simulate the middle ear function. Compared with the traditional circuit or lumped model, the finite element (FE) method has its distinct advantages over other approaches in modeling complex biological systems like the ear. The 3-D anatomic structure, ultrastructural characteristics, alterations of structural changes, and material properties of the ear can be easily modeled and interpreted in FE model. Using the technologies of 3-D reconstruction and FE analysis, we have developed one of the most complete FE models of the ear that had been reported, which includes the ear canal, tympanic membrane (TM), ossicles, ligaments/tendons, and middle ear cavity [1, 2]. With the complete middle ear cavity, it is possible to study the effect of TM perforation on middle ear function.

In this paper, the acoustic-structure-acoustic coupled FE analysis was employed to derive sound transmission from the air-filled canal to the stapes in normal and pathological ears. The structural alterations such as the TM perforations were created in the model as well as in human temporal bones. Two laser vibrometers were used to measure simultaneously the transfer function of the middle ear. The FE model results were compared with the measurements obtained in temporal bones.

2. Methods

2.1 3-D FE model and acoustic-structural coupled analysis

A 3-D FE model of human left ear (male, age 61) was created based on histological sections of a temporal bone as shown in Fig. 1. The characteristic dimensions of the ear canal, middle ear components, and middle ear cavity of the model were reported in a recently published paper [2]. The mechanical properties of the TM, ossicles, joints, and manubrium and the Young's moduli of suspensory ligaments/tendons, tympanic annulus, and stapedial annular ligament are listed in Tables 1 and 2 of that paper [2]. The ear canal was open to the atmosphere, the same situation as the experimental setup in temporal bones performed in this study.

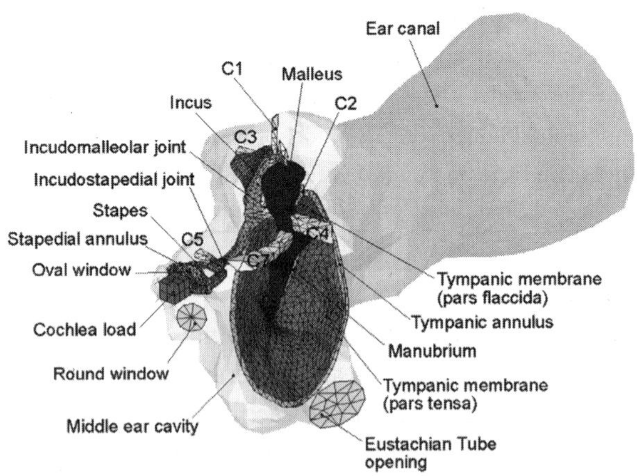

Fig. 1 FE model of human left ear including the TM, three ossicles (malleus, incus, and stapes), two joints and manubrium, ligaments and muscle tendons (C1, C2, C3, C4, C5, C7), tympanic annulus, stapedial annular ligament, external ear canal, middle ear cavity, and cochlear load, in anterior-medial view. The middle ear cavity was assumed transparent.

Modeling of sound transmission from the ear canal through the middle ear to cochlea requires multi-field coupled analysis. The air in the ear canal and inside the middle ear cavity was modeled as acoustic elements and governed by the simplified acoustic wave equation under the assumption that the fluid is compressible and inviscid with uniform mean density and pressure. The surface of acoustic elements next to the movable structure such as the TM, ossicles, and suspensory ligaments, was defined as fluid-structural interface (FSI) where the acoustic pressure distribution was coupled into structural analysis in ANSYS.

2.2 Measurement of middle ear transfer function in human temporal bones

Seven fresh-frozen cadaver temporal bones (3 male, 4 female, average age 69.4) were used in this study. The preparation of temporal bone specimen and sound delivery system were almost the same as that reported in our previous paper [3]. After facial recess on the bone, 90 dB pure tone sound signals were delivered to the TM by an insert earphone and monitored by a probe microphone placed in the canal approximately 2 mm away from the umbo. The second probe microphone was placed between the round window and stapes for measuring the middle ear pressure. The middle ear cavity was then covered by a piece of glass and closed by filling dental cement. Two laser vibrometers (Polytec, HLV-1000 and OFV 501) were used to measure vibrations of the TM and stapes simultaneously with one laser focusing on the umbo and another focusing on the stapes footplate.

The control experiment was performed first to measure the normal middle ear function. After control data were collected, two types of TM perforation were created in the temporal bones and simulated in the FE model as shown in Fig. 2. The perforation Case #1 was made in the inferior-posterior site of the TM with a perforation area of 1.4 mm^2. The perforation Case #2 was made in the inferior site with an area of 1.0 mm^2. The laser measurements of the umbo and footplate were conducted on Case #1 first and then the perforation Case #2 was made and the hole in the inferior-posterior site of the TM was patched with cigarette paper. Finally, the paper was removed and measurement was made with combination of Cases #1 and #2.

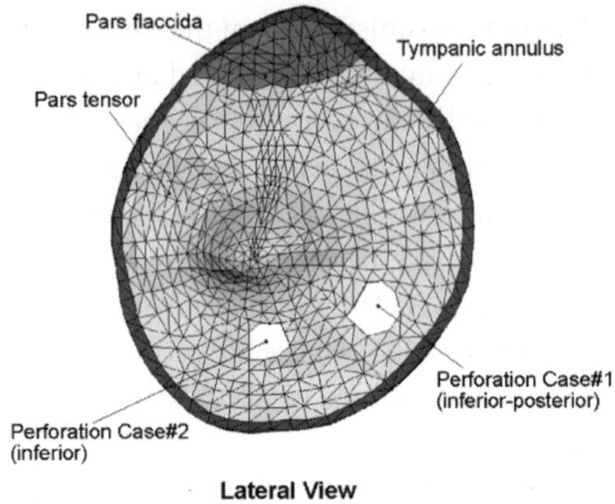

Fig. 2 Lateral view of the TM with two perforations: Case #1 – the perforation located in the inferior-posterior site of the TM; Case #2 – the perforation located in the inferior site.

3. Results

Fig. 3 shows the comparison of displacement derived from the FE model of normal ear with the data measured from 7 bones at the TM (umbo) and stapes footplate. Panels (A) and (B) display magnitude and panels (C) and (D) display phase angle. The 90 dB SPL was applied at 2 mm away from the

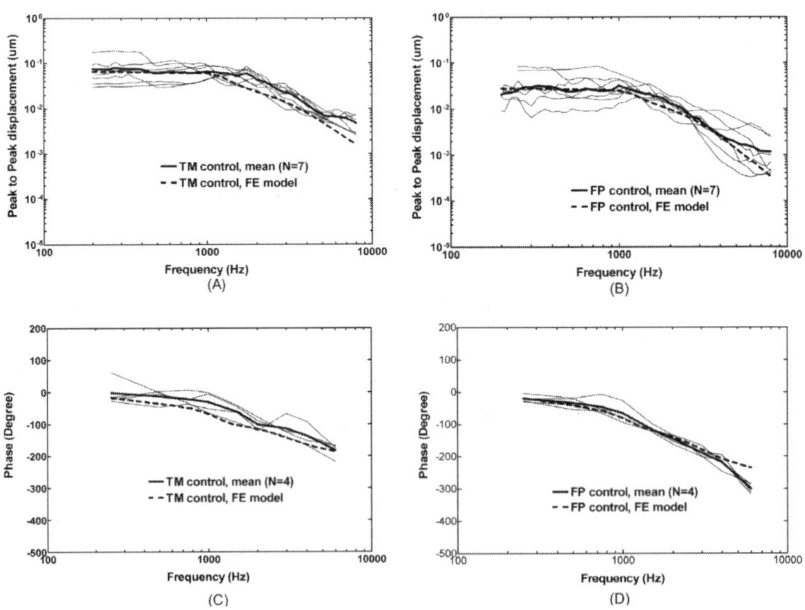

Fig. 3 Comparison of the FE model-derived TM and stapes footplate displacements with the data from 7 temporal bones in magnitude and phase angle. (A) and (C): TM displacement; (B) and (D): footplate displacement.

umbo in the ear canal of the model, which simulated the sound source in the bone experiments. A good agreement between the FE model and experimental data can be seen in Fig. 3.

Panels (A) and (C) in Fig. 4 show the mean magnitude and phase angle of the TM or umbo displacement obtained from 7 bones under control (intact TM, solid line), perforation Case #1 (Hole 1, broken-dash line), perforation Case #2 (Hole 2, dash line), and combined Holes 1 and 2 (broken line). The TM displacement curves predicted by the model are shown in panels (B) and (D). The results in Fig. 4 indicate that the model-predicted reduction of TM displacement magnitude at low frequencies (f<2 kHz) caused by perforations is consistent with the bone experimental data. A maximum of 27 dB reduction of the umbo displacement at 200 Hz was observed from the model and bone experiments. The model-predicted effect of perforation location and size on the TM displacement shows the same pattern as that measured from bones.

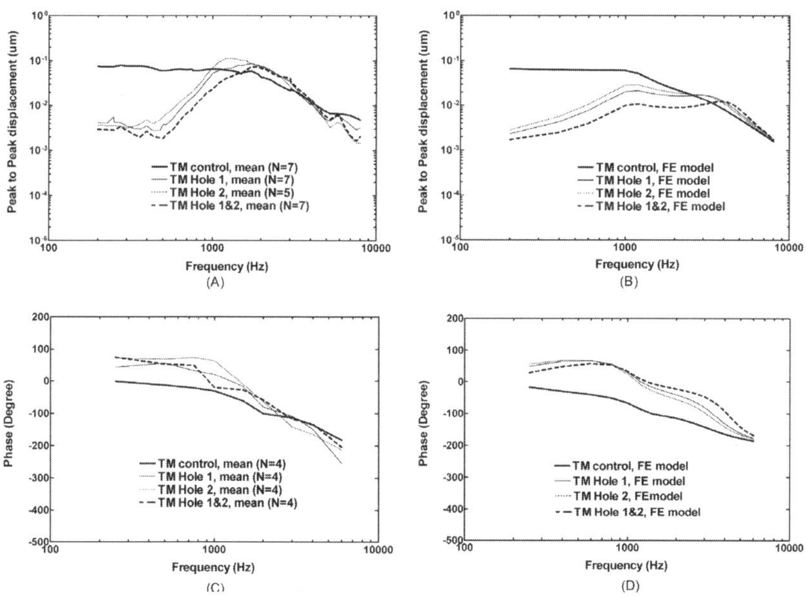

Fig. 4 Mean displacements measured at the TM and calculated from the FE model in control or intact TM (solid line), perforation Case #1 or Hole 1 (broken + dash line), perforation Case #2 or Hole 2 (dash line), and combined Holes 1 and 2 (broken line). (A) and (C): Bone experiments; (B) and (D): FE model.

Panels (A) and (C) in Fig. 5 display the mean magnitude and phase angle of stapes footplate displacement from 7 bones under control, perforation Case #1, Case #2, and combined cases #1 and #2. The model-derived footplate displacement curves are displayed in panels (B) and (D). It can be seen in Fig. 5 that the model predicted a reduction of the footplate displacement for all types of perforations at low frequencies (f<2 kHz) and a maximum of 20 dB was observed at f≤400 Hz. There were no variations of the footplate movement between different types of perforations below 500 Hz. This is different from the TM movement in either modeling or experimental data (see Fig. 4).

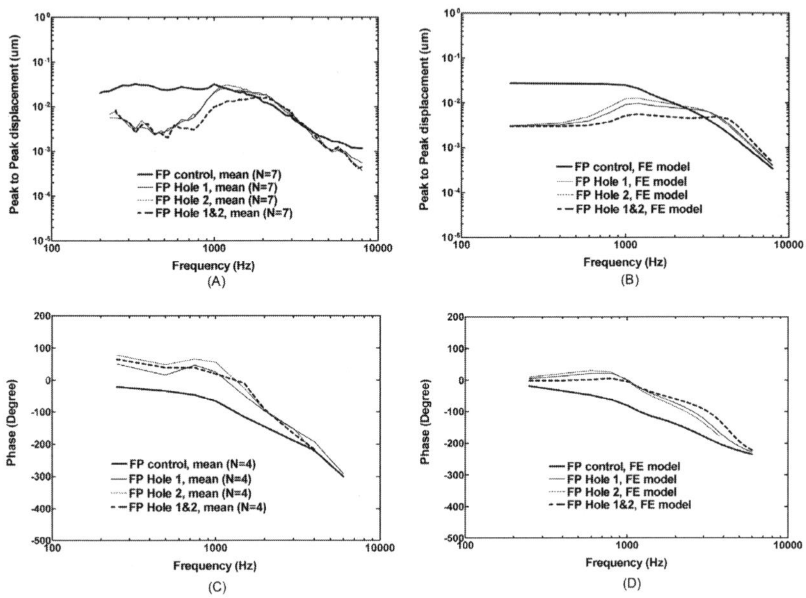

Fig. 5 Mean displacements measured at the footplate and calculated from the FE model in control or intact TM (solid line), perforation Case #1 or Hole 1 (broken + dash line), perforation Case #2 or Hole 2 (dash line), and combined Holes 1 and 2 (broken line). (A) and (C): Bone experiments; (B) and (D): FE model.

4. Discussion

In this paper, the structural alterations such as TM perforations were simulated, visualized, and computed in a 3-D FE model. The model-derived TM and footplate displacements were compared with the data measured from 7 temporal bones under the normal and TM perforated conditions shown in Figs. 3–5. This is the first time (to our knowledge) that the effect of perforations on both TM and footplate movements was measured by lasers and calculated by FE model. The frequency response curves of the displacement magnitude and phase at the TM (umbo) and footplate under various perforations are in general matching well with the temporal bone experimental data.

The FE model has predicted that there is a sound pressure difference across the TM in the normal ear. The value of pressure difference was calculated as 16 to 7 and 23 dB at frequency of 200 to 1000 and 8000 Hz. However, the pressure difference across the TM vanished at f<2 kHz when the TM was perforated and the degree of the variation in pressure difference was dependent on frequency and perforation size or location. Therefore, the sound pressure difference across the TM is the determinant factor for acoustic-mechanical transmission. This factor can be quantitatively determined in the FE model and the conclusion is similar to that reported by Voss et al. [4].

In conclusion, the study on pressure distribution and transfer function of the middle ear with the FE model has provided a complete description on the coupled acoustic-structural analysis for sound transmission through the ear. The model can be further applied to large perforations such as addressed by Mehta et al. [5] and to simulate middle ear alterations caused by middle ear diseases such as the otitis media with effusion.

Acknowledgments

The authors thank Don Nakmali, BSEE, and Kenneth J. Dormer, Ph.D., for the temporal bone experiments. This work was supported by NIDCD and NSF grants.

References

1. Gan R. Z., Feng B. and Sun Q., Three-dimensional finite element modeling of human ear for sound transmission. *Ann Biomed Eng* **32** (2004) pp. 847–859
2. Gan R. Z., Sun Q., Feng B. and Wood M. W., Acoustic-structural coupled finite element analysis for sound transmission in human ear – Pressure distributions. *Med Eng Phys* **28** (2006) pp. 395–404
3. Gan R. Z., Wood M. W. and Dormer K. J., Human middle ear transfer function measured by double laser interferometry system. *Otol Neurotol* **25** (2004) pp. 423–435
4. Voss S. E., Rosowski J. J., Merchant S. N. and Peake W. T., Middle-ear function with tympanic-membrane perforations. I. Measurements and mechanisms. *J Acoust Soc Am* **110** (2001) pp. 1432–1444
5. Mehta R. P., Rosowski J. J., Voss S. E., O'Neil E. and Merchant S. N., Determinants of hearing loss in perforations of the tympanic membrane. *Otol Neurotol* **27** (2006) pp. 136–143

EFFECTS OF MIDDLE EAR SUSPENSORY LIGAMENTS ON ACOUSTIC-MECHANICAL TRANSMISSION IN HUMAN EAR

Rong Z. Gan[1], Tao Cheng[1], Don Nakmali[2], Mark W. Wood[2]
[1] School of Aerospace and Mechanical Engineering and Bioengineering Center, University of Oklahoma, Norman
[2] Hough Ear Institute, Oklahoma City, Oklahoma, USA, Email: rgan@ou.edu

Two laser vibrometers were used to measure simultaneously the movement of the tympanic membrane and stapes footplate in human temporal bones. After control study of the normal ear, the stapedial tendon, posterior incudal ligament, tensor tympani tendon, and superior malleus/incus ligament were sectioned sequentially. The displacements of the umbo and footplate were measured repeatedly for each section. A 3-D finite element model of human ear which has accurate anatomic structure was used to mimic the middle ear structure changes and to derive the umbo and footplate vibrations in response to those alterations. The results show that the effects of ligaments on transfer function of the middle ear are frequency sensitive and vary with individual ligament.

1. Introduction

Three ossicles in the middle ear are suspended in an air-filled cavity by a complex system of ligaments and muscles, and coupled to the tympanic membrane (TM) by manubrium of the malleus. There are four ligaments and two muscle tendons which are involved in the normal function of the middle ear [1]. The locations of those ligaments and tendons are shown in Fig. 1, a 3-D finite element model of human ear created based on histological section images of a human temporal bone [2]. The superior malleus/incus, lateral malleus, posterior incus, and anterior malleus ligaments are denoted as C1, C2, C3, and C4, respectively and the stapedial tendon and tensor tympani tendon are denoted as C5 and C7, respectively.

The ligaments C1 and C4 have been reported to pathologically involve in otosclerosis which directly affect sound transmission through the ossicular chain and result in conductive hearing loss [3, 4]. The muscle tendons C5 and C7 are involved in the stapedial reflex and the inflammatory process of otitis media [5]. However, the mechanical properties of the ligaments and muscle tendons and the effects of these tissues on acoustic-mechanical transmission have not been revealed because of the extremely small size of the ligaments and complexity of the middle ear ossicles and cavity. In this paper, we report the bioengineering systems approach on middle ear ligament/tendon function using human temporal bones and finite element modeling. Two laser vibrometers were used to measure simultaneously the movements of the TM at the umbo and stapes footplate of human temporal bones upon destructions of the ligaments. A 3-D finite element (FE) model of human ear with accurate anatomic structure and mechanical properties of the ligaments was then used to mimic the middle ear structure alterations and to derive umbo and stapes footplate vibrations in response to those changes.

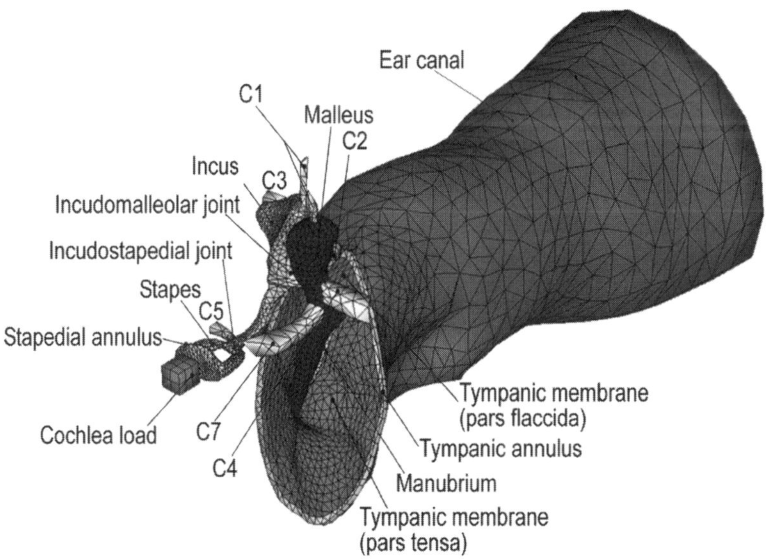

Fig. 1 Finite element (FE) model of human left ear including the TM, three ossicles (malleus, incus, and stapes), two joints and manubrium, ligaments and muscle tendons (C1, C2, C3, C4, C5, C7), tympanic annulus, stapedial annular ligament, external ear canal, middle ear cavity, and cochlear load, in anterior-medial view. The middle ear cavity wall was removed.

2. Methods

2.1 Temporal bone experiments on middle ear ligament function

Ten fresh-frozen cadaver temporal bones (3 male, 7 female, average age 64.6) were used in this study. The preparation of bone specimen and sound delivery system were almost the same as that reported in our previous paper [6]. Briefly, a canal-wall-up mastoidectomy was performed and the additus was exposed enough to view the body of the incus. After surgical preparation, two pieces of laser reflective tape were placed on the lateral surface of the umbo and the center of the stapes footplate. One laser beam was directed through the ear canal at the reflective tape on the umbo. Deviation of this laser beam varied 0° to 35° with respect to the direction of the stapes piston-like movement. Another laser beam was focused on stapes footplate with 30° to 50° deviation from the stapes piston-like movement. The 90 dB pure tone, sound signals in the frequency range of 200–8000 Hz were delivered to the TM and monitored by a probe microphone placed in the canal approximately 2 mm away from the umbo. Two laser Doppler vibrometers (Polytec, HLV-1000 and OFV 501) were used to measure vibrations of the TM and stapes simultaneously.

The control experiment with intact, nonmanipulated ossicular chain was performed first. After the control study, the middle ear ligaments and tendons were cut sequentially. The displacements of the TM and stapes footplate were measured repeatedly after each cut. Four middle ear ligaments and tendons were selected for this study: superior mallear ligament (C1), posterior incudal ligament (C3), stapedial tendon (C5), and tensor tympani tendon (C7) in the order of cutting C5, C3, C7, and C1.

2.2 3-D FE modeling of middle ear ligament function for sound transmission

A 3-D FE model of human left ear (see Fig. 1) including middle ear components, external ear and middle ear cavity, was established based on a complete set of histological sections of a human temporal bone (male, age 61) [2]. The model was characterized by (1) dimensions of the ear canal, middle ear components, and middle ear cavity; (2) mechanical properties of the TM, ossicles, joints, and manubrium; and (3) boundary conditions of the middle ear including tympanic annulus, middle ear ligaments or muscle tendons, stapedial annular ligament, and cochlear fluid. Note that all the ligaments and tendons were assumed as elastic constraints with 4-noded solid elements and dimensions [2].

The accuracy of mechanical properties of ear tissues affects the FE model-predicted middle ear function. Recently, we have completed some preliminary studies on measurement of mechanical properties of human stapedial and tensor tympani tendons and anterior mallear ligament. In this study, we employed the new Young's modulus data of 8.0, 10, and 8.0 MPa for the ligament C5, C7, and C4 which have the volume of 0.12, 1.187, and 0.563 mm^3, respectively. Following the ligament cutting sequence in bone experiments, we created the same sequence of removing ligaments in the FE model and performed the FE analysis sequentially. A 90 dB sound pressure was applied at the 2 mm away from the umbo in the ear canal. The acoustic-structural coupled FE analysis between the ear canal air column and TM or "one-chamber" coupled analysis was performed with each manipulated ossicular case. The displacements at the umbo of the TM and footplate were calculated and the results were compared with the bone experimental data.

3. Results

Fig. 2 shows mean frequency response curves of displacement at the umbo of the TM measured from 10 bones following the ligament cutting sequence: control or intact ossicular chain → C5 → C3 → C7 → C1 cut. Panel A displays the magnitude and panel B the phase angle. The results in Fig. 2 show that destruction of ligaments C5, C3, C7 and C1 affects the umbo movement at low frequencies ($f < 2$ kHz). The first cut C5 did not show much effect on the umbo vibration (< 0.5 dB) and the C7 cut showed stronger influence on TM displacement than other ligaments.

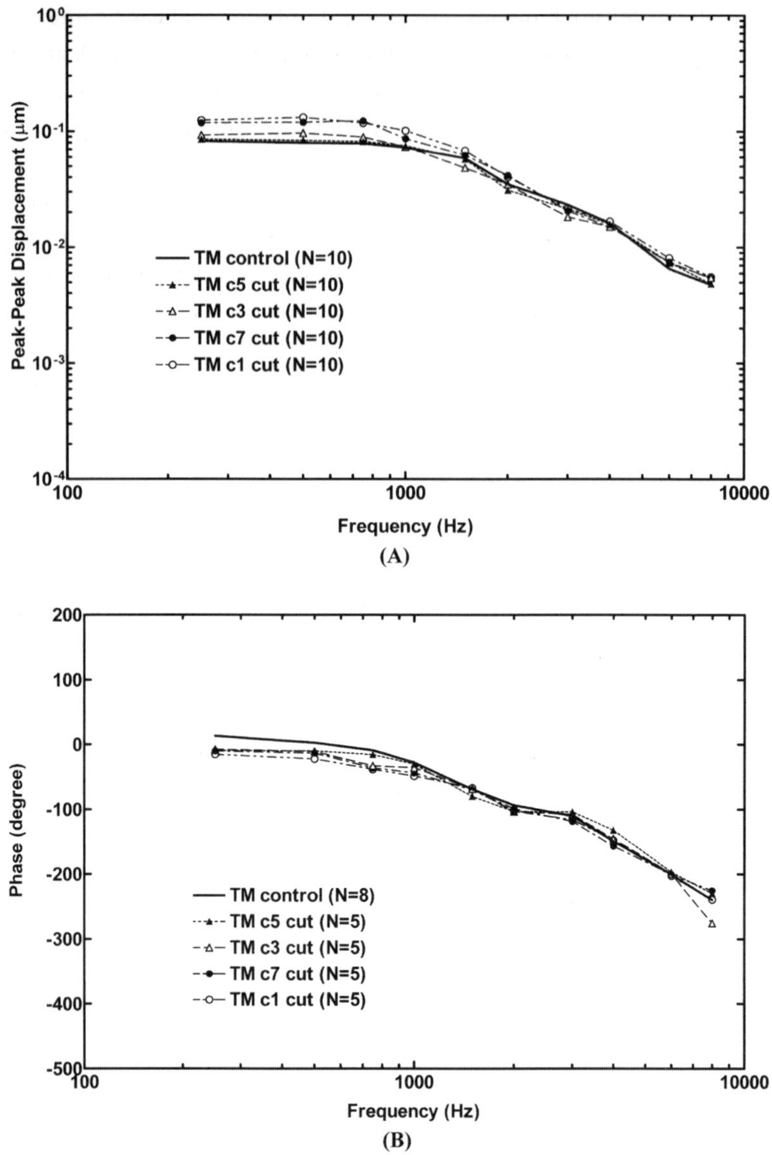

Fig. 2 Mean peak-to-peak displacement curves measured at the umbo of the TM under the control and ligament cut sequence: C5→C3→C7→C1. (A) Magnitude; (B) phase angle.

The mean displacement curves of the stapes footplate from 10 bones following the ligament cutting sequence are shown in Fig. 3. Panel A represents the magnitude and panel B the phase angle. Compared with the umbo displacement data, the destruction of ligaments limited its effect on the footplate movement at frequency below 1 kHz.

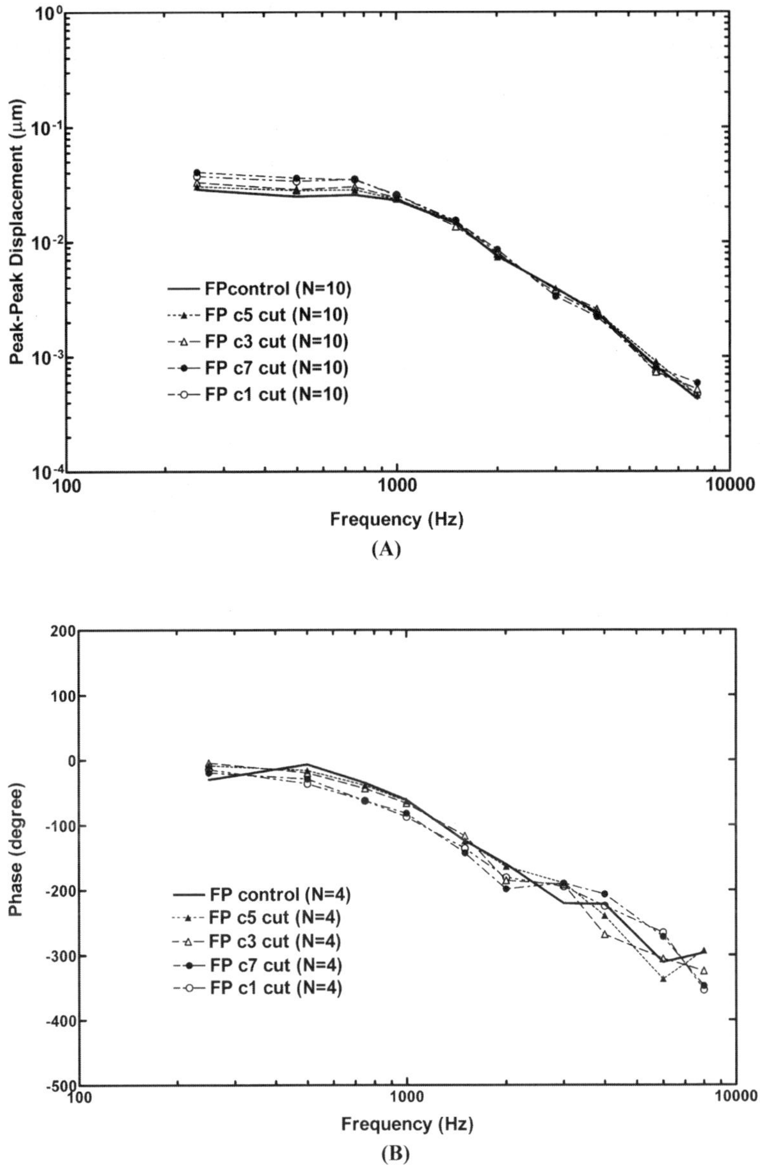

Fig. 3 Mean peak-to-peak displacement curves measured at the stapes footplate under the control and ligament cut sequence: C5→ C3→ C7→ C1. (A) Magnitude; (B) phase angle.

Fig. 4 displays the FE model-predicted displacement at the umbo of the TM with the magnitude (panel A) and phase (panel B) in response to the ligament removal sequential. The model results show that ligaments C5 and C3 did not have much effect on the umbo movement, but C7 and C1 had considerable effect on the umbo movement at low frequencies (f<2 kHz). Compared with the experimental data in Fig. 2, the model-predicted umbo displacement increased more after C7 or C1 removal at f≤1 kHz. It is also noticed that the ligament removal did not affect the umbo movement at high frequencies (f≥2 kHz) shown in the experiments (Fig. 2) and FE model (Fig. 4). However, the umbo displacement from the model decreased faster than that measured from the bones at frequencies 2 to 8 kHz.

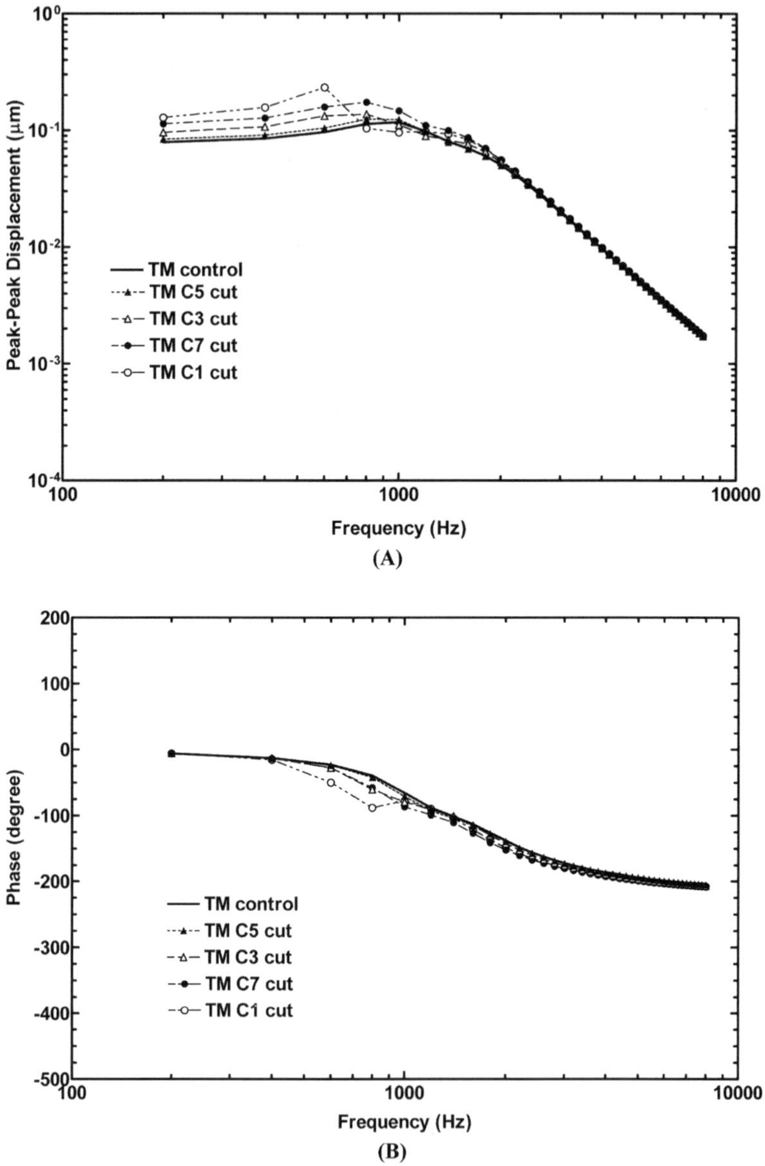

Fig. 4 FE model-derived umbo displacement curves under the normal and ligament removal sequence: C5→ C3→ C7→ C1. (A) Magnitude; (B) phase angle.

Fig. 5 shows the FE model-derived displacement curves of the stapes footplate under destruction of each ligament following the bone experimental sequence. The model results indicate that the removal of middle ear ligaments only affected the footplate displacement at f < 1 kHz and there was no obvious difference observed between ligaments. Similar to the umbo, the footplate displacement from the model decreased faster than that measured in bones at frequencies 1 to 8 kHz.

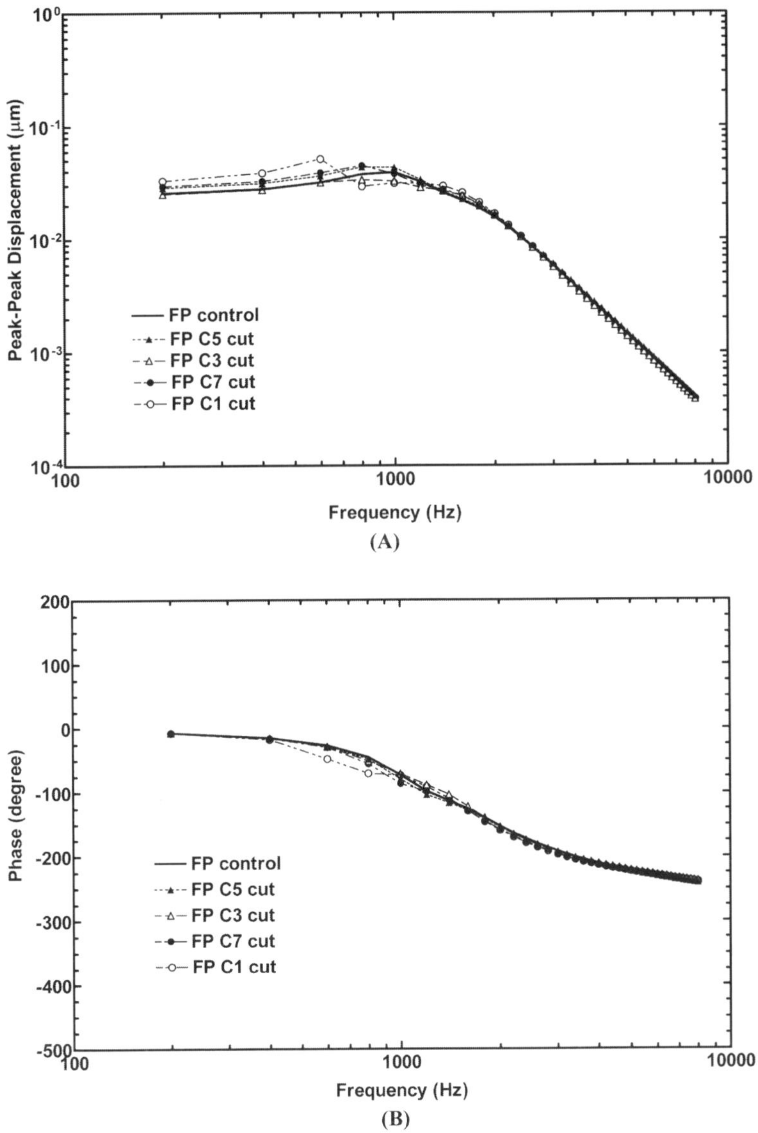

Fig. 5 FE model-derived stapes footplate displacement curves under the normal and ligament removal sequence: C5→C3→C7→C1. (A) Magnitude; (B) phase angle.

4. Discussion

Both experimental and FE modeling results show that destruction of middle ear ligaments/tendons affects the TM and stapes footplate vibrations at low frequencies (f≤1 kHz). The tensor tympani tendon and superior mallear ligament may play a more important role for acoustic-mechanical transmission compared with other ligaments. The effects of ligaments on transfer function of the middle ear are frequency sensitive and vary with individual ligaments.

To fully understand the function of middle ear ligaments on sound transmission, we must know mechanical properties of those tissues and their combined system function on ossicular chain. Our recent mechanical tests of middle ear ligaments and tendons have shown that the ear tissues are viscoelastic materials and the Young's modulus changes with stress level. In this study, we employed the preliminary data obtained from uniaxial tensile tests on tendons C5 and C7, and ligament C4 into our model (The details of material tests are not shown here and two papers are currently under review). However, the ligament mechanical property data have improved the accuracy of the model for predicting the ligament function on umbo and stapes movements as compared with our previous model predicted results reported in 2004 ARO meeting.

In conclusion, it is expected that the effect of middle ear suspensory ligaments on middle ear function is extended into several different cutting sequences in temporal bones. A more realistic model reflects middle ear ligaments and other soft tissue mechanical properties will be developed. The final conclusion on middle ear ligament function will be revealed in our future studies.

Acknowledgments

The authors thank Kenneth J. Dormer, Ph.D., for the temporal bone experiments. This work was supported by NIDCD and NSF grants.

References

1. Hüttenbrink K. B., The functional significance of the suspending ligaments of the ear ossicle chain. *Laryngorhinootologie* **68** (1989) pp. 146–151
2. Gan R. Z., Feng B. and Sun Q., Three-dimensional finite element modeling of human ear for sound transmission. *Ann Biomed Eng* **32** (2004) pp. 847–859
3. Nandapalan V., Pollak A., Langner A., and Fisch U., The anterior and superior malleal ligaments in otosclerosis. *Otol Neurotol* **23** (2002) pp. 854–861

4. Nakajima H. H., Ravicz M. E., Rosowski J. J., Peake W. T., and Merchant S. N., Experimental and clinical studies of malleus fixation. *Laryngorhinootologie* **115** (2005) pp. 147–154
5. Abdelhamid M. M., Paparella M. M., Schachern P. A., and Yoon T. H., Histopathology of the tensor tympani muscle in otitis media. *Eur Arch Otorhinolaryngol,* **248** (1990) pp. 71–78
6. Gan R. Z., Wood M. W. and Dormer K. J., Human middle ear transfer function measured by double laser interferometry system. *Otol Neurotol* **25** (2004) pp. 423–435

EVALUATION OF LASER VIBROMETRY AS DIAGNOSTIC UTILITY BY MEANS OF A SIMULATION MODEL OF THE MIDDLE EAR

Matthias Bornitz[1], Nikoloz Lasurashvili[1], Hans-Jürgen Hardtke[2], Thomas Zahnert[1]
Technische Universität Dresden
[1] Dept. of Medicine, Clinic of Otorhinolaryngology, Fetscherstr. 74, 01307 Dresden, Germany
[2] Dept. of Solid State Mechanics, 01062 Dresden, Germany
Email: matthias.bornitz@tu-dresden.de

In this study we used a Finite Element model of the middle ear to evaluate LDV (Laser-Doppler-Vibrometer) measurements of sound induced umbo vibrations. Simulations were performed for the intact ossicular chain, otosclerosis, incus luxation and malleus head fixation. Simulation results are comparable to results from clinical investigations. Incus luxation and malleus head fixation can be clearly distinguished. Results for otosclerosis range from almost unchanged to moderate changes in umbo vibrations, depending on particular middle ear morphology.

1. Introduction

Measurements of sound induced umbo vibrations (by means of Laser Doppler Vibrometry) have already been used in clinical studies to investigate their potential as a diagnostic utility [1–3]. The method is aimed to distinguish the different pathologies of conductive hearing loss and to evaluate the quality of reconstructive middle ear surgery. The clinical studies comprise patients with conductive hearing loss due to otosclerosis, incus luxation and bony malleus fixation [2]. In [3] the method was also used to evaluate post-stapedectomy results.

These measurements on patients are subject to some limitations. The measurements can only be done at one state per subject (ear), i.e. normal ear or pathologically changed ear. There is a great variance in the measurements due to individual variations. Measurements on normal ears from different individuals differ in magnitude by up to 20 dB across the whole investigated frequency range. The same holds for measurements of pathological ears. Here we also have an additional problem in terms of the classification of the pathological change. Different characteristics of one disease are normally assigned to one group. We also may have mixed pathologies where only the major one is detected.

Thus for measurements on subjects the question arises what pathologies can be reliably distinguished. And: can we observe a correlation between conductive hearing loss (from audiometric investigation) and changes in umbo vibration?

The main advantage of simulation models is that the intact ossicular chain and different pathologies can be studied at the same ear without the influence of inter-individual variations. Furthermore all parameters of the model can be modified separately, thus allowing to simulate a great variety of distinct changes of the ossicular chain. The main problem is that the model is validated against a normal ear and represents an average ear. The modifications in the model to simulate the pathological changes are sometimes very large and the validity of the model can not be assured. There may be also limitations for an adequate simulation of specific pathological changes since every model is based on simplifications. Thus simulation results and measurements should always be critically evaluated against each other.

The purpose of this work is to simulate different pathologies and their influence on the transfer function at the umbo in order to assist the clinical investigations.

2. Method

We used a Finite Element Model of the middle ear for the investigations [4,5]. It has been developed for investigations on middle ear reconstructions with focus on the acoustic transfer characteristics and the frequency range of speech. Accordingly the model is limited to the linear region (sound pressure up to 110 dB) and to frequencies up to 6 kHz.

The model consists of the ear canal (acoustic fluid), the eardrum (orthotrop-elastic shell with constant damping ratio), the ossicles (rigid bodies with mass and inertia properties), ligaments (elastic bars), joints (elastic bodies with constant damping ratio) and a spring-mass-damper model of the cochlea (values taken from [6]). The model and the calculated quantities are presented in figure 1.

Calculations were performed according to the clinical measurements to get comparable results, i.e. a harmonic analysis in the frequency range from 200 to 5000 Hz was done. A sound pressure was applied at the ear canal entrance and the reference pressure at the eardrum and the displacement of the umbo and the footplate were calculated. From that the frequency transfer function (FRF) between umbo displacement and sound pressure in front of the tympanic membrane was built (subsequently named umbo FRF). In order to consider realistic measurement conditions the umbo displacement was calculated as the mean displacement of all points within a 0.2 mm radius around the umbo. This accounts for variations in targeting the laser point to the umbo.

The calculated transfer function between stapes footplate displacement and sound pressure serves as indicator for the sound energy transfer to the inner ear. A reduction of the magnitude of this transfer function compared to the normal ear is thus comparable to a conductive hearing loss.

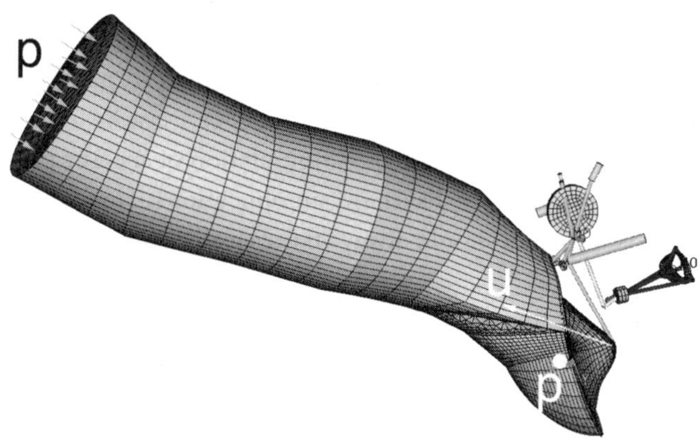

Fig. 1 Finite Element model of the middle ear. The ossicles were treated as rigid bodies and were simplified to bar structures. The calculated component of the umbo displacement is indicated by the arrow.

Calculations were done for the intact middle ear and for the following pathological changes: malleus head fixation (stiffening of the superior malleal lig. up to osseous fixation), chain interruption, stiffening of the annular ligament (otosclerosis), stiffening of the IMJ (Incudo-Malleal-Joint) and the ISJ (Incudo-Stapedial-Joint). The model parameters were also slightly varied to account for the inter-individual variations.

The calculated umbo FRF of the normal middle ear model lies within the normal range of measured transfer functions [7] (see fig. 2). Small variations of the Young's modulus of the joints (IMJ and ISJ varying between 0.4 and 40 MPa) make a difference of at most 10 dB in the FRF, which is also well within the range of individual variations.

3. Results

3.1 Ossicular chain interruption

Ossicular chain interruption leads to a shift of the first resonance peak to lower frequencies and to an increase in magnitude (fig. 2). This change can already be observed when the Young's modulus of the joint is reduced by a factor of 100 to simulate a hypermobile joint. (The Young's modulus of 0.04 MPa then corresponds to that of very weak connective tissue.)

3.2 Ossicular joint fixation

IMJ or ISJ fixation as well as the fixation of both joints do not make remarkable differences in the umbo FRF. A maximum reduction of the magnitude of up to 10 dB in the lower frequency range can be observed when the IMJ is fixed. The umbo FRF is for all these cases within the range of normal ears [7] (fig. 2).

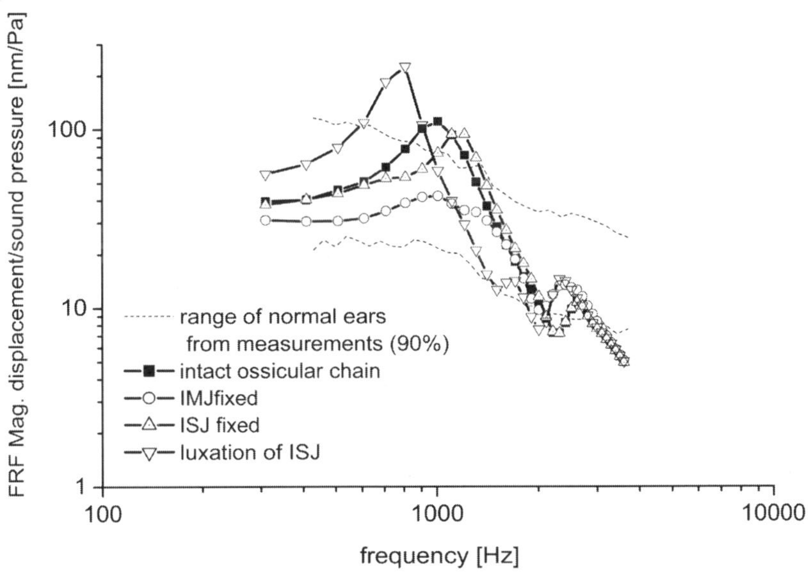

Fig. 2 Umbo FRF for intact ossicular chain and simulation of ISJ luxation, IMJ and ISJ fixation. The dashed lines indicate the 90% percentile of FRFs from measurements of normal ears [7], i.e. the normal range.

3.3 Otosclerosis, fixation of the annular ligament

Stiffening of the annular ligament leads to a reduced magnitude in the low frequency range and a shift of the resonance peak towards higher frequencies in the umbo FRF (fig. 3). The amount of these changes is strongly dependent on other parameters of the ossicular chain. When using the model with the initial set of parameters, the change in the umbo FRF was insignificant (2nd line in fig. 3), even though the Young's modulus of the annular ligament was increased by a factor of 1000, which is nearly osseous fixation.

Following that, some of the initial parameters of the model have been varied according to normal variations in geometry and material properties in normal ears. (For instance the ossicular joints, where stiffness parameters varying by at least a factor of 10 can be found across the literature.) When the ISJ stiffness was increased by a factor of 10 there was about no change in the umbo FRF. Combining this still normal ear with otosclerosis leads to remarkable changes in the umbo FRF (last two lines in fig. 3), whereas variations in the otosclerosis value do not equally show up in the umbo FRF (cp. last two lines in fig. 3).

The changes in the footplate transfer function were as expected. Reduction in magnitude is to the same degree as the increase of Young's modulus of the annular ligament (fig. 4). Changes in the ISJ hardly influence the footplate FRF.

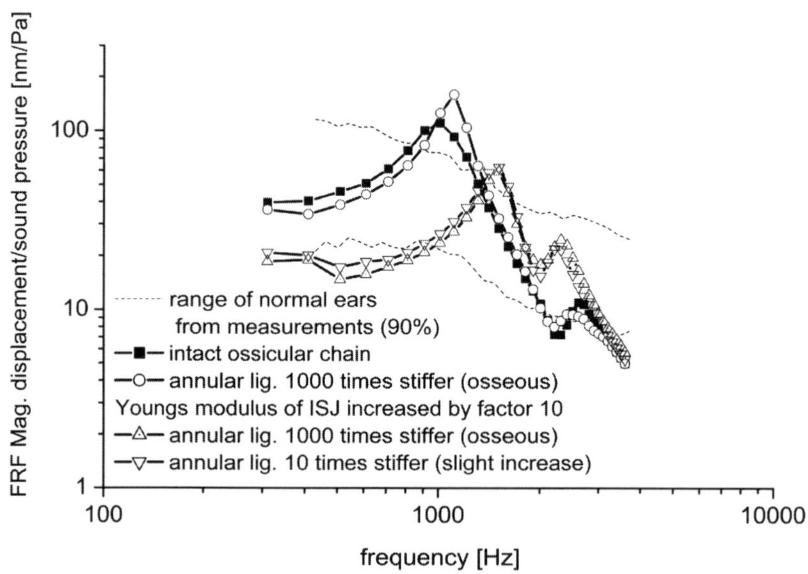

Fig. 3 Umbo FRF for simulation of otosclerosis (increasing stiffness of the annular ligament).

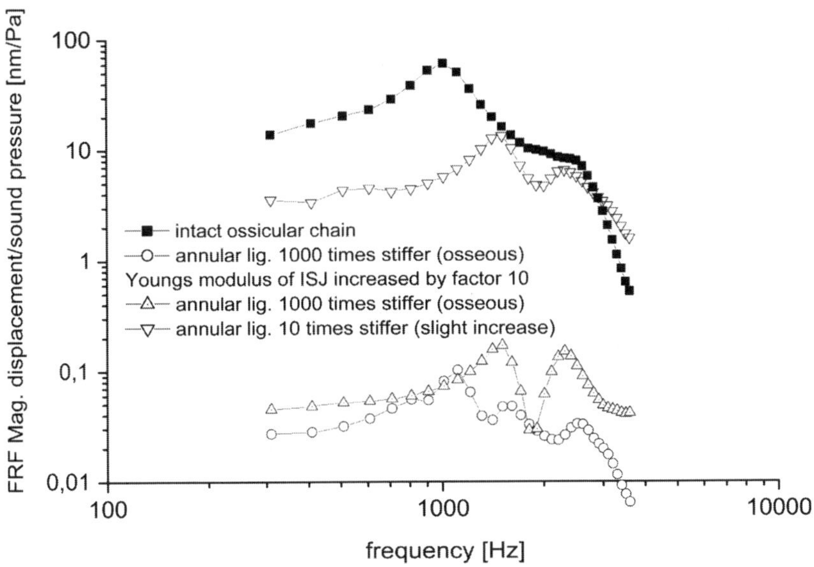

Fig. 4 Footplate FRF for simulation of otosclerosis (increasing stiffness of the annular ligament).

3.4 Malleus head fixation

Fixation of the malleus head was simulated by stepwise increasing the stiffness of the superior malleal ligament up to an osseous fixation. In case of osseous fixation the malleus is immobilized and there is a tremendous decrease in the magnitude of the umbo FRF. But this can only be observed if the FRF is calculated exactly for the umbo node (last line in fig. 5). If a mean displacement around the umbo is used the observed change in the umbo FRF is much less (3rd line in fig. 5) but it is still reliable to distinguish from a normal ossicular chain. In the case of pre-stages of an osseous fixation (2nd line in fig. 5) the umbo FRF then is within the range of normal ears.

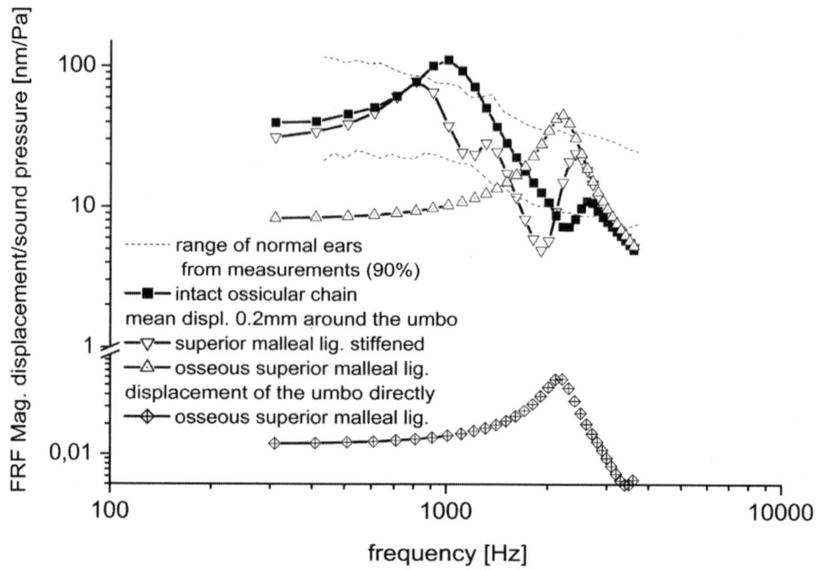

Fig. 5 Umbo FRF for simulation of malleus head fixation.

4. Discussion

The results of the simulations are in good agreement with some clinical studies using the Laser Doppler Vibrometry [1–3]. For otosclerosis, ISJ luxation and malleus fixation similar characteristic changes in the umbo FRF could be observed. This indicates that the model seems to be suitable for simulations of pathological changes of the ossicular chain.

The following conclusions can be drawn from the simulation results:

IMJ and ISJ fixation can hardly be distinguished from normal ears since the umbo FRF is within the normal range for both cases. These pathologies are also presumed to be without audiological findings because there are only minor changes in the stapes footplate FRF.

Severe changes like chain interruption and malleus head fixation can be detected and distinguished.

In case of malleus head fixation measurements are very sensitive to the location of the measurement point. Only measurements at the umbo directly show a significant reduction of the magnitude across the whole frequency range, whereas measurements at short distance from the umbo (≈ 0.2 mm) might indicate a normal ossicular chain, especially in cases where the malleus head is not totally osseous fixed.

Otosclerosis does not necessarily show up in the umbo FRF. Results can range from almost unchanged to moderate decrease in the low frequency range (for the same degree of annular ligament stiffening). The changes in the umbo FRF for otosclerotic ears depend very much on the particular morphology of the middle ear, especially the stiffness of the ISJ. A variation in ISJ stiffness by a factor of 10 determines whether otosclerosis shows up in the umbo FRF or not. These findings are in agreement with other investigations [8] where no correlation could be observed between LDV measurements on the umbo and the air-bone gap obtained from audiological investigations. For clinical diagnostics of otosclerosis this means that a comparison of amplitudes of the umbo FRF is insufficient.

References

1. Goode R.L., Ball G. and Nishihara S., Measurement of umbo vibration in human subjects – method and possible clinical applications. *Am J Otol* **14**(5), (1993) pp. 247–251
2. Huber A., Schwab C., Linder T., Stoeckli S., Ferrazzini M., Dillier N. and Fisch U., Evaluation of eardrum laser doppler interferometry as a diagnostic tool. *Laryngoscope* **111**(3), (2001) pp. 501–507
3. Rosowski J.J., Mehta R.P. and Merchant S.N., Diagnostic Utility of Laser-Doppler Vibrometry in Conductive Hearing Loss with Normal Tympanic Membrane. *Otol Neurotol* **24,** (2003) pp. 165–175
4. Beer H., Bornitz M., Hardtke H., Schmidt R., Hofmann G., Vogel U., Zahnert T. and Hüttenbrink K., Modelling of components of the human middle ear and simulation of their dynamic behaviour. *Audiology and Neuro-Otology* **4**(3–4), (1999) pp. 156–162
5. Bornitz M., Zahnert T., Hardtke H. and Hüttenbrink K., Identification of parameters for the middle ear model. *Audiology and Neuro-Otology* **4**(3–4), (1999) pp. 163–169
6. Hudde H. and Engel A., Measuring and modeling basic properties of the human middle ear and ear canal. Part III: Eardrum impedances, transfer functions and model calculations. *Acustica and acta acustica* **84,** (1998) pp. 1091–1109
7. Zahnert, T., Laser in der Ohrforschung. *Laryngorhinootologie* **82** Suppl 1, (2003) pp. 157–180
8. Merchant S. N., Nakajima H. H., Chien W. and Rosowski J. J., Six years of experience with measurements of tympanic membrane velocity by laser Doppler vibrometry as a clinical diagnostic tool. [published here]

BASILAR MEMBRANE DISPLACEMENT WITH OPENED AND OCCLUDED OVAL WINDOW AND BONE CONDUCTION

F. Böhnke[1], A. Arnold[2], T. Fawzy[1]
[1] Hals-Nasen-Ohrenklinik und Poliklinik, Klinikum rechts der Isar der Technischen Universität München, Ismaningerstr. 22, D 81675 München, Germany
[2] Univ. HNO-Klinik, Inselspital, 3010 Berne, Switzerland

PD Dr.-Ing. Frank Böhnke, Phone: +49 89 4140 4196, Fax: 49 89 4140 4971
Email: frank.boehnke@lrz.tum.de

Hearing sensations are caused by air and bone guided sound. Of course other biological materials like tendons, muscles and tissue are also involved during conduction of sound. To study the influence of bone conduction (BC) a formerly developed finite element model was excited by harmonic pressure signals at the cochlea wall. Clinical findings during middle ear surgery, namely the increase of bone conduction sensitivity with removed footplate was confirmed.

Additionally the effects of an immobile footplate and round window aplasia and bone conduction are studied. The maximum basilar membrane displacement with the closure of the oval and the round window and both with BC is examined numerically.

1. Introduction

Though bone conduction (BC) has been of clinical and scientific interest for long [1], there are still open questions concerning this acoustical phenomenon. The term BC implies hearing by the transmission of sound through bone though it does not necessarily imply that the wave propagation is entirely bone because the sound is transmitted to the organ of Corti through the bone, periosteum, lymph and other biological material. To clarify open questions to the topic of BC the wave propagation along the basilar membrane (BM) with BC stimulation must be known. Though former workers already addressed this problem, the physics was mostly covered by one-dimensional considerations [2]. These are not able to include the complex geometry of the cochlea sufficiently. Therefore we developed a 3D model of the cochlea and stimulated the bony wall surrounding the fluid by different pressure signals [3]. Herewith we are able to simulate different states in middle ear surgery.

A result, which confirms clinical findings in middle ear surgery is the increase of BM displacement with BC stimulation when the stapes footplate is removed during stapedectomy.

An evaluation and discussion of the influence of the closed round and oval window is given.

2. Modelling the Cochlea for Bone Conduction (BC)

To calculate the BC response we use a formerly developed finite element model of the cochlea [3]. Figure 1 shows the complete discretized finite element model with the stapes footplate and the round window at the base of the cochlea.

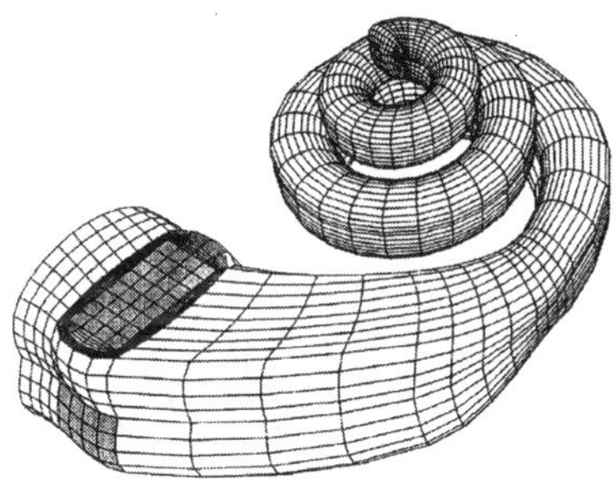

Fig. 1 3D Finite Element Model of the human cochlea showing the oval and the round windows.

The basilar membrane (BM) inside the cochlea with its characteristic gradients of width and thickness is presented in fig. 2.

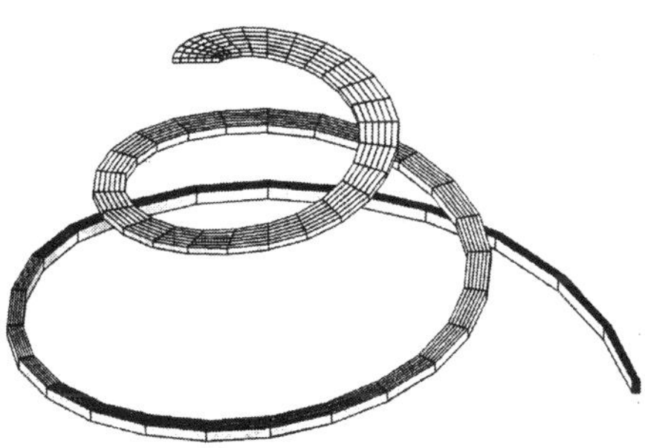

Fig. 2 The basilar membrane idealized as an elastic orthotropic shell with gradients of width and thickness.

The results shown in figs. 4 and 5 are the maximum displacements which occur with one stimulation frequency at different points along the BM. Instead of the usual stapes footplate stimulation of the middle ear the outer bony wall of the cochlea surrounding the perilymphatic fluid is stimulated (Fig. 3).

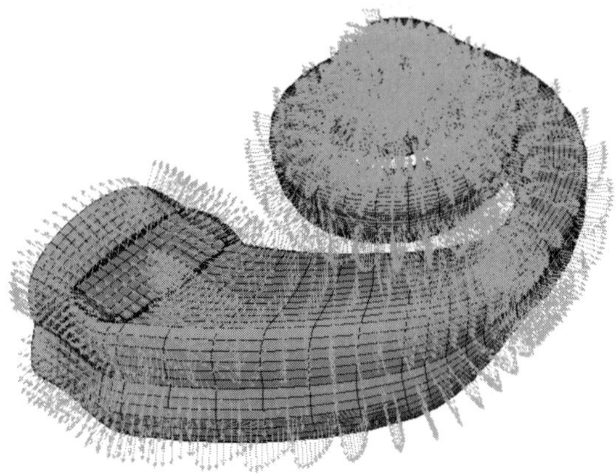

Fig. 3 Arrows represent the pressure loading of the outer cochlea wall with bone conduction.

The outer cochlea wall (OCW) is not represented by an extra material yet and therefore the pressure is applied to those areas, which confine the fluid elements. The stimulation by an external pressure is easy but the specification of an external applied displacement is not. To prescribe a displacement at the OCW, in principle the number of local coordinate systems must be as high as the number of finite elements. Because this is unrealistic an additional layer of bone might be inserted around the perilymph and stimulated on plane surfaces.

For this reason, at this point we are only able to stimulate the cochlea by pressure. According to Herzog and Krainz [4] we are merely able to study the influence of compressional BC because the middle ear is not yet included in the finite element model.

3. Results

3.1 Increase of basilar membrane displacement after footplate removal with bone conduction

During stapedectomy the complete stapes footplate is removed. Similar to the superior semicircular canal dehiscence (SCD) where BC sensitivity is increased for frequencies below 2 kHz [5] the BM displacement increases by 9 dB at f = 1500 Hz (Fig. 4) in the finite element model.

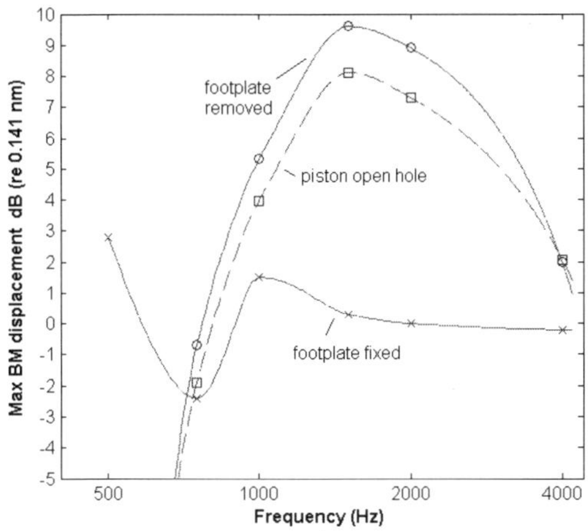

Fig. 4 The displacement of the basilar membrane is larger for an opened oval window, L_{Stim} = 94 dB(SPL).

Though there is a difference between the model presented here and the SCD, where a large amount of cerebrospinal fluid is connected, the comparison is permitted because of an experimental finding with likewise coupled air to the lymph [6]. The increase of BM displacement is larger if the area of the opening increases as it is shown in fig. 4. The smaller piston (diameter 0.6 mm) area of $A = 0.28\ mm^2$ reduces the increase up to 2 dB, depending on the frequency (Fig. 4, piston open hole). Because the BM displacement with a mobile elastic footplate does not differ considerably from the fixed state shown here it is not presented in fig. 4. The measurement of this decrease of BC threshold was done during stapedectomy with opened footplates [7].

The stimulation level of external pressure was 94 dB(SPL) in these cases. With the BC measurements the effective level at the cochlea can be lower and irregular along the cochlea wall because of anatomical conditions.

3.2 Basilar membrane displacement with aplasia of the round window and both windows fixed stimulated by compressional bone conduction

There is still a diversity of opinion how the closure of the cochlear windows affects both air conduction (AC) and BC. The results of the simulation shown in Fig. 5 give a decrease of BM displacement by 7 to 12 dB for frequencies above 1 kHz with round window aplasia. Here the bone conduction stimulation level is 70 dB(SPL).

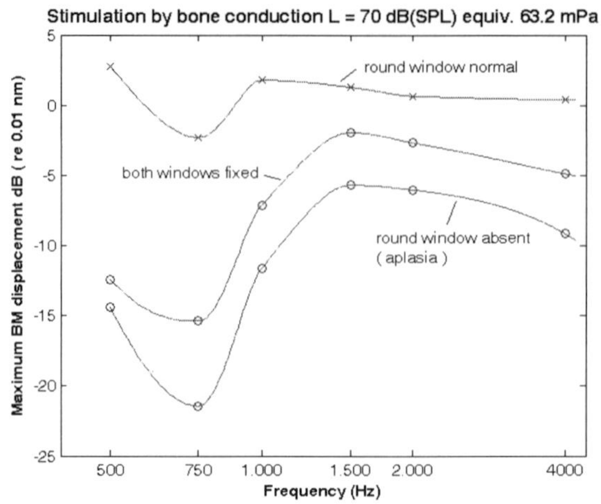

Fig. 5 The displacement of the basilar membrane for closed oval and round window, $L_{Stim} = 70$ dB(SPL).

In case of both windows fixed the BM displacement increases by 2 dB to 6 dB as a function of frequency. These results resemble the bone conduction thresholds of 15 to 35 dB with rare clinical findings of round window aplasia [11]. The differences are due to the missing middle ear in our simulation. Furthermore a comparison to experimental data by Tonndorf and Tabor [12] is possible. Closure of both windows produced a relatively small effect as to BC responses, which was not larger than that produced by closure of the oval window alone, unless the cochlear aqueduct was closed off simultaneously. Of course we are not able to study the influence of an open cochlear aqueduct with the model of the cochlea we used.

4. Discussion

The simulation of the wave propagation on the BM in the cochlea with BC excitation confirms clinical findings. In this preliminary simulation the bone was not taken into account directly. Instead of this a homogeneous pressure application on the boundary walls of the cochlea was used. Our results support recent measurements on fat sand rats, which gave a decrease of BC threshold by 7.0 dB with semicircular canal fenestration [10], though transient stimulation was used in these experiment instead of our sinusoidal stimulation.

The physical interpretation of the increase in response can be the lowering of the acoustical impedance to fluid movements and therefore the increase of fluid movement and as a consequence the increase of BM displacement.

The actual stimulation at the outer bone is in phase for all areas and has an equal amplitude along the complete outer wall. The stimulating signal which arrives at the outer wall will have a frequency dependent phase shift and might differ in its amplitude from place to place. This will be regarded in future simulations.

In further steps of modelling the ear parts of the temporal bone and particularly components of the middle ear will be included. This will enable us to study the influence of inertial BC, i.e. the contribution of the middle ear structures to BC, and the osseotympanic BC, i.e. sound energy transmitted from the external ear canal to the tympanic membrane, setting up an AC response [8]. In case of simulation of the otosclerotic ear with an immobile stapes footplate it was permissible to use the cochlea model without the middle ear because in this case it does not matter if the ossicles are present or not.

The closure of both windows and stimulation by BC further on displaced the BM because of the compressibility of the fluid representing the lymph, which had the mechanical parameters of water. Further clinical comparisons should not be drawn before a more elaborate model of the ear including the middle ear components is used.

References

1. Békésy, G. von, "Zur Theorie des Hörens bei der Schallaufnahme durch Knchenleitung (Hearing theory of acoustic perception by bone conduction),"*Ann. Phys.* (Leipzig), 1932, **13,** 111–136
2. Tonndorf J., Compressional bone conduction in cochlear models. *J. Acoust. Soc. Am.* 1962; **34,** 1127–31
3. Böhnke F., Arnold W., 3D-Finite Element Model of the Human Cochlea including Fluid-Structure Couplings. *ORL* 1999; **61,** 5, S. Karger AG Basel, 305–310
4. Herzog H., Krainz W., Das Knochenleitungsproblem. Theoretische Erwägungen. *Zeitschrift für Hals-, Nasen- und Ohrenheilkunde* 1926: 300–313.
5. Minor L.B., Superior canal dehiscence syndrome. *Am. J. Otol.* 2000; **21,** 9–19
6. Songer J., personal communication, MEMRO2006, *4th International Symposium on Middle Ear Mechanics in Research and Otolgy,* Zürich, July 2006
7. Arnold A., Fawzy T., Böhnke F. Investigations on bone conduction thresholds in otosclerosis, MEMRO2006, *4th International Symposium on Middle Ear Mechanics in Research and Otology,* Zürich, 2006, P3
8. Tonndorf J., Bone Conduction. In Tobias J.V. ed., *Foundations of Modern Auditory Theory,* New York: Academic Press, 1972; 195–237

9. Sohmer H., Freeman S., Perez R., Semicircular fenestration – improvement of bone but not air conducted auditory thresholds. *Hearing Research* 2004; **34**, 1127–31
10. Linder T., Furong M., Huber A., Round Window Atresia and its Effect on Sound Transmission, *Otology & Neurootology* 2003, **24**, 259–263
11. Tonndorf J., Tabor J., Closure of the cochlear windows: Its effect upon air and bone conduction, *Ann. Otol. Rhinol. Laryngol.*, **71**, 5–29

DEVELOPMENT OF A NEW CLIP-PISTON PROSTHESIS FOR THE STAPES

G. Schimanski, Koenigsheide 9, 44536 Luenen, ENT-practice, Germany
Email: g.schimanski@mittelohr.de
U. Steinhardt, Tuebinger Str. 3, 72144 Dusslingen, Kurz Medizintechnik, Germany
Email: usteinhardt@kurzmed.de
A. Eiber, Pfaffenwaldring 9, 70569 Stuttgart, Institute of Engineering and Computational Mechanics, University of Stuttgart, Germany
Email: eiber@itm.uni-stuttgart

275 inserted Clip-Pistons type "ÀWengen" within three years revealed difficulties in 14.5% of the cases. In those cases it was necessary to make adjustments to the clip shape (plastic deformation) before insertion due to the individual dimension of the long incudal process. During 100 middle ear surgeries the cross sections of the long incudal processes where the clip is attached was measured. This resulted in data hitherto unknown. By virtue of a Finite Element Model (FEM) these data were used for optimizing the clip shape. Design criteria were a minimal variation of the contact force for different cross-sections and to minimize the force necessary to slide the clip over the incudal process. The new clip has a lower stiffness and can therefore be applied onto different incus diameters. The lower contact force reduces the risk of arrosion. Due to its optimized shape, the maximal stress in the clip is lowered preventing plastic deformation during the application procedure. The application force was decreased by up to 45% depending on the application points. This leads to easy and safe application reducing the risk of damaging the ossicular chain.

1. Introduction

For several years now, the titanium Clip-Piston type "ÀWengen" (manufacturer: KURZ Medizintechnik , Dusslingen, Germany) has been a tried-and-tested stapes replacement in otosclerosis surgery. Its advantage is its standardized manner of fixation to the long incudal process [1].

Otosurgical practice has shown that pushing the Clip-Piston "ÀWengen" (following called Clip"ÀW") onto the incudal process can be problematic in cases when the incudal process is either too thin or too thick. For this reason, the cross-section of the incudal process in the area of the piston fixation was intraoperatively measured. As a result, the authors developed a new clip (following called Clip"new") aiming at changing the piston geometry in order to make it less stiff, and thus to provide a Clip-Piston prosthesis which can be implanted regardless of the wide variety of diameters the long incudal process may be.

2. Method

2.1 Evaluation of stapes surgical reports with Clip"ÀW"

On the basis of the surgical records 275 stapes surgeries implanting a Clip"ÀW" were evaluated retrospectively. The surgeries were done by author 1 within a period of three years. The question was, how often problems occurred when pushing Clip"ÀW" onto the incudal process.

2.2 Cross sections of the long incudal process

By means of a measuring device developed from a regular microsurgical instrument (author 1) 100 incudes were measured at the application site of a stapes piston prosthesis. It allows intraoperative measurement during middle ear surgery with intact ossicular chain. The lateral width of the gauge is 0.2mm and thus corresponds to the lateral width of the titanium clip prosthesis. 2 diameters were examined: $D_{a\text{-}p}$ (anterior-posterior) and $D_{l\text{-}m}$ (lateral-medial). $D_{a\text{-}p}$ describes the horizontal axis from the malleus handle to the posterior part of the middle ear; $D_{l\text{-}m}$ describes the vertical axis from the level of the tympanic membrane to the footplate and corresponds to the clip aperture (Fig. 1).

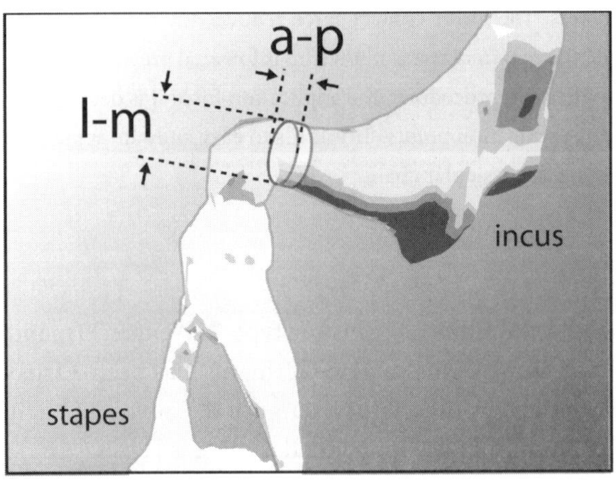

Fig. 1

2.3 Computer modeling

On the basis of the results, the geometry of Clip"new" was designed, analyzed, and optimized by Finite Element Model (FEM) using ANSYS software [2].

2.4 Laboratory tests

A special test station was developed in the laboratory (author 3). The key components of the test station were: load cell, type KYOWA LVS-20GA (range 0–200mN), motor controlled translation stage type "Physik Instrumente" M-126.DG (accuracy 0.1 μm, adjustable stroke 18mm), 1-D Laser-Doppler-Vibrometer Polytec type OFV-303 and light-optical microscope for optical control. In this manner, reproducible results were achieved. The test procedure was controlled by the software COCKPIT [3].

The stiffness of Clip "ÀW" and Clip"new" was compared by measuring the pushing force F_a for various diameters of an "artificial" incudal process (wire pin).

In the first test the force F_a was applied at the knob provided at the upper branch of the clips. In the second test with Clip"ÀW" F_a was applied just below the clip and with Clip"new" at the notch of the posterior area (Fig. 4).

3. Results

3.1 Stapes surgery reports

Evaluating the 275 surgical records, 3 cases (1.1%) showed an incudal process which is too thin for Clip"ÀW", and 37 cases (13.5%) showed an incudal process which is too large in diameter: In 14.5% of all cases, implantation of Clip"ÀW" was suboptimal or not possible at all.

3.2 Cross-sections of the long incudal process

The 100 incudes were measured intraoperatively in 75% of the cases while performing tympanoplasty-surgery and in 25% during otosclerosis surgery. Both measured diameters varied by 0.5 to 0.9 mm (Fig. 2).

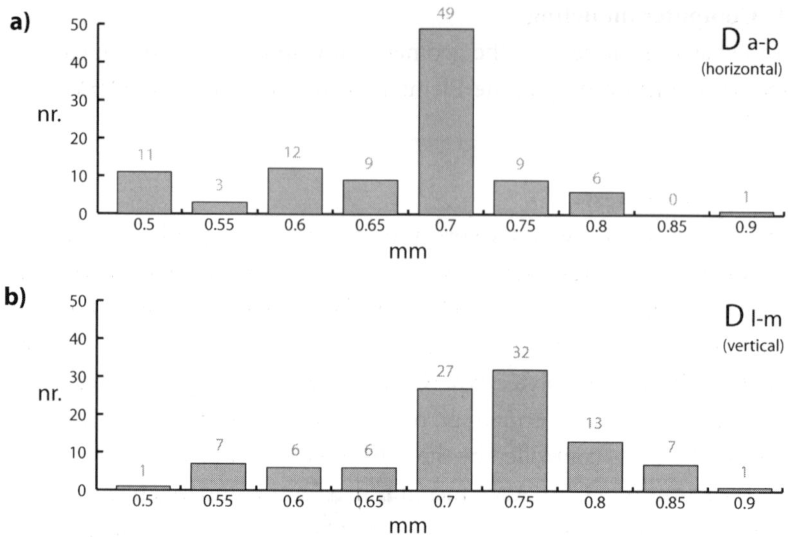

Fig. 2a) and 2b)

The measurements of $D_{a\text{-}p}$ showed that most cases (49 cases) are 0.70 mm, and that the majority is within the lower diameter range. The measurements of $D_{l\text{-}m}$ showed that most cases are above 0.70 mm with the maximum of the cases at 0.75 mm (32 cases). Table 1 combines both diameters, thus the cross-section can be read: 71 cases are vertically oval, 23 cases are round, and 6 cases are of a horizontally oval cross-section. The thinnest incudal processes are those of 6 children (below the age of 16, marked with*). Circled are two cases marking the bottom and top ends of the range. These are stapes surgeries in a female patient (0.55 × 0.55 mm) and a male patient (0.9 × 0,85 mm).

Table 1

diameter D a-p (vertical)

diameter D l-m (horizontal)

	.50	.55	.60	.65	.70	.75	.80	.85	.90	
.50	1*	5*	3			1	1			total 71
.55		1			2					
.60		1	2	4	4		1			
.65			1	1	4	3				
.70				1	15	26	6		1	
.75					2	2	4	1		
.80							1	5		
.85										
.90								1		
	total 6									23

3.3 Simulation

The FEM method facilitated the investigation of a multitude of different geometry variants regarding deformation behavior, stiffness, application force, and clamping force [3]. For the practical tests a suitable model was chosen, named Clip"new" (Fig. 3) and produced (author 2).

Clip "ÀWengen" and Clip "new"

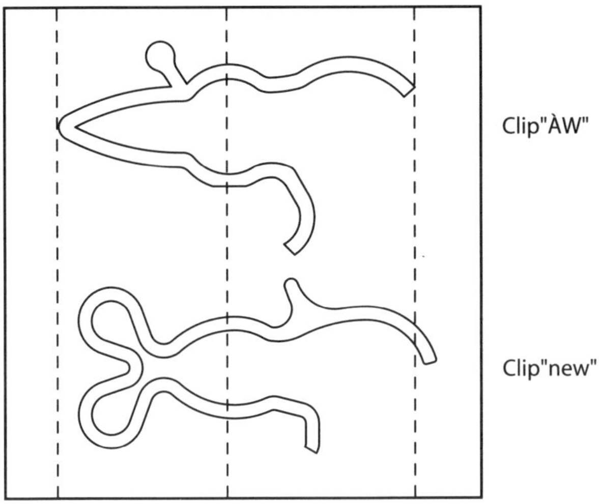

Fig. 3

In comparison with Clip"ÀW" the stiffness of this Clip"new" was reduced by 25%. The maximal stress is 30% lower, considerably reducing the risk of plastic deformation.

3.4 Measurement of application force F_a

When pushing by the knob (Fig. 4a, marked by arrows), for an incus diameter of 0.8 mm a force of 170 mN for Clip"ÀW", and 127 mN for Clip"new" were measured. This is 30% less F_a in favor of Clip"new". When using the second application point below the clip of Clip"ÀW" respectively at the rear end in the area of the notch of Clip"new"(Fig. 4b), 110 mN for Clip"ÀW" and 60 mN for Clip"new" were measured, which means 45% less application force F_a for Clip"new".

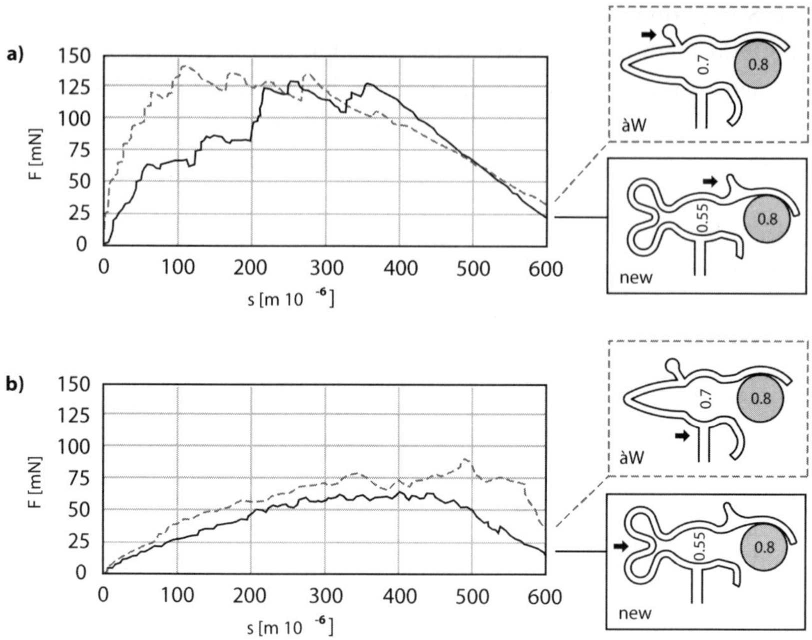

Fig. 4a) and 4b)

4. Discussion

Otosclerosis surgery is affected by prostheses of a broad variety of materials and various methods of fixation to the long incudal process [4] [5]. The widespread crimping of the prosthesis is a risky manner of fixation both for the incus and the inner ear. Moreover, it does not provide a constant quality in sound transmission [6] [7] [8] [9]. Insofar, Clip"ÀW" constitutes a milestone in the development of stapes prostheses, as it abolishes the crimping process and safeguards a constant, standardized fixation to the incus. The bone compatible titanium Clip"ÀW" contacts the incus only partially sparing the incudal process from arrosion and necrosis, which have been described with other types of prostheses [10] [11]. The Clip"àW" with an aperture of 0.7 mm was developed for surgical procedures with normal incus diameter and shape in the application area.

The considerable surgical practice of author 1 with more than 10,000 middle ear operations in 23 years (among them more than 2,000 stapes surgeries), has tested the limits of Clip"ÀW" in 275 otosclerosis patients in a period of three years: In 14.5% of the cases, Clip"ÀW" was either too loose at the incudal process (3 cases), because the incudal process was too thin, or pushing Clip"ÀW" was difficult or impossible due to an incudal process which was too thick. Postoperatively, an incudal process too thin for the aperture of Clip"ÀW" leads to loose contact with poor acoustical function, distortion and/or remaining air-bone-gap in the pure tone audiogram. During placement onto a thick incudal process, the Clip"ÀW" – due to its stiffness – requires a high application force. This increases the risk of luxating the incus especially for surgeons with little experience.

To date, there have not been any broad investigations into the cross-section of the incudal process. Apart from a general description of the incus [12], there has been a measurement of 11 extracted incudes [13]. Thus, intraoperative measurement is a novelty. The result of 100 incudes measured at the application site of the stapes prosthesis shows a larger variety than to date assumed or described. It is remarkable that two cases of otosclerosis limit the top and bottom variety range. They are circled in Table 1 presenting the cross-section of the long incudal process.

Concluding, a new clip prosthesis must have a geometry resulting in a lower stiffness. Consequently this means a lower application force and a more stable clamping force even with the most different incus cross-sections. The six smallest cross-sections marked with * in Table 1 (0.5×0.5 and 0.55×0.5 mm) can be disregarded, because those cases are children below the age of 16 and otosclerosis is not a disease typical of that age.

To this end computer modeling by means of FEM [14] [15] resulted in the fact that all parts of the clip were re-designed and optimized, leading to the development of Clip"new" (Fig. 3): compared to Clip"ÀW" the rear section (spring area) is more elastic due to the different shape with its longer titanium band. In the middle section (final incus position after application procedure) the clearance is less, corresponding to the small diameters Dl-m of 0.55 mm. The horizontal axis in this section has a larger diameter Da-p according to the measured value of 0.85 mm. The latter is also true for the application area (anterior part of the clip for application onto the incus). Finally, the angles of the insertion area ("bottleneck" for the incus) have been adapted for a better handling for the otosurgeon.

From several laboratory tests, two significant examples were selected for this publication. If pushing is done at the provided knob at the upper part of the clips, F_a of Clip"ÀW" has a relatively steep slope compared with Clip"new" and reaches a 30% higher value (Fig. 4a). Figure 4b shows for both clips that the maximum values are lower than those in Fig. 4a. So, rather than pushing the clip as shown in Figure 4a by the arrows, it is preferable to push the clip from the bottom (Clip"ÀW") or at the notch of the rear end (Clip"new"). With a maximum value of 60mN, Clip"new" has a 45% lower F_a than Clip"ÀW" (Fig. 4b). A direct comparison of the application force is not possible due to the different pushing points. Yet this value is remarkably low in favour of Clip"new".

Another positive outcome is the fact that with the incus diameter of 0.8 mm used in testing, the aperture of clip"new" is only 0.55 mm and thus clearly smaller than the aperture of Clip"ÀW" (0.7 mm). The reduced stiffness, resulting from the different geometry, can be clearly felt in practice. Even when there is a thick incudal process, Clip"new" can be pushed onto it gently without the risk of luxation of the malleus-incus joint. In case of a thin incudal process, there is still enough clamping force to avoid "loose contact".

5. Conclusions

Based on the data of 100 intraoperatively measured incudal processes, the tried-and-tested Clip-Piston "ÀWengen" was modified by further development of the clip design in all sections in such a manner that the result was a considerably lower stiffness with a sufficiently stable clamping force. In this process the computer simulation by means of FEM has proved itself a precondition for effective laboratory tests [16]. In cases of extreme incudal process diameters, the design of Clip"new" offers improved handling even for less experienced otosurgeons and thus more benefit for the patients.

References

1. ÀWengen, D.F., Die neue selbsthaltende Clip-Stapes-Prothese aus Titan: erste klinische Erfahrungen. *Schweiz Med. Forum* 2003; **11:** 14–16
2. Kohnke P. Ansys Theory Manual – Release 5.7. SAS IP 2001
3. Hildenbrand M.: Zum Steifigkeitsverhalten von Steigbügelprothesen. Studienarbeit STUD-218, Universität Stuttgart, Institut B für Mechanik Februar 2005
4. Häusler R. Advances in Stapes Surgery (in Jahnke K., Editor) *Middle Ear Surgery: Recent Advances and Future Directions.* Thieme 2004; **5:** 95–139

5. Hüttenbrink KB. Biomechanics of Stapesplasty: A Review. *Otology & Neurotology* 2003; **24:** 548–559
6. De Bruijn, AJG. *Clinical and audiological aspects of stapes surgery in otosclerosis.* Academisch Proefschrift, Universität Amsterdam 2000; Chapter 9: 115–131
7. Huber AM., Furong M., Felix H., Linder, T. Stapes Prosthesis Attachment: The Effect of Crimping on Sound Transfer in Otosclerosis Surgery. *The Laryngoscope* 2003; **113:** 853–858
8. Kwok P., Fisch U., Strutz J., May, J. Stapes Surgery: how precisely do different prostheses attach to the long process of the incus with different instruments and different surgeons? *Otology & Neurotology* 2002; **23:** 289–295
9. Skinner M., Honrado C., Prasad M., Kent N., Selesnick SH. The Incudostapedial Joint Angle: Implications for Stapes Surgery Prosthesis Selection and Crimping. *The Laryngoscope* 2003; **113:** 647–653

10. Schimanski G. Die Arrosion und Nekrose des langen Ambossschenkels nach Otoskleroseoperation. *HNO* 1997; **45:** 682–689
11. Schimanski G. Die Steigbügeloperation bei Otosklerose. *HNO* 1998; **46:** 289–292
12. Lang J. *Klinische Anatomie des Ohres.* Springer 1992
13. Kwok P., Fisch U., Gleich O., Achhammer K., Strutz J. Stapes Surgery: The Diameter of the Long Process of the Incus. *Otology & Neurotology* 2006; **27:** 469–477
14. Meissner U., Menzel A. *Die Methode der finiten Elemente.* Springer 1989
15. Müller G., Groth C. FEM für Praktiker. *Expert* 1997
16. Eiber A., Kauf A. Berechnete Verschiebungen der Mittelohrknochen unter statischer Belastung. *HNO* 1994; **42:** 754–759

ON THE OPTIMAL COUPLING OF AN IMPLANTABLE HEARING AID – MEASUREMENTS AND SIMULATIONS

Albrecht Eiber and Christian Breuninger, Institute of Engineering and Computational Mechanics, University of Stuttgart, Pfaffenwaldring 9, 70550 Stuttgart, Germany
Email: eiber@itm.uni-stuttgart.de

Jesus Rodriguez Jorge, Hans P. Zenner, Marcus M. Maassen
Department of Otolaryngology, Head & Neck Surgery, University Hospital of Tübingen, Germany, Email: Jesus.Rodriguez@uni-tuebingen.de

The sound transfer is strongly dependent on the coupling of the prosthesis to the ossicles. This holds for both passive but in particular for active implants. Various principles of coupling and different designs of attaching the implant to ossicle are in use showing a different mechanical behavior concerning stiffness and damping. Pressing a driving rod against the ossicles means a unilateral coupling which needs a particular prestress. Due to the nonlinear transfer behavior of the coupling region and ossicular chain, the actual motions, e.g. of actuator, stapes and umbo are dependent on that prestress. An optimal coupling should allow a stapes motion sufficient to compensate a hearing loss, but should avoid a distorted sound transfer or feedback due to sound radiation from ear drum. The static adjustment influences the sound transfer of the dynamical system essentially. To find an optimal adjustment of the actuator, the dynamical behavior of the actuator itself, of the coupling region and the individual ossicular chain has to be regarded. During surgery the stiffness of the individual chain has to be estimated and the configuration when the actuator touches the ossicles has to be detected very carefully.

1. Introduction

Beside the conditions of the individual hearing, the sound transfer characteristics of a reconstructed middle ear essentially depend on the mechanical behavior of the coupling between passive or active implant with the ossicular chain. The entire system has to be considered to describe the dynamical behavior and to give directives for the optimal coupling of an implant. Simulations have to be carried out with computational models of the middle ear with its adjacent structures and the actuator. The simulations are based on modeling techniques such as Finite Elements and Multibody Systems approach known from dynamical analysis of mechatronical systems. Static pressure variations [1–4] or preloads from middle ear prostheses and scar tissue displace the ossicles and change stiffness and damping of the visco-elastic elements which directly changes the dynamical properties of middle ear.

1.1 Problem

The Otologics Middle Ear Transducer (MET) is a partially implantable electro-magnetic middle ear hearing device to excite the ossicular chain mechanically. The driving rod of the MET is pushed against the incus using an adjustment screw between the body of MET and the skull. A general guideline for the adjustment travel of the screw was given by Waldmann et al. [5] without considering the individual stiffness of the middle ear. Therefore, mechanical characteristics of the entire system have to be regarded for the investigation of the motion of stapes, the distortion in the sound transfer and the risk of feedback or ringing. Mechanically, the rotation φ at the screw with the pitch h results in a static adjustment travel which causes a static preload in the contact region between driving rod and incus. The effective forces in this area and in the ligaments depend on the static adjustment φ and the internal stiffness of the actuator but also on the compliance of the individual middle ear.

The problem is to find an adjustment position of actuator that applies a sufficient amplitude of displacement to the ossicular chain, that gives a proper coupling between actuator and ossicle without distortion, maintains this coupling in case of external or internal pressure changes and avoids attenuated or nonlinear sound transfer or shifted natural frequencies.

2. Methods

Investigations of the dynamical behavior of a given system start normally with measurements on the original system or on experimental models of it. Rodriguez Jorge et al. have found different transfer behavior for different stiffness of ossicular chain [6] using Laser Doppler Vibrometry (LDV). In Fig. 1 the measured amplitudes of stapes displacement y_s are shown for a stiff, a normal and a compliant ossicular chain of temporal bones. The ossicular chain was driven by a MET inserted with different static adjustment travels φ. The angle can be controlled by the surgeon, together with the pitch $h = 250\mu m$ of the adjustment screw it leads to the displacement $h\varphi$ of the actuators housing.

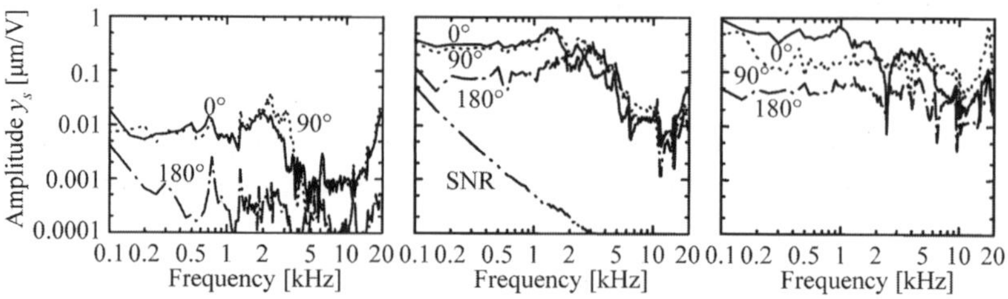

Fig. 1 Measured amplitudes of stapes for different adjustment travels $\varphi = 0°$, $90°$ and $180°$ related to 1 V excitation at MET. Ossicular chain stiff (left), normal (middle) and compliant (right).

For the interpretation of these findings simulations have been carried out. The used spatial models of the middle ear contain the ossicular chain, the actuator with its adjustment screw as well as the nonlinear behavior of the ligaments and of the coupling region. A simplified representation of it is shown in Fig. 2.

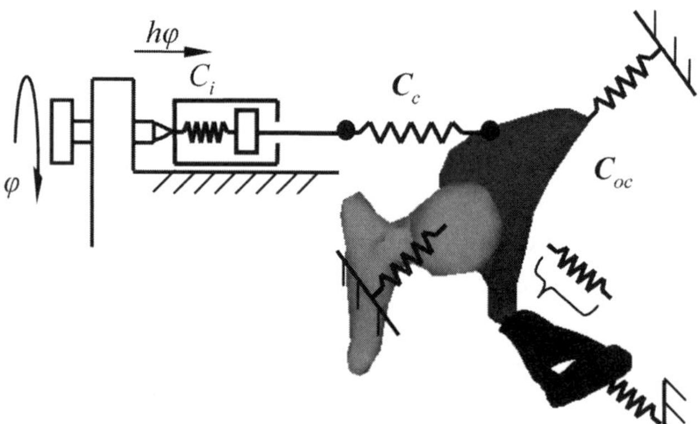

Fig. 2 Simplified representation of ossicular chain with actuator. The turn angle of adjustment screw is denoted by φ, h is the pitch of the adjustment screw, C_i is the internal stiffness of the actuator and C_c and C_{oc} are the individual stiffness matrices of the coupling region and ossicular chain, respectively. Note: C_c and C_{oc} are dependent on φ due to nonlinear properties of coupling region and ligaments.

The simulations show, in agreement with the measurements, that the static adjustment φ of the actuator influences the amplitude of stapes and the amplitude of umbo depending on the stiffness of the chain. In a first step at these investigations the working position of the ossicular chain due to the static adjustment φ was calculated regarding the nonlinear characteristics of the ligaments and of the coupling region [7]. Subsequently, the sound transfer was simulated using a model linearized with respect to this working position. The results considered here are derived from a particular parameter set of a normal ear, but the same qualitative behavior can be observed for other parameter sets as considered in Fig. 1.

Two of the state variables are of interest: The amplitude y_s of stapes determining the hearing impression and the motion of umbo y_u leading to sound radiation into the outer ear canal. It can be used for the detection of contact but may cause a feedback of excitation. Due to the nonlinear behavior of the ligaments, in particular of the stiffening annular ring, the ossicular chain becomes increasingly immobile with increasing static adjustment. Increasing the adjustment travel of the MET causes a shift of the natural frequencies to higher values and is followed by a progressive nonlinear drop in stapes amplitude particularly in the lower frequency range up to 3 kHz. For the umbo motion this effect is not so distinct because the ear drum shows a wider range of mobility than the annular ring, Fig. 3.

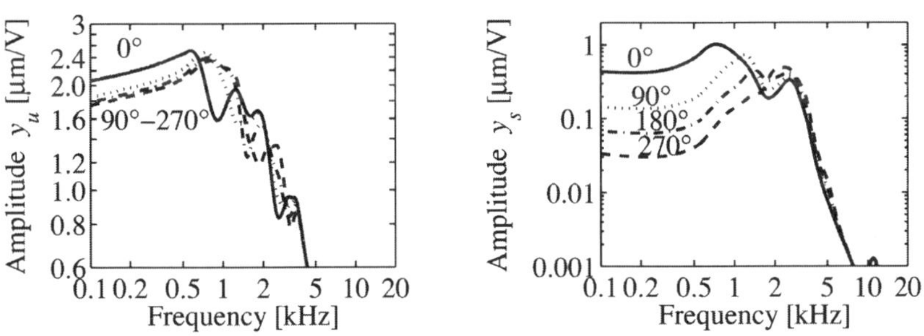

Fig. 3 Dynamical amplitudes of displacements for different working positions related to 1 V excitation at MET. Left: Displacement of umbo. Right: Displacement of stapes.

In the coupling region it may occur for a certain adjustment that pushing the driving rod against the incus (forward motion) has a higher stiffness than the retraction. This leads to a distorted motion of the stapes even for an excitation in the range of physiological sound pressure.

Further, the effective displacement amplitudes y_a of actuator's rod are dependent on the load, i.e. on the stiffness of the ossicular chain and the static adjustment as it can be seen for the lower frequency range in Fig. 4 left. Looking at higher frequencies above 3 kHz, this effect is less distinct.

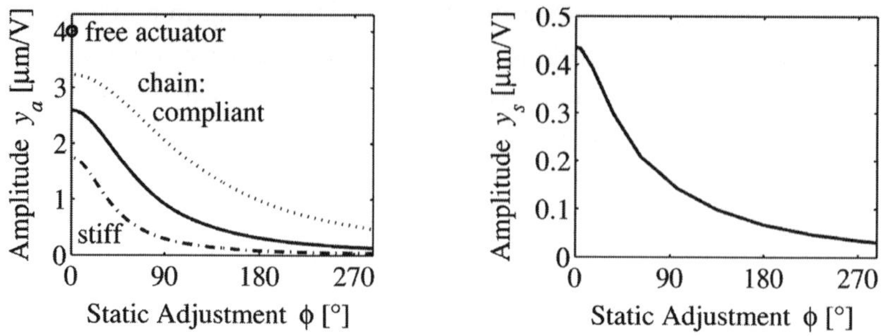

Fig. 4 Dynamical amplitudes of displacements for different working positions in the low frequency range related to 1 V excitation at MET. Left: Actuator amplitude for the free actuator and different stiffness of chain. Right: Amplitude of stapes.

3. Results and Discussions

To avoid nonlinear transfer effects, the static force in the coupling region must be higher than the amplitude of the dynamic force which has to be applied for the required hearing impression.

A too high static position adjustment travel leads to unphysiological high tension in the incudo-stapedial joint. Consequently, the joint becomes very compliant with a reduced sound transfer and there is an increased risk of joint separation.

3.1 Surgery process

During surgery the surgeon has only limited possibilities of intervention. To avoid feedback and distortion, the static adjustment should be kept low. To an optimal compensation for an actual hearing loss to a large extent, several steps can be done by the surgeon:

The compliance of the individual ossicular chain should be estimated. For this, a static or dynamic excitation, e.g. from the actuator itself can be applied and the response measured by Laser Doppler Vibrometry at the umbo or by microphone in the ear canal. In addition, results from tympanometry can be evaluated.

Next, when approaching the actuator, the state when the driving rod comes into contact with the incus should precisely be detected by observing the response of the chain at the umbo as described above or checking the reaction of the actuator itself, e.g. measuring its electrical impedance. The adjustment travel to apply should take into account the individual compliance of the middle ear. Compliant chains need a higher position adjustment travel than stiff ones.

3.2 Assessment of coupling

Because of restricted access to the stapes during surgery the coupling conditions can be assessed by measuring the umbo motion using a microphone or LDV. An estimation of the motion of stapes can be derived by using the transfer function between motion of umbo and stapes as shown in Fig. 5 for an ear reconstructed with a MET. In the lower frequency range, the attenuation of stapes motion increasing with static adjustment can clearly be seen and the risk of giving a too high static adjustment by exclusively considering the motion of umbo becomes obvious.

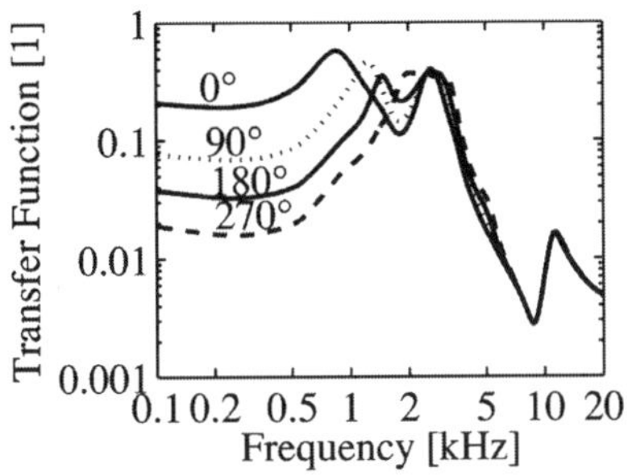

Fig. 5 Transfer function between motion of umbo and stapes, i.e. amplitude of displacement of stapes if that of umbo is equal 1.

4. Conclusions

Optimal coupling of an actuator with an ossicle depends on the design of the coupling region, the mechanical properties of the actuator itself as well as on the dynamical behavior of the ossicular chain. Appropriate criteria for optimization may be good sound transfer, low distortion and no ringing. The realization must be "robust", i.e. not sensitive to changes in the parameters of the system. This is essential because pressure in the tympanic cavity or inner ear may vary and biological structures undergo alterations due to time. Particularly the given prestress of ligaments and static pressure are time-variant.

For the determination of an optimal coupling, the mechanical properties of the actuator as well as the dynamical behavior of the ossicular chain have to be considered.

A static adjustment travel of the actuator leads to a static prestress in the ossicular chain. Due to the nonlinear behavior and the large deformations in the ligaments the mechanical properties like stiffness and thus the dynamical behavior of the middle ear are altered.

Intraoperative measurements give more information about the mechanical properties and a deeper insight into the dynamical behavior of the middle ear. This enables the surgeon to better adjust active or passive middle ear prostheses.

An excitation of high intensity leads to displacements of the ossicles which have to be calculated from nonlinear models by applying time integration procedures. For normal hearing with physiological excitation the transfer process through the middle ear can be described with linear models.

Acknowledgments

These investigations have been partially financed by the German Research Council (DFG).

References

1. Hüttenbrink K.B., The mechanics of the middle ear at static air pressures. *Acta otolaryngol.* **451** (1988) pp. 1–35
2. Dirckx J. J., Decraemer W., Area change and volume displacement of the human tympanic membrane under static pressure. *Hearing Research* **62** (1992) pp. 99–104
3. Densert O., Ivarsson A., Pedersen K., The influence of perilymphatic pressure on the displacement of the tympanic membrane. *Acta otolaryngol.* **84** (1977) pp. 220–226
4. Gaihede M., Kabel J., The normal Pressure-Volume Relationship of the Middle Ear System and its biological Variation. In J. Rosowski and S. Merchant (eds.) *The function and mechanics of normal, diseased and reconstructed middle ears.* Kugler Publications, The Hague, Netherlands (2000) pp. 59–70
5. Waldmann B., Maier H., Leuwer R., Indicator for Efficient Coupling of the Otologics MET™ Ossicular Stimulator. In K. Gyo. H. Wada, N. Hato and T. Koike (eds.) *Middle Ear Mechanics in Research and Otology.* (World Scientific, Singapore 2004) pp. 377–383
6. Rodriguez Jorge J., Pfister M., Zenner H.P., Zalaman I., Maassen M., *In Vitro* Model for Intraoprative Adjustment in an Implantable Hearing Aid. *Laryngoscope* **116** (2006) pp. 473–481
7. Eiber A., Breuninger C., Nonlinear Properties of the Middle Ear: Some Influences on Hearing and Diagnosis, In K. Gyo. H. Wada, N. Hato and T. Koike (eds.) *Middle Ear Mechanics in Research and Otology.* (World Scientific, Singapore 2004) pp. 19–26

THE EFFECT OF COCHLEAR IMPLANT ELECTRODE INSERTION ON MIDDLE EAR FUNCTION AS MEASURED BY IN VIVO LASER DOPPLER VIBROMETRY

N. Donnelly Mrcs[1], **A. Bibas** Msc Drmed Frcs (Otol)[1,3], **D. Jiang** Phd Frcs (Orl)[1], **C. Santulli** Phd[1,2], **A. Fitzgerald O'Connor** Frcs[1]

[1] Dpt. of Otolaryngology – Head & Neck Surgery, Guy's and St Thomas' Hospitals, London, UK

[2] School of Construction Management and Engineering, University Reading, UK

[3] Dpt. of Otolaryngology – Head & Neck Surgery, Hippokrateio Hospital, University of Athens, Greece

Email addresses for correspondence:
neildonnelly@doctors.org.uk, hanosbibas@hotmail.com
danjiang@doctors.org.uk, c.santulli@reading.ac.uk, afoc@globalnet.co.uk

Keywords: cochlear implantation, residual hearing, middle ear, transfer function, Laser Doppler Vibrometry

Background: Preservation of residual low-frequency hearing can substantially improve the speech perception abilities and hearing in noise of cochlear implant users.

Aim: The aim of this study is to investigate the impact of cochlear implant electrode insertion on middle ear low frequency function.

Patients and methods: Stapes displacement was measured intra-operatively using Laser Doppler Vibrometry before and after electrode insertion in seven patients undergoing cochlear implantation.

Results: In three patients, there was little change in stapes displacement following the electrode insertion. In two patients there was a significant increase, while in a further two there was a significant reduction in stapes displacement. This variability may reflect alteration of cochlear impedance associated with the electrode insertion.

Conclusion: Insertion of a cochlear implant electrode can produce a change in stapes displacement at low frequencies, which may have an effect on residual low-frequency hearing thresholds.

1. Introduction

Cochlear implant (CI) selection criteria have recently expanded to include individuals with residual low-frequency hearing. The aim is to use a cochlear implant to stimulate the basal turn of the cochlea where high-frequency hearing has been lost and a conventional acoustic hearing aid to stimulate the apical residual low frequency hearing. This is termed combined electrical acoustical stimulation (CEAS). Results have demonstrated improved speech perception abilities and hearing in noise with combined stimulation compared to acoustic and electrical stimulation in isolation [1]. Additionally, music appreciation and quality of sound is maintained due to residual hearing providing finer spectral resolution than is possible with current CI speech-processing algorithms [2]. To utilise the preserved low frequency hearing requires an intact middle ear conductive mechanism. Although there are many studies in the literature on the traumatic effects of cochlear implantation on the cochlea, there is no study as yet on the possible effect of cochlear implantation on middle ear mechanics. Laser Doppler Vibrometry (LDV) is a tool that has frequently been employed in middle ear research on animals, human temporal bones and live humans [3, 4, 5, 6]. Huber et al examined intra-operative stapes movement in seven patients undergoing cochlear implantation; however no post-implant measurements were taken [7]. They established that LDV was practical for taking measurements during live surgery and the results obtained were comparable to findings in temporal bone preparations. The aim of this study is to explore the effect of the cochlear implant electrode insertion on the function of the middle ear. This could have implications on future development of cochlear implant electrodes or insertion techniques.

2. Methodology

Subject recruitment and method protocols were approved by the National Health System (NHS) Research Ethics Committee. Subjects recruited for the study were sequential paediatric and adult cochlear implant cases already on the NHS waiting list. The aetiology of the hearing loss included congenital causes, post-meningitis hearing loss, severe presbyacusis and idiopathic causes. None of the patients were undergoing implantation with a view to combined electrical and acoustic stimulation. The exclusion criteria for the study were evidence of middle ear disease as assessed preoperatively by otoscopy and tympanometry or intraoperatively by inspection and palpation. None of the patients approached needed to be excluded. Stapes displacement was measured in seven patients undergoing cochlear implantation. Intraoperative measurements were carried out before and after electrode insertion via the round window membrane. Sound was delivered into the ear canal via an ER-2 earphone and calibrated via an ER-7C probe microphone (Etymotic Research) approximately 3mm from the tympanic membrane. The speaker and probe microphone were integrated into an individually made ear mould, which was made preoperatively in the adult patients and intraoperatively in children. The mould was fashioned from the impression material used to make hearing aid moulds and the technique used was the same. A punch biopsy instrument made a hole through the mould large enough to accommodate the tubing for the loud speaker and the microphone.

The measurement system consisted of a sound delivery and calibration system, and an operating microscope mounted LDV system. Sound was delivered through an ER-2 earphone (Etymotic Research) coupled to the customised ear mould which was inserted into the ear canal. The output was calibrated at approximately 3 mm from the tympanic membrane using an ER-7C probe microphone (Etymotic Research), which was also incorporated within the ear mould with an ER7-14C probe tube. The ER-7C probe microphone was calibrated against a standardised calibrator at the beginning of each experiment. The sound stimulus was digitally synthesized using the Vibsoft software and was outputted to a digital-analog converter. A multisine stimulus was used consisting of tones at 0.25, 0.5, 1 and 2 kHz with each frequency having an intensity of 80dB SPL. A commercial HLV-1000 Laser Doppler Vibrometer System (Polytec) was used to measure stapes velocity at the stapes head. This was mounted over the lens of an operating microscope and the helium-neon laser beam was focused on the head of the stapes through the posterior tympanotomy, without using reflective paint. The reflected signal was detected and decoded by the vibrometer controller to produce an output voltage proportional to the stapes velocity. It is estimated that the measurement angle between the LDV beam and the direction of the piston-like stapes motion is between 65–80 degrees [8]. Since each patient served as his own control and the angle of measurement was constant for each patient, no cosine corrections were made.

3. Results

The results presented display the difference in dB between the displacement responses of the stapes before and after electrode insertion to the same stimuli for each patient (Figure 1).

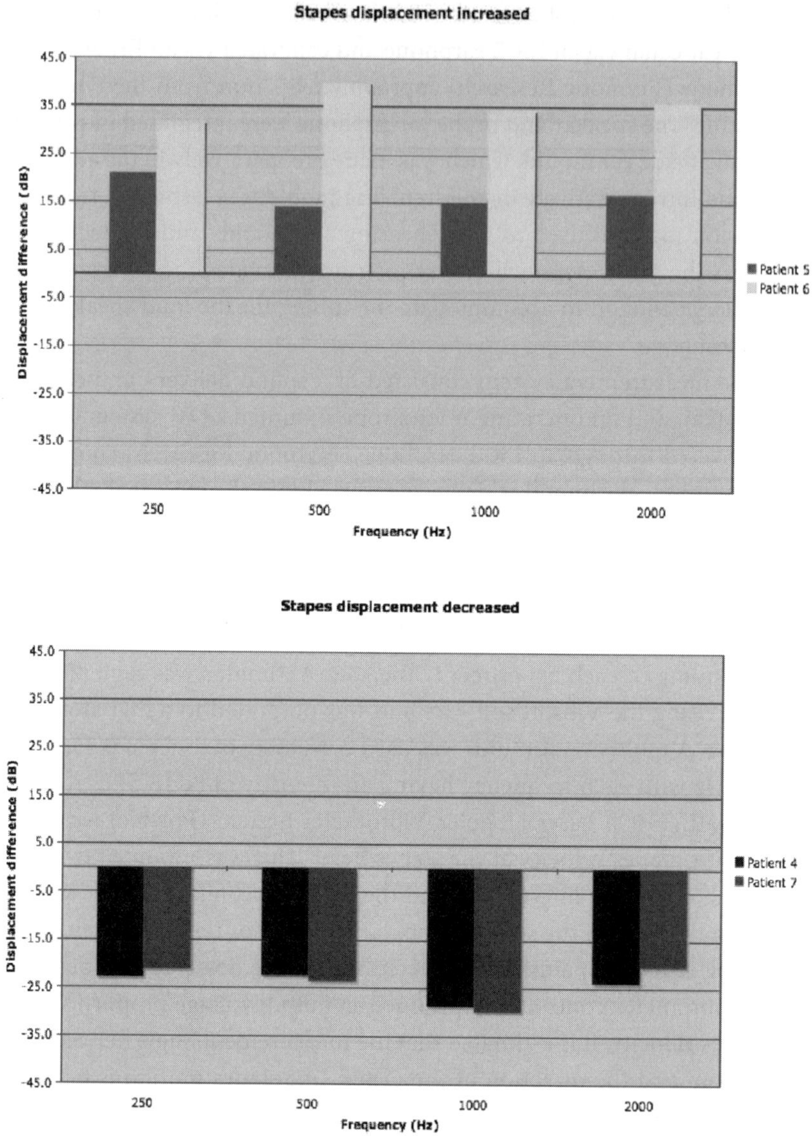

Fig. 1 Difference in dB in stapes displacement amplitude before and after electrode insertion to the same stimuli for each patient.

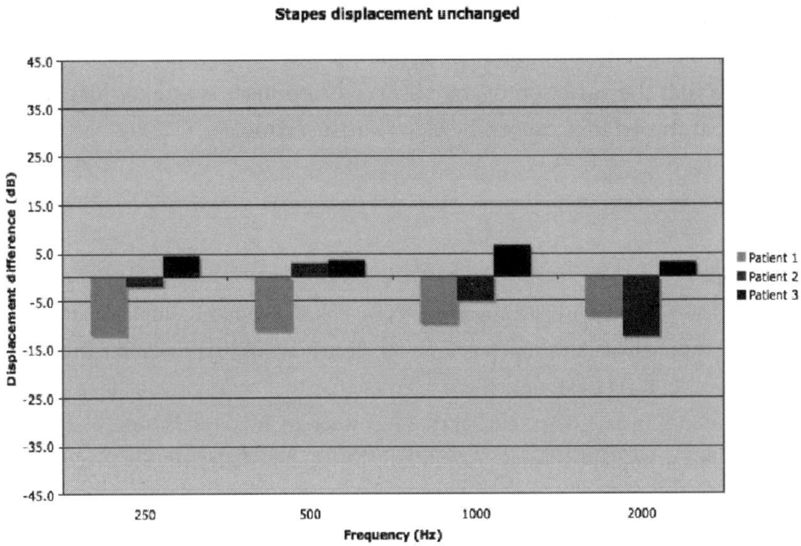

Fig. 1 (*continued*)

The responses fall into three categories: increased displacement (patients 5 and 6), decreased displacement (patients 4 and 7) and no significant change (patients 1, 2 and 3). At 1 kHz, the average decrease in stapes displacement in patients 4 and 7 was 22.8 dB (maximum of 27 dB in patient 7). In patients 5 and 6 the increase in displacement was 15.2 dB and 34.5 dB respectively.

4. Discussion

The effect of opening the scala vestibuli has little effect on middle ear transfer function [9]. Research has shown that an increase in inner ear pressure results in a reduced amplitude of stapes velocity, with greater effects at lower than higher frequencies [10]. Temporal bone studies that have drained the cochlea have demonstrated varied stapes displacement with the largest effect being at frequencies greater than 1 kHz [11, 12]. The effect of cochlear implant insertion on cochlear impedance is unknown. The volume effect of a cochlear implant electrode is likely to increase cochlear impedance, while perilymph loss or introduction of air bubbles in the perilymph will reduce impedance. By increasing cochlear impedance one would expect a decrease in stapes displacement. In contrast, a reduction in cochlear impedance due to varying quantities of perilymph loss would reduce the stapes displacement accordingly. No two insertions will be identical and it is therefore possible that the discrepancy between the observed responses is a reflection of this. As a consequence of perilymph homeostasis, one would expect this effect to be short-lived.

5. Conclusions

Insertion of a cochlear implant electrode can alter stapes displacement. We speculate that the variation of the observed responses is due to the change in cochlear impedance caused by electrode insertion.

References

1. Gstoettner W., Kiefer J., Baumgartner W.D., Pok S., Peters S., Adunka O., Hearing preservation in cochlear implantation for electric acoustic stimulation. *Acta Otolaryngol.* **124(4)** (2004) pp. 348–52
2. Gantz B.J., Turner C.W., Gfeller K.E., Lowder M.W., Preservation of hearing in cochlear implant surgery: Advantages of combined electrical and acoustical speech processing. *Laryngoscope* **115** (2005) pp. 796–802
3. Goode R.L., Ball G., Nishihara S., Nakamura K., Laser Doppler vibrometer (LDV) – A new clinical tool for the otologist. *Am J Otol* **17** (1996) pp. 813–822
4. Heiland K., Goode R., Asai M., Huber A., A human temporal bone study of stapes footplate movement. *Am J Otol* **20** (1999) pp. 81–86
5. Gan R.Z., Wood M.W., Dormer K.J., Human Middle ear Transfer Function Measured by Double Laser Interferometry System. *Otol Neurotol* **25** (2004) pp. 423–435
6. Needham A.J., Jiang D., Bibas A., Jeronimidis G., Fitzgerald O'Connor A., The Effects of Mass Loading the Ossicles with a Floating Mass Transducer on Middle Ear Transfer Function. *Otol Neurotol* **26** (2005) pp. 218–224
7. Huber A., Linder T., Ferrazzini M., Schmid S., Dillier N., Stoeckli S., Fisch. Intraoperative assessment of stapes movement. *Ann Otol Rhinol Laryngol* **110** (2001) pp. 31–35
8. Chien W., Rosowski J.J., Ravicz M.E., Merchant S.N., Measurements of stapes velocity in live humane ears *MEMRO 2006*
9. Aibara R., Welsh J.T., Puria S., Goode R.L., Human middle-ear sound transfer function and cochlear input impedance. *Hearing Research* **152** (2001) pp. 100–109
10. Murakami S., Gyo K., Goode R.L., Effect of increased inner ear pressure on middle ear mechanics. *Otolaryngol H N Surg* **118** (1998) pp. 703–708
11. Gyo K., Aritomo H., Goode R.L., Measurement of the ossicular vibration ratio in human temporal bones by use of a video measuring system. *Acta Otolaryngol* **103** (1987) pp. 87–95
12. Lord R.M., Abel E.W., Wang Z., Effects of draining cochlear fluids on stapes displacement in middle-ear models. *J Acoust Soc Am* **110** (2001) pp. 3132–3139

MIDDLE EAR MORPHOMETRY FROM CADAVERIC TEMPORAL BONE MICRO-CT IMAGING

S. Puria[1,2,4], J.H. Sim[1,4], M. Shin[2,4], J. Tuck-Lee[1,4], C.R. Steele[1,2]
[1] Stanford University, Department of Mechanical Engineering, 496 Durand Building, Stanford, CA 94305
[2] Stanford University, Department of Otolaryngology-HNS, 801 Welch Road, Stanford, CA 94304
[3] Stanford University, Department of Aeronautics and Astronautics, 496 Durand Building, Stanford, CA 94305
[4] Department of Veterans Afairs, 3801 Miranda Avenue, Palo Alto, CA 9430
Email: puria@stanford.edu

An anatomically based three-dimensional (3D) compuational model requires detailed morphometry of middle ear structures. We report methods and results using the microCT imaging modality for the middle ear. Stacks of images were obtained from cadaveric temporal bone ears of human, cat, chinchilla and guinea pig. The images were segemented and 3D structures reconstructed. The structures include the eardrum (thickness map and 3D shape), volumes of each of the three middle ear bones, and suspensory ligaments and tensor tympani tendon. The volume reconstruction of the malleus indicates that it has a solid rod-like shape in human, is a hollow cylinder in cat, and has an I-beam like shape in guinea pig and chinchilla. From the ossicle volumes, principal axis of rotation and principal moments of inertia, both around the center of gravity, were calculated. The results indicate that for the guinea pig and chinchilla, where the malleus-incus joint is fused, the clasical axis of rotation through the malleus and incus heads holds. However, the data also indicate a new mode of operation at high frequencies in animals where the malleus-incus joint is mobile (human and cat). We hypothesize that the malleus shape, along with a mobile joint, provides optimal transfer of energy to the cochlea at high frequencies through a rotation motion (torsion) around the long axis (superior-inferior) of the malleus.

1. Introduction

The eardrum transduces acoustic energy into mechanical motions, which is the first of many transducers in the auditory system. The sensitivity and frequency range of the eardrum depends on its shape, collagen fiber layer thickness profile, overall thickness profile, and material properties [1, 2]. Motions of the eardrum result in motion of the malleus-incus complex (MIC) of the middle ear. The MIC consists of the malleus and incus bones suspended from the surrounding middle ear cavity walls by ligaments and tensor tympani tendon. From the morphometry data of the MIC simple deductions can be made regarding middle ear dynamics. For example the ligaments and tendons, which are soft tissues and thus spring-like, dominate at low frequencies. On the other hand moments of interia due to mass dominate at high frequencies. Motion of the incus drives the stapes which in turn generates a fluid pressure in the cochlea. Structure and function are often easier to explore using mathematical models.

To develop anatomically based biocomputational models of middle ears, morphometry data is critical. To obtain morphometry of the ear, histological methods have been the primary technique. However, this technique is destructive and has other disadvantages such as stretching distortions and long preparation time [3]. One of the most recent advances for obtaining anatomical information is computed-tomography with μm resolutions (microCT). Here we describe methods to determine parameters, needed for computational models, from the microCT imaging modality. Morphometry measurements include: (1) Eardrum shape and thickness profile, (2) principal axes and principal moments of inertia of the malleus, incus and stapes, (3) dimensions and angles of suspensory ligament and tendon attachments relative to the principal axis, (4) malleus-incus joint separation (if any), and (5) middle ear cavity shape. The morphometry data presented illucidate the dynamical behaviour of the middle ear sub components. Cadaveric temporal bones of human, cat, chinchilla and guinea pig were studied. However, not all of these types of analysis were performed on a single species and not all of the results are reported here due to lack of space.

2. Methods

Cadaveric temporal bone ears of human (4), cat (1), chinchilla (1) and guinea pig (1) were scanned using a Scanco VivaCT 40 scanner (www.scanco.ch). The bore diameter ranged from 20.5 to 39 mm depending on the size of the core. Each temporal bone core was dissected to fit into as small a bore size as possible while keeping all structures of interest intact. The temporal bone was wrapped in cellophane before placement into the scanner bore. The scan resolution was 2048 × 2048 which resulted in an image resolution ranging from 10 to 19 μm (both in plane and out of plane). The beam intensity was set to 50 kV, with a current of 145 μA, and integration time of typically 300 ms. The scan time ranged from 6 to 12 hours depending on the number of slices in a given specimen. The high-resolution images (1000 to 2000 slices) were used for 3D reconstructions of the ossicles, suspensory ligaments and tensor-tympani tendon, tympanic membrane eardrum curvature and its relative position in the ear canal, tympanic membrane thickness, and middle ear cavity dimensions. The vivaCT software and RainDrop geomagic were used for the 3D reconstructions.

3. Results

Figure 1 shows sample slices from human and chinchilla ears. These images demonstrate that the density of the eardrum, ossicles, and middle ear cavity walls are distinguished from each other and more import from the lower density of the air surrounding these structures. The contrast difference between desired structures and air, or bone, allows drawing of contours around regions of interest. The regions of interest are stacked and joined together to obtain a 3D volume of interest.

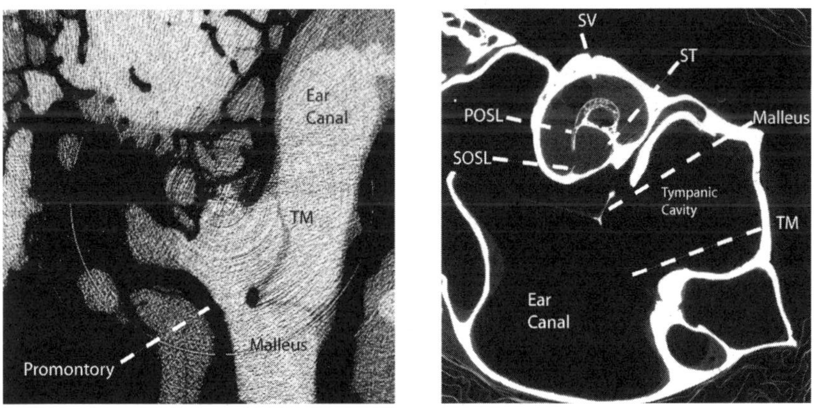

Fig. 1 Example microCT slices from human (left) and chinchilla (right) temporal bones. In the left panel highest density is in black while the lowest density is in white. The cone-shaped eardrum and malleus just above the cochlea promontory are visible. In the right panel, the reverse is true: highest density in white and lowest in black. A section of the cochlea within the middle ear cavity is clearly delineated.

3.1 Eardrum thickness

MicroCT images were used to resconstruct the eardrum shape and thickness for the cat eardrum. Figure 2 (left panel) shows the thickness profile as a color map. These results are compared with measurements reported by Kuypers et al (right panel) with the confocal microscopy approach [4]. They measured the thickness along several lines (along the x-axis at y = 0,2,4.5 and below the umbo along the y-axis) and interpolated the thickness at the other points, which explains why the results look very uniform. Although the results by the two approaches look similar there are differences. The superior portion of the eardrum is thicker than the inferior portion and the asymetry in the anterior and posterior sections is observed (Fig. 2, left panel). In the thinnest region the thickness values with the μCT approach is about 20 μm while the thinnest values obtained by Kuypers et al are about 15 μm. In general the μCT approach appears to yield thickness values that are more than that with the confocal approach.

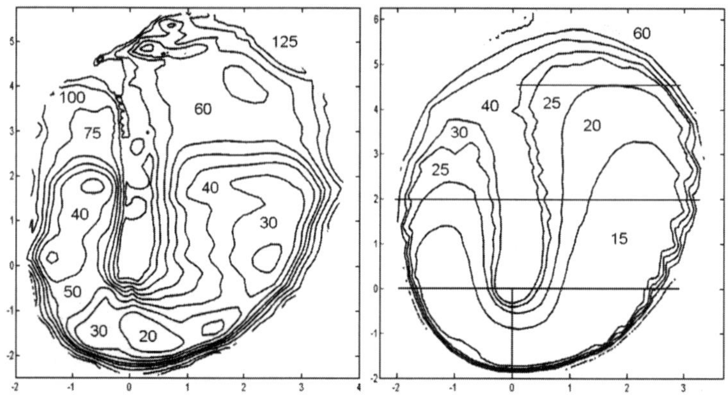

Fig. 2 Contour map of eardrum thickness obtained from micro-CT imaging based reconstruction (left) and from confocal microscopy approach (right) measured at the indicated four straight lines and then interpolated and projected onto an eardrum [4].

3.2 Malleus structure

It is well known that the malleus is directly attached to TM. Consequently, the structure of the malleus may play an important role in integrating the motion of the TM [1, 5] and efficiently transfering TM vibration to the incus and stapes. From microCT images (Fig. 3 center column) and corresponding 3-D reconstructions (Fig. 3, left column), significant structural differences are observed between the four species. Human and cat have solid and hollow structures respectively while chinchilla and guinea pig have similar structure which is I-beam like (Fig. 3, right column). The hollow structure is stronger against torsion and bending than the solid structure for a given mass. The I-beam like structure is stonger against one directional bending than the solid structure for a given mass. This structural property can be also beneficial in transfering the high frequency vibration since it could have the same strength in one directional bending with less mass. Thus it is possible to deduce that the umbo vibration is mostly one-directional at least in guinea pig and chinchilla.

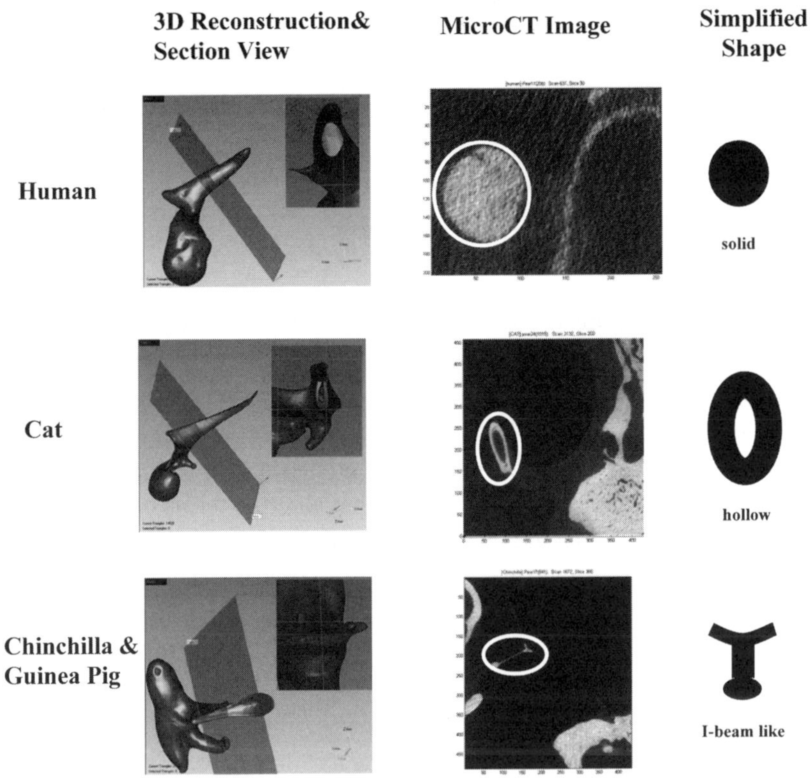

Fig. 3 Left column: 3-D reconstruction of malleus and its section (inset) view. Middle column: microCT slice image showing the section shape of each malleus. Right column: Simplified shape description in terms of a solid rod, a hollow cylinder, and I-beam like shapes.

3.3 Malleus-incus joint

From the scanned images and 3D reconstruction of the four species, the malleus-incus joints for human and cat appear separated while the malleus-incus joint for chinchilla and guinea pig appear to be fused. This is consistent with previous observations regarding joint separation [6,7].

3.4 Principal axes and moments of inertia

Moment of inertia along the x-axis was calculated as follows:

$$I_{xx} \approx \sum_{i=1}^{N_L} (y_i^2 + z_i^2)\Delta m_L + \sum_{i=1}^{N_H} (y_i^2 + z_i^2)\Delta m_H \quad (1)$$

The other two moments along the y and z axis (I_{yy} and I_{zz}) were similarly calculated. The x and y –axis cross term inertia was calculated as:

$$I_{xy} \approx -\sum_{i=1}^{N_L} x_i y_i \Delta m_L - \sum_{i=1}^{N_H} x_i y_i \Delta m_H \qquad (2)$$

The other cross terms (I_{xz} and I_{yz}) were similarly calculated. Here, m_L and m_H represent the lower density mass of the fluid space (i.e., blood vessels) and higher density mass of bone respectively. Once the 3×3 moment of inertia matrix that includes the diagonal terms (I_{xx},I_{yy}, and I_{zz}) and the cross terms is calculated, it is pivoted to obtain an orientation of coordinate system relative to a given rigid body such that all cross terms of inertia (Eq. 2) are zero. This results in a diagonal matrix. The principal directions and corresponding three principal moments of inertia are calculated using eigenvalue decomposition.

The 3D reconstruction along with priniciple axes of rotation of each ossicle are shown in Figure 4 for all four species. The moment of inertia for each bone that has a minimum is shown by blue lines while the maximum moment is shown by red lines. The axis in between is indicated by green lines. The calculated principal moments of inertia (Table 1) can be compared to those reported by Weistenhöfer and Hudde for human [8]. For the malleus the moments of inertia are within 13%. For the incus they are within 21%. On the other hand differences between our calculations for stapes are different by 20%. For comparison of the other species we studied, inertial moments are not available.

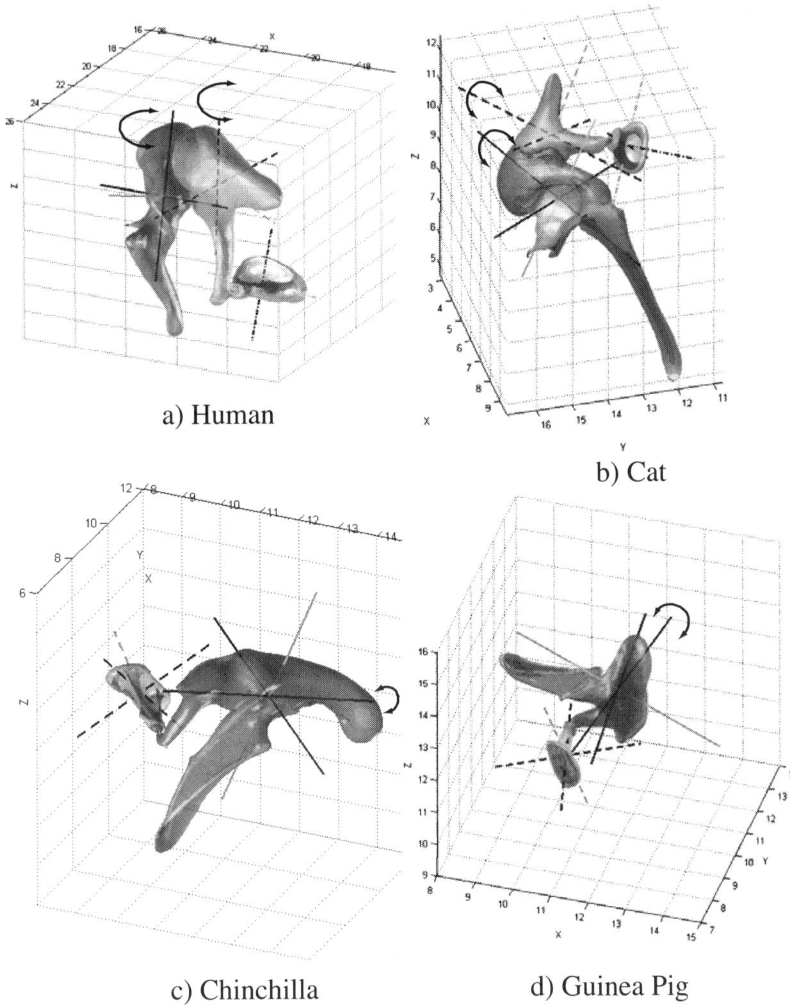

Fig. 4 Middle ear bones of four species (human, cat, chinchilla and guinea pig) and their principal axes of rotation (see Table 1). The circular arrows point to the axis with the minimum moment of inertia (MI). The minimum MI is approximately around the superior-inferior axis for human (a) and cat (b), both with mobile incudo-malleal joint. For chinchilla (c) and guinea pig (d) the mallues-incus joint is fused and the minimum MI axis is through the fused joint.

Figure 4 shows that the minimum moment of inertia (MI) is along the long axis (circular arrows) of the malleus and incus for both human and cat. However, for guinea pig and chinchilla the minimum moment of inertia is through the fused malleus incus heads. The minimum moment of inertia for the human and cat malleus are a factor 5–6 smaller than the maximum moment of inertia (Table 1).

Table 1 Comparison of moments of inertia (mm⁵), normalized by density ρ, across the four species.

		Human	Cat	Chinchilla	Guinea Pig
I_{MIN}/ρ	Malleus	5.33	2.23	4.30 [fused]	1.22 [fused]
	Incus	14.65	0.62		
	Stapes	0.95	0.05	0.07	0.03
I_{MID}/ρ	Malleus	31.38	11.45	13.81 [fused]	2.00 [fused]
	Incus	22.31	0.73		
	Stapes	1.77	0.11	0.12	0.04
I_{MAX}/ρ	Malleus	33.37	12.40	17.21 [fused]	2.84 [fused]
	Incus	32.47	1.02		
	Stapes	2.48	0.14	0.16	0.07

We can deduce the high frequency behavior of ossicle motion if we assume that all ligaments and tendons are passive springs. For deducing the high frequency behavior, we need two statements in mechanics. 1) In spring-mass system, high frequency motion is mass dominated, if we neglet damping which is justified. In this case, since the model is 3-D model, inertia in 3D space, instead of mass, is dominant. 2) If there is no energy supply, any physical phenomenon goes to the minimum energy state. From 1), we can say that the inertia of malleus and incus have a more dominant role than ligaments and tendons. Thus, we can neglect the angle and attachement of ligaments and tendon at high frequencies. From 2), we can say that if the TM attachement to the malleus does not constrain the whole vibration of malleus, then malleus rotates around the minimum principal axis whose direction is rotation about the superior-inferior axis for the case of the mobile incus-malleus joint.

3.5 Suspensory ligaments and tendon

When modelling 3-D ossicles, the shape and the attached positions of ligaments and tendon in middle ear cavitiy are important, particularly at low frequencies. After 3D reconstruction from the images, we obtain the shape and attached position on ossicles. The shapes of malleus ligaments and tendon are represented as tapered cylinders while the posterior ligament of the incus is represented as a polygon (see Sim and Puria, this volume). By comparing model calculations using microCT with experimental data, we can estimate the mechanical properties of the ligaments and tendon.

3.6 Human malleus-incus joint thickness map

Human malleus-incus joint thickness varies from 0.075mm to 0.275mm and it has a saddle shape. From the geometry information of malleus-incus joint, we can add the joint effect on the motion of ossicles. However, there are some difficulties in modeling this joint with a one-directional spring.

One of them is that we can not decide the attached position if we assume this joint as a spring because the joint has wide attachment area to both malleus and incus compared to its thickness. Since we have also observed sticky fluid inside of the joint (unpublished), we have started to work on a mathematical model using lubrication theory. This mathematical model can be compared with the experimental data. Then, we expect the elucidation of the role of the joint.

4. Discussion

Many of the middle ear structures, including the tympanic membrane cone shape and thickness, ossicles, and suspensory soft tissue (not shown), can be visualized because there is often good density contrast between these structures and air in the ear canal and middle ear cavity. Because they provide the best resolution, histological methods remain the standard. However, microCT imaging offers some distinct advantages [3]. These include: (1) elimination of stretching distortions commonly found in histological preparations, (2) use of a non-destructive method, (3) shorter preparation time (hours rather than 12–16 months), and (4) results already in digital format. After scanning, the ossicles and soft tissue attachments were segmented and their 3D volume reconstructed.

The malleus handle structure is linked to its function. At low frequencies, the suspensory ligaments and tendon attachments determine ossicle dynamics which is similar to the classical mode where rotation is hinged through the malles-incus center of gravity (orthogonal to the minimum MI in Figs. 4 a and b). At high frequencies the dynamics are determined by moments of inertia. The minimum moment of inertia is through the long axis of the fused malleus and incus in both guinea pig and chinchilla (Fig. 4 c and d). Thus the hinged motion is maintained even at high frequencies. The I-beam like shape is consistent with motion in one dimension.

However, in both human and cat the minimum moment of inertia is rotational vibration along the long axis of the malleus. We hypothesize that the reason why the malleus has a cylindrically shaped manubrium (Fig. 3), which is strong against torsion and why the joint is mobile (human and cat), is that it provides a mechanism to transfer energy to the incus with minimum inertia which is important for high frequency sound transmission to the inner ear. Possible asymmetrical anatomy (Fig. 2) and material properties [1, 2] of the eardrum can result in asymetrical motions at high frequencies which in turn can lead to rotational motion of the manubrium. It is our hypothesis that the asymetrical motions leading to torsion of the malleus require in-plane propogation of the eardrum. This is one reason why the wave speed on the eardrum is slow in comparison to air and why there is delay on the eardrum [2, 9, 10].

Acknowledgments

Work supported by grant No. DC 05960 from the NIDCD of NIH. We thank Chris Jacobs (Ph.D.) for use of the micro-CT scanner and Derek Lindsey for technical support.

References

1. Fay J. P., Puria S., and Steele C. R., The discordant eardrum. *Proc Natl Acad Sci USA*, 2006. 103(52): pp. 19743–19748
2. Fay J. P., Puria S., and Steele C. R., Three approaches for estimating the elastic modulus of the tympanic membrane. *J Biomech*, 2005. 38(9): pp. 1807–1815
3. Decraemer W. F., Dirckx J. J., and Funnell W. R., Three-dimensional modelling of the middle-ear ossicular chain using a commercial high-resolution X-ray CT scanner. *J Assoc Res Otolaryngol*, 2003. 4(2): pp. 250–263
4. Kuypers L. C. *et al.*, Thickness Distribution of Fresh Eardrums of Cat Obtained with Confocal Microscopy. *J Assoc Res Otolaryngol*, 2005: pp. 1–11
5. Funnell W. R., Decraemer W. F., and Khanna S. M., On the damped frequency response of a finite-element model of the cat eardrum. *J Acoust Soc Am*, 1987. 81(6): pp. 185–189
6. Amin S. and Tucker A. S., Joint formation in the middle ear: lessons from the mouse and guinea pig. *Dev Dyn*, 2006. 235(5): pp. 1326–1333
7. Vrttakos P. A., Dear S., and Sanders J. C., Middle ear structure in the chinchilla: a quantitative study. *J Otolaryngol*, 1988. 9: pp. 58–67
8. Weistenhöfer C. and Hudde H., Determination of the shape and inertia properties of the human auditory ossicles. *Audiol Neurootol*, 1999. 4(3–4): pp. 192–196
9. Puria S. and Allen J. B., Measurements and model of the cat middle ear: evidence of tympanic membrane acoustic delay. *J Acoust Soc Am*, 1998. 104(6): pp. 3463–3481
10. Olson E.S., Observing middle and inner ear mechanics with novel intracochlear pressure sensors. *J Acoust Soc Am*, 1998. 103: pp. 3445–3463

INVESTIGATION OF BONE CONDUCTION THRESHOLDS IN OTOSCLEROSIS

Andreas Arnold[1,2]**, Tamer Fawzy**[2]**, Frank Böhnke**[2]
[1] Dept. of Otorhinolaryngology, Inselspital, Universität Bern, 3010 Bern, Switzerland, Email: andreas.arnold@insel.ch
[2] Dept. of Otorhinolaryngology, Klinikum rechts der Isar, Technische Universität München, Ismaninger Straße 22, 81675 München, Germany

Keywords: otosclerosis, bone conduction, Carhart notch, finite element model, basilar membrane displacement

Introduction: Comparing bone conduction thresholds before and after stapes surgery in most cases reveals a reduction of preoperative bone conduction loss not only around 2 kHz (Carhart notch) but in the entire audio range. Postoperatively, a maximum threshold rise in the low and middle frequencies (500–3000 Hz) is seen.

The present study was devised to determine if there is an increase in bone conduction after removal of a fixed stapes footplate without a prosthesis in place.

Methods: Stapedectomy under local anaesthesia was performed in 24 patients with otosclerotic stapes fixation. We compared the bone conduction of preoperative audiograms with intra-operative thresholds measured directly after removing the footplate using a bone conduction transducer at test frequencies of 0.5, 1, 2 and 4 kHz.

Results: Our data showed a clear improvement at 0.5, 1 and 2 kHz, but not at 4 kHz. Threshold rise is best at 2000 Hz, corresponding to the Carhart notch. Pure-tone averages (PTA) were calculated from the collected data and statistically analyzed. The improvement was significant for PTA from 0.5 to 2 kHz. No significant improvement was found for PTA from 0.5 to 4 kHz.

To investigate the underlying cochlear mechanisms, a finite element model of the cochlea was used. It suggests an increased amplitude of the basilar membrane displacement with an open oval window due to a lower impedance compared to the situation with a fixed footplate.

Discussion: These results provide evidence that optimal basilar membrane movement depends on the integrity of the cochlear windows. In a cochlea with a totally fixed stapes, there is mechanically "captured energy" which cannot properly act on the basilar membrane during bone conduction stimulation. This is the first investigation in which audiometry was performed with an opened oval window during stapedectomy.
Conclusion: After total removal of the fixed stapes footplate, bone conduction thresholds improve immediately, corresponding to an increase of basilar membrane displacement.

1. Introduction

The comparison of pure-tone bone conduction thresholds before and after stapes surgery reveals in most cases a significant improvement over the preoperative bone conduction loss in addition to the expected closure of the air-bone gap. This reduction of preoperative bone conduction loss not only occurs in the range around 2000 cycles per second, known as the Carhart notch [1], but in the entire audio range with a maximum postoperative threshold rise in the low and middle frequencies (500–3000Hz). (Fig. 1)

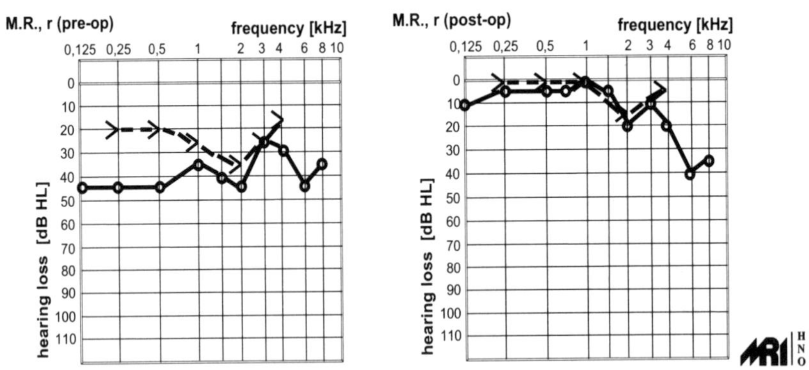

Fig. 1 Pre- and postoperative pure tone audiogram with maximum postoperative bone conduction threshold rise in low and middle frequencies (500–3000Hz).

The aim of this study was to determine if there is an increase in bone conduction after removal of a fixed stapes footplate without a prosthesis in place.

2. Patients and Methods

2.1 Clinical study

Stapedectomy under local anaesthesia was performed on 24 patients (14 female, 10 male, age 25–74) with stapes fixation due to otosclerosis. All patients underwent the regular preoperative audiological assessment with a pure-tone audiogram and speech tests using Aurical Audiometers (Madsen/GN Otometrics) calibrated to EN ISO 389 in a soundproof chamber. Intra-operative thresholds were measured directly after removing the footplate using a bone conduction transducer JKG 96 (CB-Elmec), certified for audiological measurements (Physikalische Technische Bundesanstalt) at test frequencies of 0.5, 1, 2 and 4 kHz. In order to avoid a bias, the first 10 patients were measured with both systems preoperatively. No difference between the results was found. Masking of the contralateral ear during intra-operative testing showed no difference compared to the results without masking on the same subject.

Finally, we compared the bone conduction of preoperative audiograms with intra-operative thresholds and did statistical analyses (Friedman test). The patients gave their written consent for the intra-operative measurement.

2.2 Finite element (FE) model

Using a FE model of the human cochlea, previously set up in ANSYS finite element software [2], the amplitude of the basilar membrane displacement was computed. In our model, the stimulation was done via bone conduction. A pressure signal with different frequencies (500–4000Hz) and constant sound pressure amplitude of 1 Pa equivalent to 94 dB (SPL) was applied to the total outer cochlear wall. The round window was presumed to be normal with mobile membrane structures. Basilar membrane displacement was calculated in a cochlea with a totally fixed stapes, in a cochlea with a piston hole in the stapes footplate (stapedotomy) and in a cochlea with a totally removed stapes (stapedectomy).

3. Results

Comparing the pre-operative and intra-operative averaged frequency values from all 24 patients, the rise in bone conduction thresholds at 500–2000 Hz is evident. This is not the case at 4 kHz. Corresponding to the Carhart notch, threshold rise is best at 2000Hz (Fig. 2). Pure-tone averages (PTA) were calculated from the collected data and statistically analyzed. The intra-operative improvement was significant for PTA from 0.5 to 2 kHz. (Fig. 3) No significance was found for PTA from 0.5 to 4 kHz. (Fig. 4)

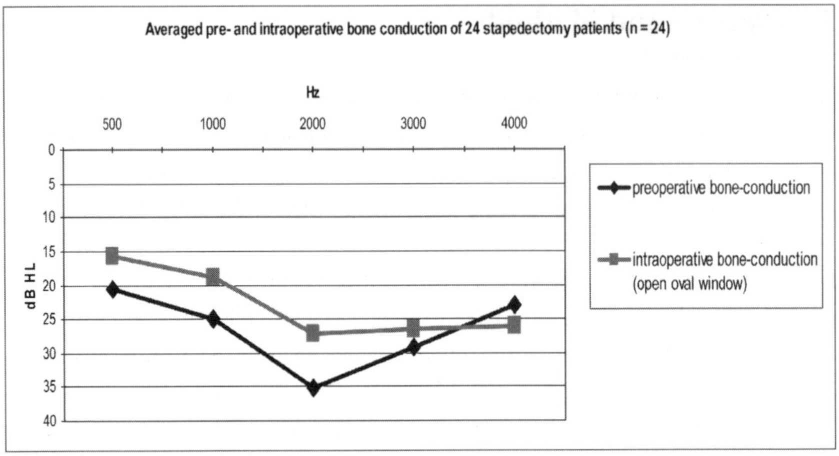

Fig. 2 Averaged frequency values from all 24 patients: the rise of intra-operative bone conduction thresholds at 500–2000 Hz is evident.

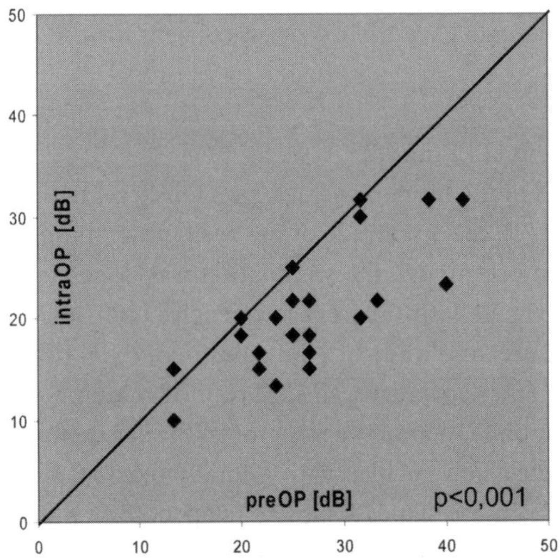

Fig. 3 Change of bone conduction pure-tone averages (PTA) for every patient (=dot) after removal of the fixed stapes footplate: For PTA from 500 to 2000 Hz, a clear intra-operative improvement is visible and found statistically significant.

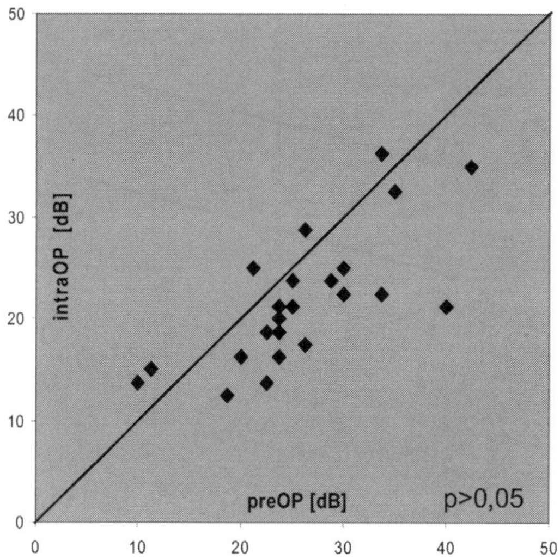

Fig. 4 Change of bone conduction pure-tone averages (PTA) for every patient (=dot) after removal of the fixed stapes footplate: For PTA from 500 to 4000 Hz, the overall tendency for intra-operative improvement is also visible but without statistical significance.

The investigation of the underlying cochlear mechanisms with the finite element model of the human cochlea computed an increased amplitude of the basilar membrane (BM) movement with an open oval window due to a lower impedance, compared to the situation with a fixed footplate. In the otosclerotic case with totally fixed footplate the BM displacement is about 0,141 nm for relevant frequencies between 1–4 kHz. In contrast to this the opened oval window (footplate removed) shows an increase of BM displacement by up to 0,523 nm. The increase of BM displacement is largest for the frequencies between 1–4 kHz.

The total removal of the stapes footplate produced a slightly greater effect than a piston hole. (Fig. 5)

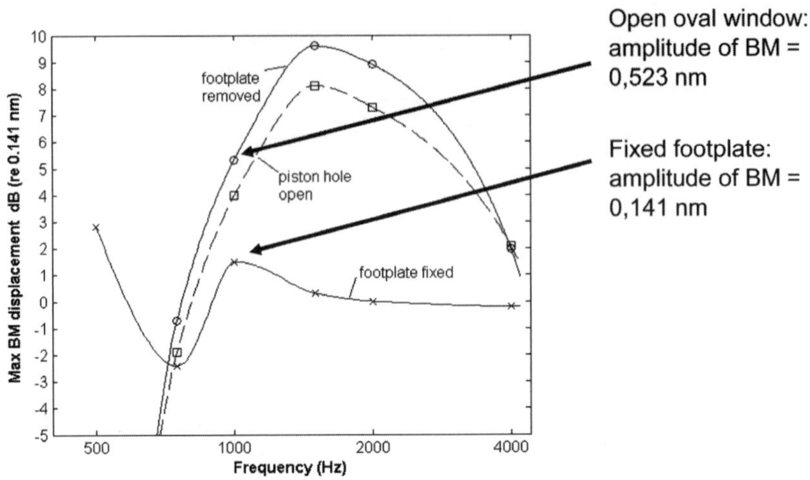

Fig. 5 FE-model of the human cochlea: the increase of basilar membrane (BM) displacement after removal of the fixed stapes footplate is nearly 5-fold at 1000 Hz and is largest for the frequencies between 1–4 kHz.

4. Discussion

These results show that bone conduction thresholds increase immediately after removal of the fixed stapes footplate. This sudden rise in bone conduction threshold must have a mechanical cause (e.g. Carhart`s cochlear reserve) [1]. It is not of sensorineural origin. A fixed footplate leads to a dissipation of parts of the energy applied to the cochlear fluid system by bone conduction stimulation, even with a mobile round window membrane. This gives evidence that optimal basilar membrane movement depends on the integrity of the cochlear windows. In other words, in a cochlea with totally fixed stapes there is "captured energy" which cannot properly act on the basilar membrane during bone conduction stimulation. By removing the fixed footplate, additional energy becomes available for basilar membrane displacement, corresponding to a better bone conduction threshold. Physically, a cochlea with an opened oval window has a lower impedance.

The averaged intra-operative bone conduction frequency values improve up to 2000 Hz. The value at 4000 Hz shows an opposite trend. This may be caused by the known variability of bone conduction audiometry at higher frequencies [3]. For the same reason the values of PTA from 500 to 4000 kHz do not improve in a statistically significant manner.

This is the first investigation in which audiometry was performed with an opened oval window during stapedectomy. It directly explains the mechanical cause of parts of the depression of bone conduction in otosclerosis as already suspected by Carhart.

5. Conclusion

After total removal of the fixed stapes footplate, bone conduction thresholds improve immediately, corresponding to an increase of basilar membrane displacement.

References

1. Carhart R., Assessment of sensorineural response in otosclerotics. Arch Otolaryngol. 1960 Feb; 71: 141–149
2. Böhnke F., Arnold W., Bone conduction in a three-dimensional model of the cochlea. ORL J Otorhinolaryngol Relat Spec. 2006; 68(6): 393–396
3. Laukli E., Fjermedal O., Reproducibility of hearing threshold measurements. Supplementary data on bone-conduction and speech audiometry. Scand Audiol. 1990; 19(3): 187–190

TRANSCRANIAL TRANSMISSION OF BONE CONDUCTED SOUND MEASURED ACOUSTICALLY AND PSYCHOACOUSTICALLY

Sabine Reinfeldt, Dept. of Signals & Systems, Div. of Biomedical Engineering, Chalmers University of Technology, SE-412 96 Göteborg, Sweden
Email: sabine.reinfeldt@chalmers.se
Stefan Stenfelt, Dept. of Neuroscience and Locomotion, Div. of Audiology, Linköping University, SE-581 85 Linköping, Sweden, Email: stefan.stenfelt@inr.liu.se
Bo Håkansson, Dept. of Signals & Systems, Div. of Biomedical Engineering, Chalmers University of Technology, SE-412 96 Göteborg, Sweden
Email: boh@chalmers.se

The transcranial transmission is important in bone conduction (BC) audiometry and for fitting BC hearing aids. In BC audiometry, the BC hearing threshold depends on the stimulation position, and the transcranial transmission determines the relative amount of the sound that reaches the contralateral cochlea when fitting BC hearing aids. Previously reported transcranial transmission results seem to depend on the method used. Here, a comparison between the transcranial transmission, measured with BC hearing thresholds and ear canal sound pressure (ECSP), is performed for both open and occluded ear canals. The transcranial transmission was similar for BC hearing thresholds and ECSP above 800 Hz; this indicates that the ECSP can be used to estimate changes of the BC hearing perception produced by alterations of the stimulation. The transcranial transmission results are also similar to vibration measurements of the cochleae made in earlier studies. Hence, vibration measurements of the cochleae can also estimate relative BC hearing.

1. Introduction

The transcranial transmission is normally defined as the bone conduction (BC) transmission to the contralateral cochlea compared with the ipsilateral one. This difference between the cochleae is important when testing BC thresholds clinically; the transcranial transmission determines the amount of masking necessary to isolate the ear of interest. Also, it is important for BC hearing aids, e.g. it provides an estimate for the effectiveness of using BC hearing aids for unilaterally deaf persons. So far, the transcranial transmission (sometimes referred to as transcranial attenuation) has been estimated by BC hearing thresholds or skull bone vibration measurements [1,2]. The most extensive investigation of BC hearing thresholds reported a nearly frequency independent average transcranial transmission of around –10 dB [2]. The aim of this study is to estimate the transcranial transmission. We also investigated whether the transcranial transmission can be estimated from ear canal sound pressure (ECSP) measurements.

2. Method

20 normal hearing persons between 23 and 43 years old participated in the study. A BC transducer was used to stimulate at three positions of the skull bone, one at a time. The stimulation positions were at the center of the forehead and at the mastoid portion of both temporal bones. The BC hearing threshold of the test ear was obtained using a pulsed Békésy procedure, while the other ear was masked with pink noise 10 to 20 dB above the individuals' hearing thresholds. The ECSP was measured with a probe microphone close to the eardrum. All measurements were conducted with open and occluded ear canals. The ear was occluded by a foam earplug.

The transcranial transmission was calculated as the BC hearing threshold or ECSP for contralateral stimulation relative to the same measure with ipsilateral stimulation (Fig. 1a). The transmission from the forehead was calculated as the BC hearing threshold or ECSP for stimulation at the forehead relative to the same measure with ipsilateral stimulation (Fig. 1b). Also obtained was the occlusion effect that was calculated for the three stimulation positions as the relation between BC hearing thresholds or ECSP with an occluded and open ear canal.

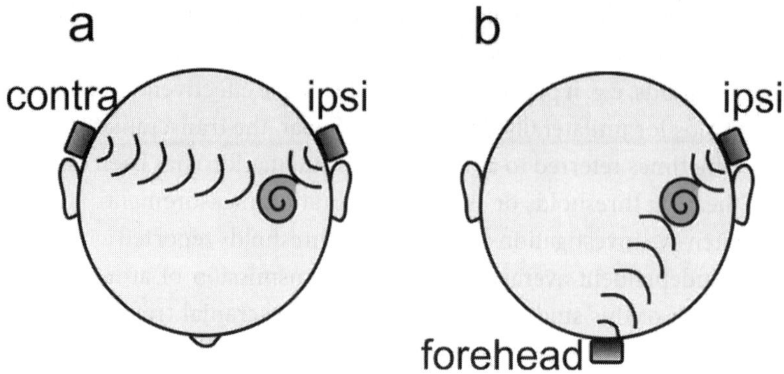

Fig. 1 Definitions for (a) the transcranial transmission and (b) the transmission from the forehead.

3. Results

The transcranial transmission results for the ECSP and BC hearing thresholds, both with open and occluded ear canal, are shown in Fig. 2. At low frequencies, there are some differences in the results between open and occluded ear canal. But above 800 Hz, the results from the BC hearing threshold and ECSP measurements are similar. The standard deviations are almost frequency independent with somewhat higher values for the ECSP measurements with open ear canal.

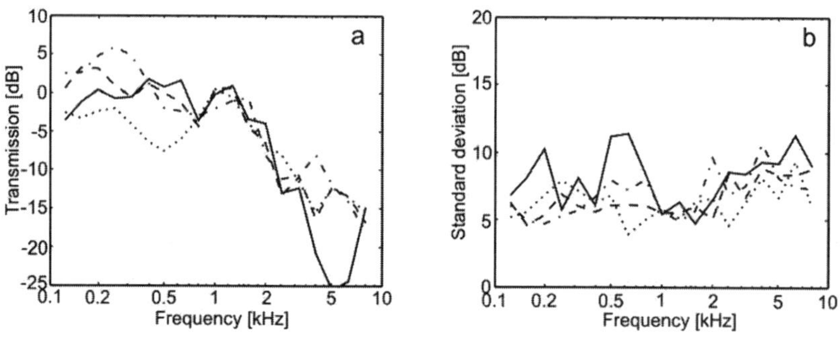

Fig. 2 The transcranial transmission results; (a) is the median results and (b) is the standard deviations. The ECSP measurement results are the solid and dashed lines from open and occluded ear canal, respectively. The BC hearing threshold results are the dotted and dash-dotted lines from open and occluded ear canal, respectively.

The results for the transmission from the forehead are shown in Fig. 3 for all methods. As for the transcranial transmission, open and closed ear canal produced different transmission at low frequencies, but at higher frequencies, the results from the four methods gave similar results. As for the transcranial transmission, the standard deviations are close to frequency independent.

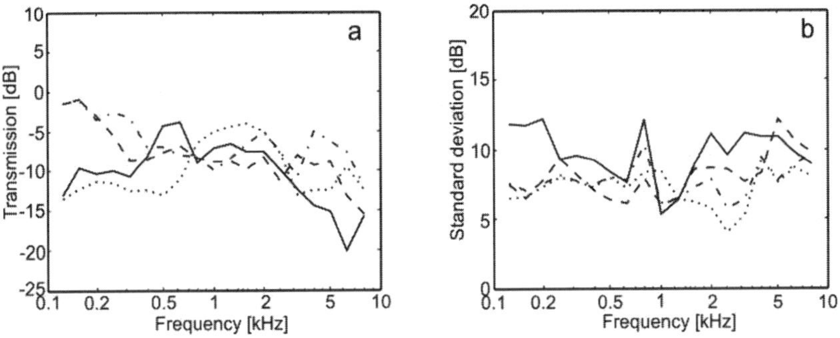

Fig. 3 The results for the transmission from the forehead; (a) is the median results and (b) is the standard deviations. The ECSP measurement results are the solid and dashed lines from open and occluded ear canal, respectively. The BC hearing threshold results are the dotted and dash-dotted lines from open and occluded ear canal, respectively.

The occlusion effects from the different stimulation positions are given in Fig. 4, both for ECSP measurements (a) and for BC hearing thresholds (b). The low-frequency occlusion effects from the ECSP measurements were greater than from the threshold measurements because other BC pathways contribute to the BC perception. Ipsilateral stimulation resulted in a lower threshold occlusion effect. The standard deviations, shown with thin lines, are essentially frequency independent.

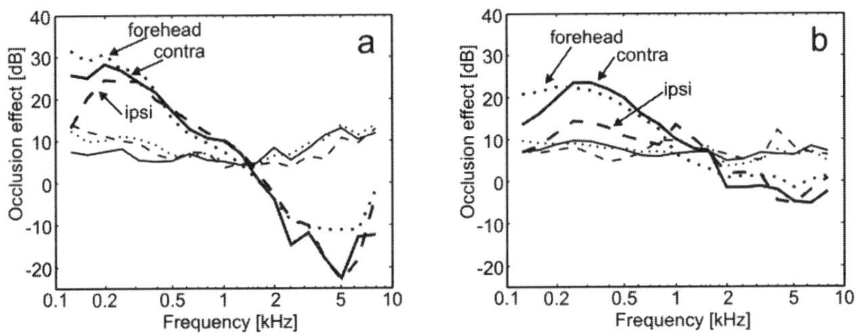

Fig. 4 The results for the occlusion effect measured with (a) ECSP and (b) BC hearing thresholds. The thin lines are the standard deviations for the different positions.

4. Discussions and Conclusions

The transcranial transmission was found frequency dependent. When measured with an occluded ear canal, the contralateral ear shows 5 dB greater excitation than the ipsilateral (positive transcranial transmission) at low frequencies. The transcranial transmission decreases with frequency and is about –15 dB at 8 kHz (attenuation = 15 dB). The transcranial transmission is similar whether obtained by hearing thresholds or by ECSP. This means that the ECSP can be used to estimate relative BC hearing. When the results are compared with the BC vibration study by Stenfelt and Goode [1] (Fig. 5), who measured the three-dimensional vibrations of both cochleae while stimulating at several positions of the skull bone, similar results are seen when the stimulation position is similar as here. This indicates that vibrations of the cochlea can provide a good measure of the relative BC hearing, at least for the difference in BC hearing between two stimulation positions. Nolan and Lyon [2] used BC hearing thresholds to estimate the transcranial transmission, but their results are lower and frequency independent (Fig. 5).

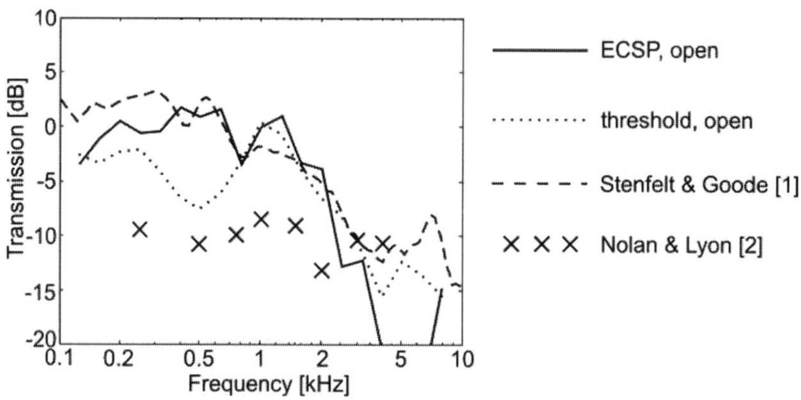

Fig. 5 Comparison of the transcranial transmission with results from earlier studies, [1] and [2].

There is no clear explanation for the differences at low frequencies between open and occluded ear canals. One obvious explanation is that the BC transmission routes to the cochlea depend on the stimulation position causing the relative difference. However, a similar phenomenon was discovered in loudness measurements where Keidser et al. [3] present a comparison between different loudness studies with open and occluded ear canals; the problem is discussed but the source for the discrepancies is not found. The lower occlusion effect with ipsilateral stimulation is also related to the differences for open and occluded ear canals at low frequencies.

References

1. Stenfelt and Goode, Transmission properties of bone conducted sound: Measurements in cadaver heads, *J. Acoust. Soc. Am.* **118** (2005) pp. 2373–2391
2. Nolan and Lyon, Transcranial attenuation in bone conduction audiometry, *J. Laryngol. Otol.* **95** (1981) pp. 597–608
3. Keidser, Katsch, Dillon, and Grant, Relative loudness perception of low and high frequency sounds in the open and occluded ear, *J. Acoust. Soc. Am.* **107** (2000) pp. 3351–3357

HIGH-RESOLUTION 3-D IMAGING OF MIDDLE EAR OSSICLES AND THEIR SOFT TISSUE STRUCTURES IN INTACT GERBIL TEMPORAL BONES, USING ORTHOGONAL FLUORESCENCE OPTICAL SECTIONING

J.A.N. Buytaert, J.J.J. Dirckx
Laboratory of Biomedical Physics, Department of Physics, University of Antwerp
Groenenborgerlaan 171, B 2020 Antwerp, Belgium, Email: Jan.Buytaert@ua.ac.be

Detailed models of middle ear morphology are an important input to improve realism of computer models of middle ear mechanics. Established imaging techniques all have their specific limitations. Orthogonal-plane fluorescence optical sectioning or OPFOS, is an important additional technique which, after adequate specimen preparation, produces high quality, perfectly aligned sectional images in nearly real-time of both bone and soft tissue simultaneously. The technique was introduced by A. Voie with a slicing resolution of 14μm. Using improved optical design and adding motorized scanning along a direction of the image plane, we were able to reduce slicing thickness to 2μm, thus creating a high-resolution OPFOS (HROPFOS) technique. Sections from HROPFOS data show histological detail, f.i. the hollow structure of the stapes head, cavities within the body of the ossicles, etc. From the section data, we reconstructed accurate 3-D models of the middle ear ossicles and its soft tissue structures, such as the stapedial muscle and artery which are nearly invisible with X-ray CT. By imaging bone as well as soft tissue, these models are an important input for finite-element modeling. Measurements were obtained in preparations of intact temporal bones of gerbils, as the technique allows region-of-interest scanning.

1. Introduction

To generate 3-D models of biomedical structures, several well established techniques are available. On the one hand, there is optical imaging of actual physical sections. On the other hand, there are tomographic techniques which deliver 3-D data on intact specimens.

Physical sectioning of an object, followed by imaging with light microscopy, delivers very high resolution (< 1μm) data, and can easily be combined with functional staining techniques. The preparation methods and especially the sectioning itself can introduce important shape artefacts and are extremely work intensive.

Tomography leaves the specimen intact: virtual sections are obtained which are auto-registered, and slicing can be repeated along several directions. Magnetic Resonance Imaging essentially detects differences in water content in a specimen. Imaging of structures with little water content, such as bone, is difficult. Resolutions down to 10μm can be obtained in biomedical specimens. Calculations are needed to obtain the image information and high-resolution measurements take long. X-ray Computer Tomography (CT) is based on contrast differences in X-ray absorption. μCT images mainly bone (resolution ±5μm) but has difficulty to visualize soft tissue. Back-projection calculations are necessary and region-of-interest (ROI) imaging can only be applied to some extent. Confocal Microscopy generates images of a specimen by focusing a laser beam to a small diffraction limited point (< 1μm) within the tissue, and detecting the fluorescent light which emerges from that same point. To obtain a complete image, point-by-point scanning is needed, resulting in long measurement times. Functional staining is possible, but the imaging depth is limited to ±100μm.

In 1993, Voie introduced the OPFOS-technique: Orthogonal-Plane Fluorescence Optical Sectioning microscopy [1]. In this paper, we will demonstrate a high-resolution OPFOS method (HROPFOS) with a strongly reduced slicing thickness, so that axial resolution is much more adapted to in-plane resolution.

2. Materials and Method

2.1 Conventional OPFOS

In conventional OPFOS [2,3], a plane of laser light is projected through a transparent and fluorescent specimen, and the light emitted from this plane within the object is observed in orthogonal direction. The spectacular advantage of the OPFOS technique is that virtual sections through the object of bone as well as soft tissue are generated in real-time.

In reality it is impossible to generate a plane of laser light: a small numerical aperture cylindrical lens focuses a broadened laser beam along 1 dimension to a hyperbolic light pattern (cross section in *Fig.1A*). In the vicinity X_R of the minimal focus d_1 created by this lens, the hyperbolic light pattern is approximated to a plane of constant thickness $d = \sqrt{2}\, d_1$, in which one records the virtual intersections orthogonally with a CCD-camera. Using a large numerical aperture lens, a finer focus d_2 can be obtained, but the imaging zone corresponding with the approximated plane becomes very small. Hence in conventional OPFOS a trade-off exists between image width and slice thickness d. In previous work [2], foci of $d_1 = 10\mu m$ (at the centre of an OPFOS-image) were obtained, causing the approximated thickness of the slicing plane at the edges of the image to drop to $d = 14\mu m$.

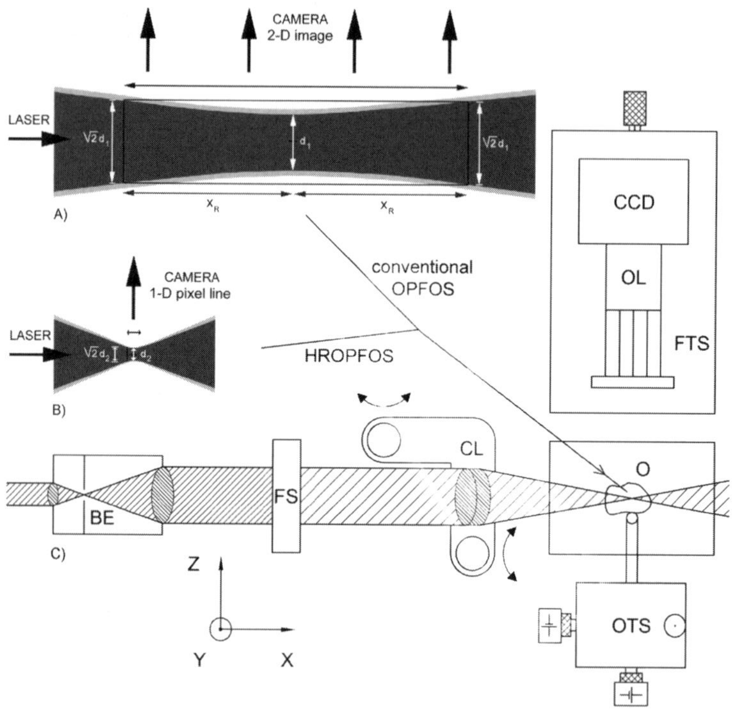

Fig. 1 A) Focusing profile of a small numerical aperture cylindrical lens (OPFOS). In the zone < $\sqrt{2}d_1$ (~plane) a 2-D image is taken. **B)** Focusing profile of a large numerical aperture cylindrical lens (HROPFOS). Images are built by scanning and recording 1-D pixel lines in the thin focus. **C)** Schematic drawing of the HROPFOS setup: laser light passes through a beam expander (BE) and a cylindrical achromat (CL) which focuses the laser along 1 dimension in the transparent and fluorescent object (O). A two-axis motorized object translation stage (OTS) scans the specimen along X and Z. A CCD on a focusing translation stage (FTS) with microscope objective lens (OL) and colour filter records a Y-pixel column.

2.2 Improved optical setup: HROPFOS

In HROPFOS we no longer record 2-D images, but we scan the object through a line of best focus, created by a large numerical aperture cylindrical lens causing a much smaller focus d_2 and corresponding tight imaging width (*Fig. 1B*). The CCD therefore only records 1 Y-pixel column of his imaging array in the focus d_2, and an entire image is built by line-scanning the specimen through the focus by means of a motorized translation stage along the X-axis (*Fig. 1C*). Next, the object is moved with a second motor to image a next section along Z. HROPFOS no longer causes the sectioning thickness to be a compromise with image width, and makes this thickness in theory only diffraction limited.

2.3 Specimen preparation

To apply (HR)OPFOS, the plane of laser light needs to pass through the object without scattering or refraction, and the object needs to emit fluorescent light. The technique of clearing biomedical specimens is well established and was proposed many years ago by Spalteholz [4]. In short, the gerbil temporal bone is first decalcified in a water solution of 10% EDTA (accelerated by exposing it to low power microwave radiation). After all calcium has been removed, the ear is gradually dehydrated and made completely transparent by putting it in Spalteholz fluid. Finally the ear is stained by submerging it in fluorescent dye. After this preparation procedure, the temporal bone and middle ear are completely transparent and fluorescent, which makes it compatible with OPFOS.

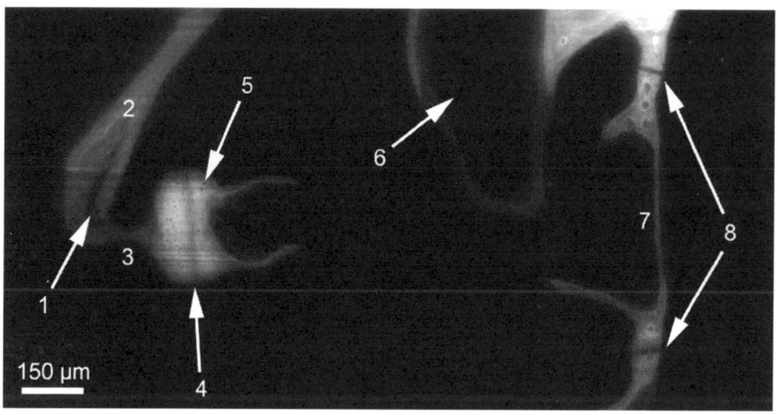

Fig. 2 HROPFOS-scan of 2500 × 1280 pixels (1.88 × 0.96 mm) through a right gerbil stapes showing histological detail: 1) channel within incus, 2) incus, 3) lenticular process, 4) articulation, 5) calcified cartilage in stapes head, 6) stapedial artery through the cruras, 7) stapes footplate, 8) footplate annular ligament. 1×1 µm in-plane and 2µm slicing resolution.

3. Results

We have improved the sectioning or axial resolution of OPFOS with a factor of 7. HROPFOS obtains a (constant) slicing resolution of 2μm over the entire image because of the improved optical design and line-scanning, while conventional OPFOS performs sectioning with a slicing thickness varying from 10μm in the center to 14μm at the edges of the image. Within the sectioning plane, the resolution is only limited by diffraction of the imaging lens. Because of the line-scanning principle in HROPFOS, there is no longer a limitation in image width, as the slicing thickness is maintained along a scan. Extended sections can now be made of a region-of-interest inside a bigger object. *Fig.2* demonstrates an example of a scan of 2500 columns with a height of 1280 pixels, showing histological detail of a right gerbil stapes still inside its temporal bone. *Fig.3* shows a right gerbil cochlea, in which we can even distinguish the Reissner's membrane.

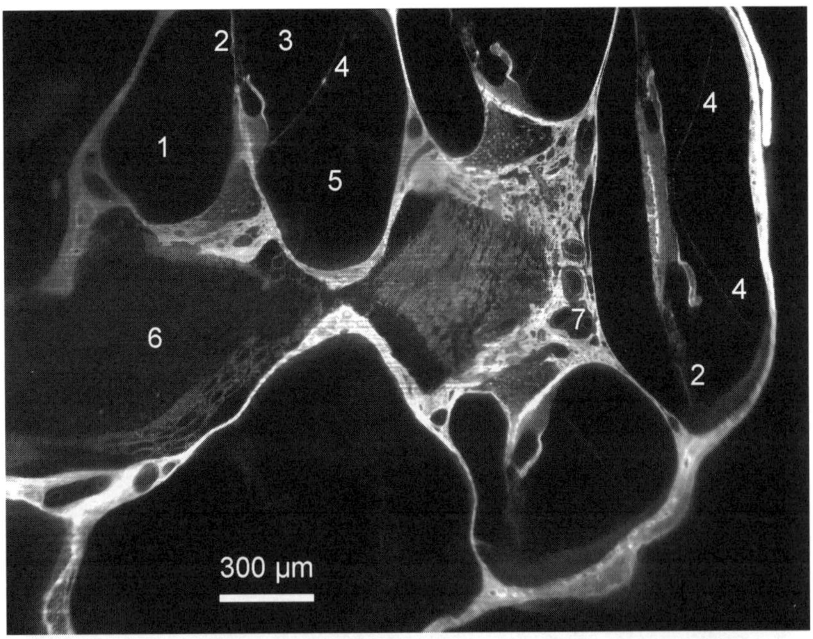

Fig. 3 HROPFOS-scan of 1700 × 1280 pixels (2.55 ×1.92 mm) of a right gerbil cochlea: scala tympani, 2) basilar membrane, 3) cochlear duct or scala media, 4) Reissner's membrane, 5) scala vestibuli, 6) modiolus nerve, 7) blood vessels. Lateral & axial resolution 2μm.

From a series of auto-aligned sectional images obtained with HROPFOS, we can produce accurate 3-D models, e.g. of the incudo-stapedial joint and the exact location and morphology of the stapedial muscle, tendon and artery (*Fig. 4*).

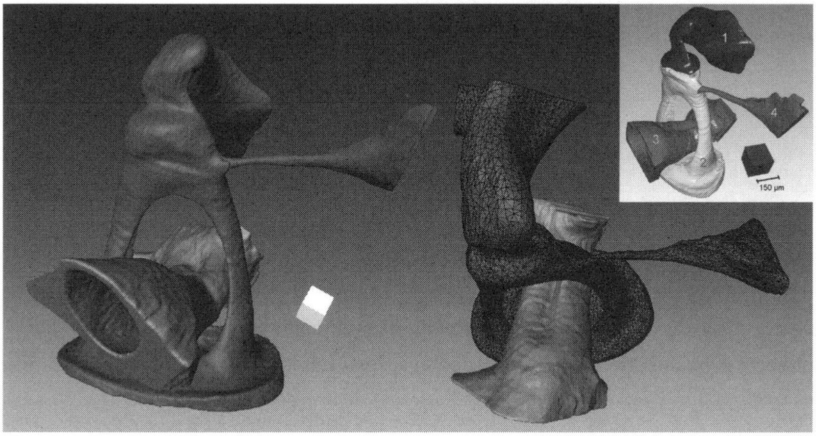

Fig. 4 3-D models from HROPFOS-data showing: lenticular process of the incus & stapes (purple), stapedial artery (orange), stapedial muscle (red) of a right gerbil middle ear. These models are obtained from raw data without smoothing. Voxel: 3 × 3 × 3 μm.

4. Conclusion

We have introduced a high-resolution optical technique, HROPFOS, which allows to generate images of virtual sections through biomedical specimens. We achieved image resolution < 2μm in slicing direction, and down to 1μm in the slicing plane. Slicing thickness is independent of object or image size, and high axial resolution is maintained over the entire image width. Specimens need to be cleared, refractive index matched and stained.

Despite conceptual simplicity, HROPFOS generates high-resolution images of bone as well as soft tissue in nearly real-time, without the need of calculations, and a region of interest can be imaged with high-resolution within a much larger specimen under a variety of orientations, all of which is impossible with μCT (*Fig. 5*). There also is no out-of-focus fluorescence, which is typical for light microscopy. Hence, our technique fills a gap not yet covered by existing imaging techniques. From HROPFOS-sections, full 3-D shape data are obtained, which are important input for finite-element modeling, as they not only give the shape of the ossicles, but also the exact morphology and position of soft tissue elements, such as arteries, muscles and tendon.

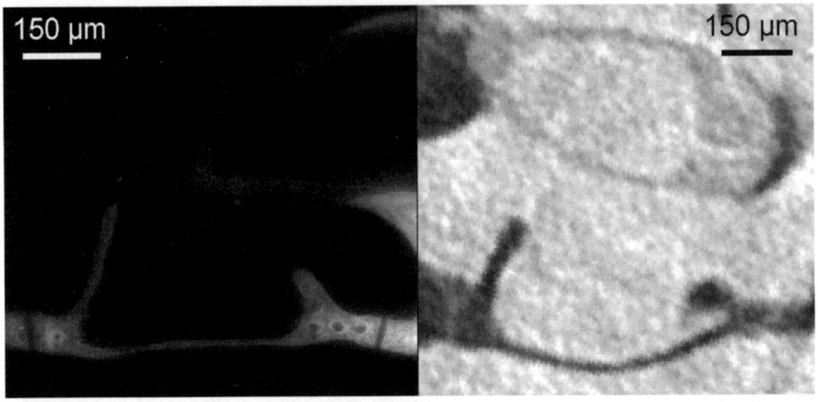

Fig 5 A) HROPFOS image of a gerbil stapes with clearly visible artery. Lateral resolution 1μm. Axial resolution 2μm. B) Image obtained with μCT-tomographic device (Skyscan 1072) of a gerbil stapes in a comparable orientation, after back-projection of an entire dataset recorded in several hours. Lateral resolution 8μm.

References

1. Voie A. H., Burns D. H., Spelman F. A., Orthogonal-plane fluorescence optical sectioning: three-dimensional imaging of macroscopic biological specimens. *J. Microsc.* **170** (1993) pp. 229–236
2. Voie A. H., Imaging the intact guinea pig tympanic bulla by orthogonal-plane fluorescence optical sectioning microscopy. *Hear. Res.* **171** (2002) pp. 119–128
3. Valk W. L., Wit H. P., Segenhout J. M., Dijk F., van der Want J. J. L., Albers F. W. J., Morphology of the endolymphatic sac in the guinea pig after an acute endolymphatic hydrops, *Hear. Res.* **202** (2005) pp. 180–187
4. Spalteholz W., *Über das Durchsichtigmachen von menschlichen und tierischen Präparaten und seine theoretischen Bedingungen*, S. Hirzel, Leipzig (1914)

HYPERELASTIC WARPING APPLIED TO X-RAY MICRO-CT IMAGES FOR THE STUDY OF HUMAN MIDDLE EAR CHAIN DEFORMATIONS UNDER STATIC PRESSURE LOAD

S.L. Gea[1], S.A Maas[2], W.F. Decraemer[1], H. Maier[3], J.J.J. Dirckx[1]
[1] University of Antwerp, Dept. Biomedical Physics
[2] University of Utah, Dept. Bioengineering
[3] HNO UNI-Klinik, Eppendorf Hamburg University
Email: Stefan.gea@ua.ac.be

In everyday life the human ear is subject not only to sound but also to slow, quasi-static pressure variations with amplitudes in the order of tenths of a mm. In the present study we investigated how the ossicular chain deforms and changes its 3-D configuration when acted upon by large static pressures. To determine with good precision the small deformations of the ossicular chain we use 'hyperelastic warping', a deformable image registration method. In this relatively new technique a 3-D finite element model, based on careful segmentation of a template dataset, is deformed until it aligns with a target dataset at a different pressure. 3-D displacement of the ossicles will be shown and expressed mathematically by plotting the displacement of a few landmark points as a function of pressure. We will also describe the 3-D changes in configuration and show how the slippage in the ossicle joints performs as a protecting mechanism of the middle ear.

1. Introduction

The middle ear provides a mechanism to protect the inner ear from excessive static pressures while at the same time it conserves the capability to process sound signals. Early research by Helmholtz already pointed out that the incudo-malleal (IM) joint merely behaves as a gliding joint when acted upon with static pressures, while an acoustic stimulus results in a functionally fixed joint [1]. Hüttenbrink was amongst the first who quantitatively described the movement of the ossicles at static pressures [2]. In his study, the umbo (MU) showed a pronounced movement in the medial-lateral direction while the lenticular process (LP) and stapes head (SH) described a predominant superior-inferior displacement. It became clear that the IM joint and incudo-stapedial (IS) joint play a major role in reducing the magnitude of the displacements from the malleus to the stapes footplate, hence protecting the fragile inner ear. However, despite the complex deformations of the middle ear ossicle chain, not much effort was further made to describe the movement of the ossicles three-dimensionally. Hüttenbrink used microscopic and radiographic techniques, which lead to one- and two-dimensional measurements. In the present study we investigated how the ossicular chain deforms and changes its configuration when acted upon by large static pressures. All our results are 3-dimensional and provide a precise insight in the position and displacements of the ossicles and their rotation axes. Moreover, the use of x-ray tomography allowed us to leave the complete middle ear cavity intact.

2. Methods

We present results of experiments performed on a fresh human temporal bone which was prelevated within 24h post-mortem. It was stored at a temperature of 5°C and measured within 48 hours post-mortem. A tympanogram, obtained directly after prelevation of the temporal bone, showed that the ear had a normal response. The pressure applied on the external ear canal stepped between –490daPa and +490daPa and scans of the entire temporal bone were recorded using an in-vivo x-ray micro-CT scanner (Skyscan 1076) with an isotropic voxel size of 35μm. The temporal bone was wrapped in parafilm during the entire experiment to prevent it from drying out.

Accurate 3-D models of the ossicles were created in Amira (Template Graphics Software, Inc.) with a region growing tool. The contours were determined in section images in one orientation and verified and corrected in perpendicular sections. A 3-D smoothing filter finally removed most of the remaining small imperfections.

To determine with good precision the small deformations of the ossicular chain we need a transformation which aligns the different models at each pressure step. This alignment can be done by methods such as the iterated closest point algorithm (ICP). However, ICP needs an accurate 3-D model of every ossicle at every pressure step to be segmented. First of all, this is a very time-consuming process. And second, because of a manual segmentation the models are always subject to personal interpretations of the section images. Thus, it is difficult to manage an objective segmentation. This could be done using a relatively new technique, hyperelastic warping (HEW) [3], which is a deformable image registration method. To find a transformation that aligns the features of two datasets, a 3-D tetrahedral finite element model at zero pressure (template) is being displaced and deformed (warped) until it aligns with a dataset at a different pressure (target). With this method only one model needs to be segmented from the dataset at zero pressure.

The kinematics of the ossicles are determined by comparing the complete nodal lists of the computer models at successive pressures. The deformation of the middle ear chain will be described quantitatively in two ways. (a) As deformation was found to be small we could assume rigid body behaviour and described the ossicle's motion between two successive pressure steps as a translation along and a rotation around an 'instantaneous screw axis' (ISA) [4]. (b) By means of displacements of some typical landmarks, the MU, the LP and the SH.

3. Results

3.1 Individual ossicle movements

To describe the direction of movement a reference frame was chosen similar to that used by Hüttenbrink, as shown in Figure 3. The movement of the SH and LP towards the oval window is represented by the parameter a, while b and c are the transversal components, lying in the intersecting plane of the IS joint.

Figure 1 shows the position and orientation of the ISA of the ossicles at each pressure step, while the angle of rotation α is given in Table 1. For the malleus the ISAs are roughly parallel to the axis between the *lig. mal. lat.* and the *corpus incudis*. Compared to positive pressures the ISAs at negative pressures have opposite orientation, as can be expected, and they are located closer to the lateral side of the malleus neck. Two axes (+300 and –490daPa) behave differently and are located much farther away from the other ISAs. However, the corresponding angles (0.06° and 0.34°) are relatively small, indicating that the malleus displacement is mainly translational. The umbo describes a predominantly inward-outward movement with maxima of 190µm (+490daPa) and –369µm (–490daPa).

The movement of the incus (Fig. 1b and e) is more complex as there is no predominant orientation of the rotational axis. The ISA at +50daPa has the largest rotation angle (0.42°) exceeding the other rotations greatly. The LP thus becomes almost motionless at pressures larger than +50daPa, as can be seen in Fig. 1b. Even at +490daPa the LP only moves over a total distance of 19μm compared to zero pressure, which is due to the small lever arm between the ISA and the LP. On the other hand, negative pressures exceed this value greatly, up to 122μm at –490daPa. But nevertheless, at every pressure the displacement is predominantly in-plane (*b* and *c*).

The SH is pulled outward (–*a* direction) to a maximal extend of 23μm at –490daPa while the in-plane component is significantly larger (78μm). The SH mainly describes a transversal motion, rather than a piston-like one. At positive pressure the IS gap is being reduced, while at negative pressures it is enlarged.

It is clear from Table 1 that there is a substantial reduction of movement between the manubrium and the stapes. The ratio between static displacement of the MU and the in-out component of the LP and SH is 23:1.2:1 at +490daPa and 16:2.6:1 at –490daPa.

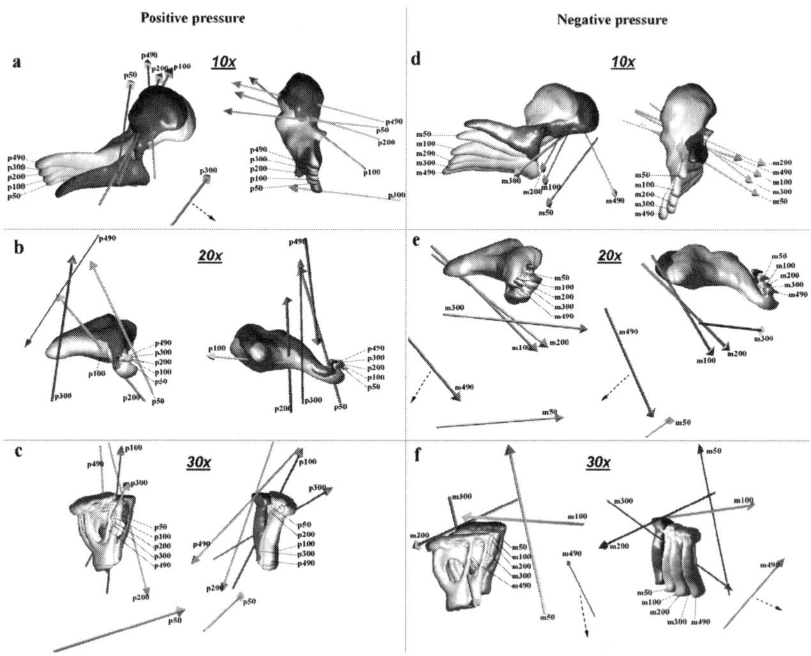

Fig. 1 The ISAs shown here represent the rotation of models between two successive pressure steps; the rotation angle α (°) can be found in Table 1. The ossicles at positive (left) and negative (right) pressure are displayed in two directions to get a better 3-D insight in the position of the ISAs. However, to clearly observe the motion, the displacements were enlarged 10x (Malleus), 20x (Incus) and 30x (Stapes). The dark model represents the reference model at zero pressure. Note that the tiny displacements of the stapes causes the ISAs to be very different with successive pressures, both in orientation and position.

Table 1 Displacement parameters (μm) of some landmarks (for axis orientation see Fig. 3); *a*: inward-outward movement, *b* and *c*: in-plane movement. The total transversal motion is given by $\rho = \sqrt{b^2 + c^2}$. The umbo shows a primarily unidirectional motion, given by *d*. The instantaneous rotation angles α (°), e.g. between +200daPa and +490daPa, around their respective ISA are given as well.

p	Umbo		Lenticular process					Stapes head					MI joint	SI joint
(daPa)	d	α	a	b	c	ρ	α	a	b	c	ρ	α	α	α
50	78	0.96	0	13	-8	15	0.42	-16	-8	-13	15	0.28	0.83	0.62
100	105	0.54	3	14	-7	16	0.08	-11	-4	-14	15	0.19	0.50	0.27
200	143	0.46	6	18	-6	19	0.09	-11	-8	-14	16	0.15	0.38	0.21
300	152	0.06	7	17	2	17	0.08	-8	-1	-4	4	0.47	0.08	0.48
490	190	0.40	10	16	-3	16	0.05	-8	-11	-13	17	0.27	0.37	0.27
-50	-109	0.89	-15	-6	-31	31	0.15	-14	-11	-22	25	0.37	0.67	0.38
-100	-219	1.11	-37	-20	-56	59	0.41	-20	-8	-39	40	0.14	0.68	0.48
-200	-280	0.64	-47	-25	-67	72	0.22	-22	-15	-47	49	0.18	0.43	0.38
-300	-317	0.46	-49	-19	-73	75	0.08	-19	-2	-50	50	0.35	0.39	0.35
-490	-369	0.34	-60	-42	-98	107	0.10	-23	-18	-76	78	0.10	0.26	0.17

3.2 Joint kinematics

The motions of the joints are the key concept in understanding the protecting properties of the middle ear chain. If the joints are functionally rigid e.g. due to ankylosis, the protection mechanism vanishes and the stapes is greatly pushed in and out of the oval window, as was demonstrated by Hüttenbrink.

In figure 2 we pointed out two bulges of the saddle-shaped articulation of the incus, and named them the *inferior* and the *superior bulge*. The figure shows the kinematics of the MI joint at successive pressure steps. We look at the 3-D models from the side of the ear canal, so the manubrium is pointed upward. The models were moved to the reference frame of the incus at zero pressure in order to visualize relative motions. It shows that the malleus glides over the surface of the incus, and rotates roughly around the superior bulge of the incus. From table 1 it can be seen that the largest

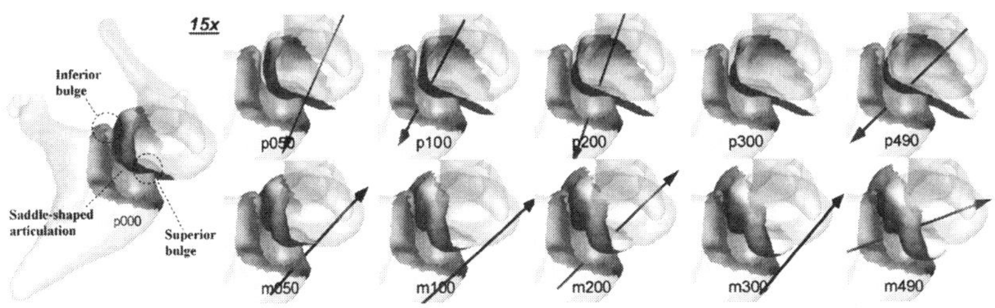

Fig. 2 The relative motion (enlarged 15×) of the saddle-shaped articulation at positive (top) and negative (bottom) pressures in the MI joint. The ISAs are shown for the malleus relative to the incus; but one can observe that the ISAs are orientated roughly through the superior bulge.

relative rotation occurs at pressures up to ±100daPa. The ISA at +300daPa is situated outside the upper-right corner of the image, however, its rotation angle is negligible (0.08°).

The IS joint shows a gliding motion as well. At positive pressures the ISA is roughly pointed to the right in the direction of *b*, hereby rotating the stapes head to an upward position (direction of +*c*), while at negative pressure the rotation is reversed (direction of −*c*). This rotational motion of the stapes can be found in figure 1c and 1f as well. These gliding motions of the MI and IS joints cause the above mentioned decoupling of ossicular movement, which is exactly the origin of the protecting properties of the ossicular chain.

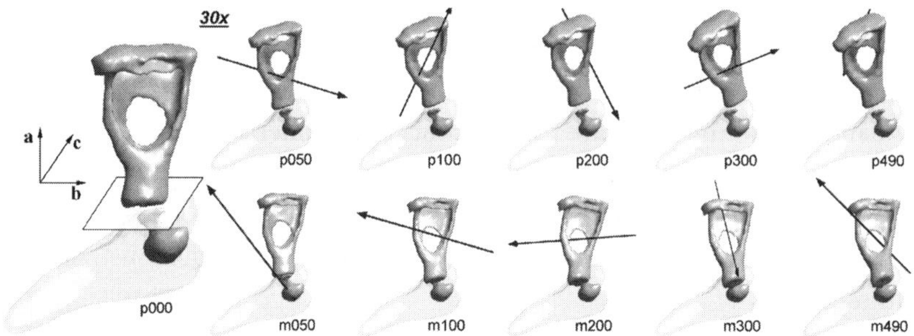

Fig. 3 The enlarged (30x) relative motion of the incus and stapes, as well as the ISAs are given at positive (top row) and negative (bottom row) pressure. The model at zero pressure (left) shows the orientation of the axes, *a* being the inward motion towards the cochlea and *b* and *c* the in-plane components. The apparent opening of the gap at positive pressures is misleading as it depends on the viewpoint and the 30 times enlargement of the movement.

References

1. Helmholtz H. The mechanics of the ossicles of the ear and tympani. *Pflügers archiv,* **1** (1886) pp. 1–60
2. Hüttenbrink K.B. The mechanics of the middle ear at static ear pressures. The role of the ossicular joints, the function of the middle ear muscles, and the behavior of stapedial prostheses. *Acta Oto-laryngologica,* **Suppl. 451** (1988) pp. 1–35
3. Bowden A.E., Rabbitt R.D., Weiss J.A. Warping template finite element models into alignment with subject specific image data. *Proc ASME Winter Annual Meeting,* BED-**39** (1998) pp. 289–290
4. Selvik G. Roentgen stereophotogrammetry. A method for the study of the kinematics of the skeletal system. *Acta Orthop. Scand. Suppl.* **232** (1989) pp. 1–51

REAL-TIME OPTO-ELECTRONIC HOLOGRAPHIC MEASUREMENTS OF SOUND-INDUCED TYMPANIC MEMBRANE DISPLACEMENTS

J.J. Rosowski[1,2], C. Furlong[3], M.E. Ravicz[1], M.T. Rodgers[3]
Email: John_Rosowski@meei.harvard.edu
[1] Eaton-Peabody Lab., Massachusetts Eye & Ear Infirmary, Boston MA USA
[2] S.H.B.T. Program, Harvard-M.I.T. Division of Health Sciences and Technology, Cambridge MA USA
[3] Worcester Polytechnic Institute, Worcester MA USA

Computer-aided Opto-Electronic Holography (OEH) was used to measure the sound-induced displacement of the tympanic membrane (TM) of cadaver cats and chinchillas. Real-time time-averaged holograms (gathered at video rates) were used to roughly determine the frequency dependence of TM displacements as tone frequency was swept from 0.4 to 20 kHz. Stroboscopic holography was used at selected frequencies to measure the difference in displacement between condensation and rarefaction phase of the pressure stimulus and enable discrimination of inward and outward displacements of the TM surface with nanometer resolution. The time-averaged holographic data demonstrate standing wave patterns on the cat's TM surface, which move from simple uni-modal or bi-modal patterns at low frequencies, through complicated multi-modal patterns above 3 kHz, to highly ordered arrangements of displacement waves with tone frequencies above 15 kHz. The frequency boundaries of the different wave patterns are lower in chinchilla (simple patterns below 0.6 kHz, ordered patterns above 4 kHz) than cat. The stroboscopic holography measurements indicate wave-like motion patterns on the TM surface, where the number of wavelengths captured along a transect of the TM increased with stimulus frequency with as many as 11 wavelengths visible on the chinchilla TM at 16 kHz. Counts of the visible number of wavelengths on TM transects with different sound stimulus frequency provided estimates of wave velocity along the TM surface that ranged from 5 m/s at frequencies below 8 kHz and increased to 25 m/s by 20 kHz.

1. Introduction

The tympanic membrane (TM) is the initial structure involved in the middle-ear's acousto-mechanical transformation of environmental sounds to sound pressure and velocity within the inner ear. While some basic facts are known about the mechanics of the healthy TM at low frequencies, there are many unresolved issues: e.g., the effect of TM shape and pathology on function, the effect of large differences in TM mechanical properties across species, the nature of TM function at higher frequencies, and the hypothesized presence of standing or traveling surface waves on the surface of the TM [1].

Many of these issues can be addressed by measuring the motion of the entire TM surface in response to sound. Most of the few extant measurements of TM motion were obtained with time-averaged laser holography using photographic plates [2]. Displacements were estimated by counting fringes in the interference pattern. New opto-electronic techniques [3,4] that take advantage of fast high-resolution digital cameras and advanced signal processing techniques can generate holographic images in real time at rates up to 500 frames/second.

In this study, we measured sound-induced motion of the TM surface in cat and chinchilla using two new opto-electronic techniques: Real-time time-averaged holography, which gives displacement amplitude and resolution data comparable to the earlier technique but is much faster; and stroboscopic holography, which rapidly determines the magnitude and phase of displacements over the entire TM surface with nanometer resolution [3,4]. We (1) demonstrate the utility of the new techniques; (2) validate them by comparing to other measurements; (3) present new data that suggest fundamental differences in the mechanics of the chinchilla and cat TM; and (4) show new evidence of standing waves in TM motion in cat and chinchilla.

2. Methods

2.1 Opto-electronic holography system (OEH)

Our OEH system [3] uses a frequency doubled Nd:YAG laser (wavelength $\lambda = 532$ nm) and is operated in two modes:

(1) Time-average mode, used for rapid identification (at video rates) of TM resonant frequencies and corresponding mode shapes. Displacement resolution ~130 nm (λ / 4).

(2) Stroboscopic mode, used for rapid quantification of the magnitude and phase of dynamic deformations of the TM surface. Displacement resolution ~1 nm (λ / 500).

2.2 Deformations and shape measurements with OEH

Images acquired by the digital camera of the OEH are processed by computer to provide quantitative measurements of deformations and shape of the samples of interest through determination of the fringe-locus function $\Omega(x,y)$. Processing is based on spatial intensity distributions In(x,y) defined at the imaging plane (x,y) and recorded by a high-resolution digital camera, i.e.,

$$I_n(x,y) = I_0(x,y) + I_r(x,y) + \sqrt{I_0(x,y)\, I_r(x,y)}\, \cos[\Delta\phi(x,y) + \theta_n + \Omega(x,y)], \quad (1)$$

where Io(x,y) and Ir(x,y) represent intensities of the (reflected) object beam and the reference beam, respectively, $\Delta\varphi$ (x,y) represents the optical phase difference between the two beams, and θn are n known phase steps introduced by varying the reference beam path length with a piezoelectric actuator.

In time-averaged mode, an image is acquired during a camera exposure of duration Δt to provide intensity distributions of the form

$$I(x,y) = \frac{1}{\Delta t} \int_t^{t+\Delta t} I_t(x,y,t)\, dt \quad (2)$$

In stroboscopic mode, quantitative measurements are obtained by determining $\Omega_i(x,y)$ in various states of deformation (e.g., over 2 or more instants or phase points within a period of a tonal stimulus). The difference,

$$\Delta\Omega(x,y) = \Omega_i(x,y) - \Omega_{i+1}(x,y) \quad (3)$$

provides a direct measurement of deformations between each pair of states or instants. This technique is similar to the speckle interferometry technique described by Wada et al. [4].

2.3 Animal preparation

The heads of a cat and two chinchillas used in other physiological experiments were harvested after euthanasia. The bilateral bullae were exposed and much of the bullar walls removed to expose the tympanic cavity. The cartilaginous ear canals were resected, and the bony external auditory canals were drilled away until at least 90% of the TM surface was visible. The TMs were painted with white ink. The head was oriented in the object beam of the OEH system with the surface of the TM perpendicular to the beam. The reflected object beam was focused in the interferometric head. A glass-backed sound coupler was placed over the TM. A probe-tube microphone was integrated into the coupler. A Beyer DT-48 was used as the sound source.

3. Results

3.1 Time-averaged holography: Iso-displacement contours in cat and chinchilla 400 Hz –19 kHz

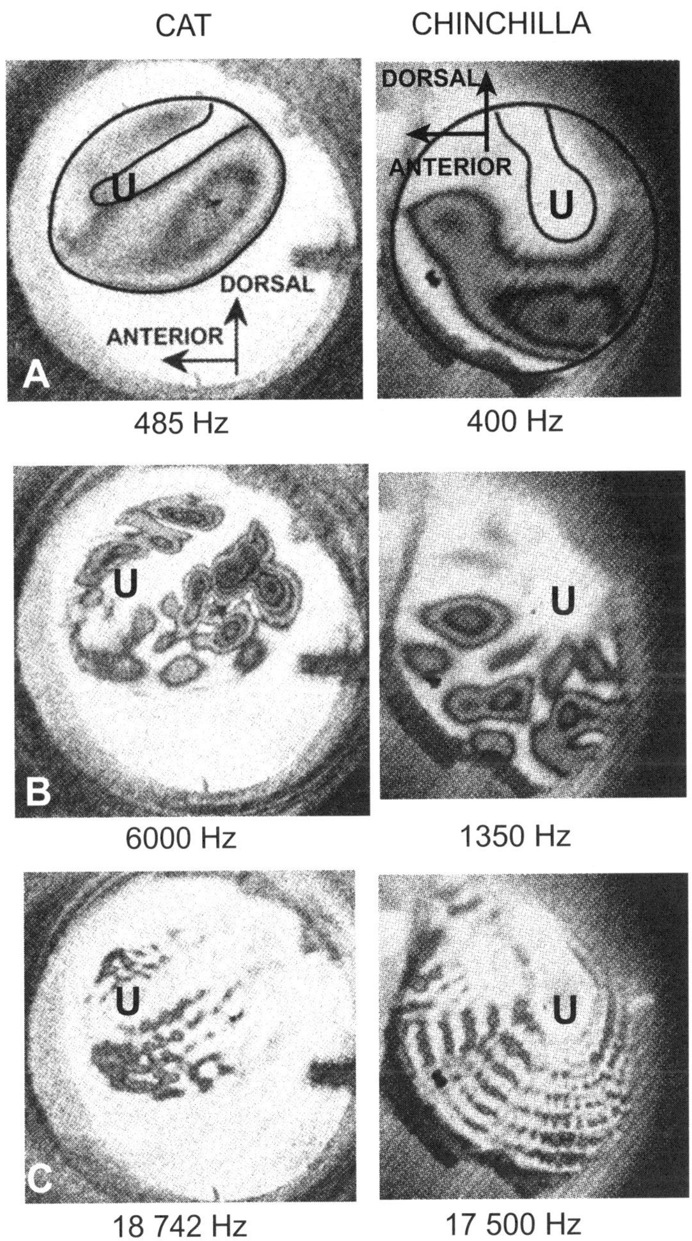

Fig. 1 Time-averaged holograms in cat (left) and chinchilla (right) at selected frequencies showing *simple* (A), *complex* (B), and *ordered* (C) displacement patterns. The TM and manubrium are outlined in Panel A, and the umbo is marked "U".

Time-averaged holograms that describe the sound-induced displacements of the TM of a cat (left) and chinchilla (right) are shown in Figure 1 at selected frequencies and sound levels. Increasing displacement is indicated by alternating dark and light bands. At low frequencies, the TM displacement patterns in cat and chinchilla are *simple* (Fig. 1A): There are one or two regions of maximal displacement.

At medium frequencies, the TM displacement patterns are *complex* (Fig. 1B): There are multiple areas of maximal displacement separated by areas of small displacement. In cat, the transition from simple to complex occurs near 3,000 Hz; in chinchilla, at a much lower frequency, near 600 Hz. The simple and complex displacement patterns in cat are similar to those seen previously [2].

At high frequencies, the TM displacement patterns show an *ordered* arrangement (Fig. 1C): Many small areas of maximal displacement are arranged in concentric rings surrounding the manubrium. Radial patterns of rays can also be seen, especially in chinchilla. In cat, the transition from complex to ordered occurs near 15,000 Hz; in chinchilla, at a much lower frequency, near 4,000 Hz. The *ordered* patterns of rings and rays in these time-averaged holograms are *indicative* of standing waves on the TM (Sec. 4.2).

3.2 Stroboscopic holography: Sub-fringe displacements in cat and chinchilla – complex and ordered displacement patterns

Stroboscopic holography allows measurements of smaller displacements than time-averaged holography and allows discrimination of inward motions from outward motions. Figures 2 and 3 show the difference in TM displacement between the condensation and rarefaction phases of the sound stimulus. (Similar images in response to lower-frequency stimuli in guinea pigs were presented by Wada et al. [4]).

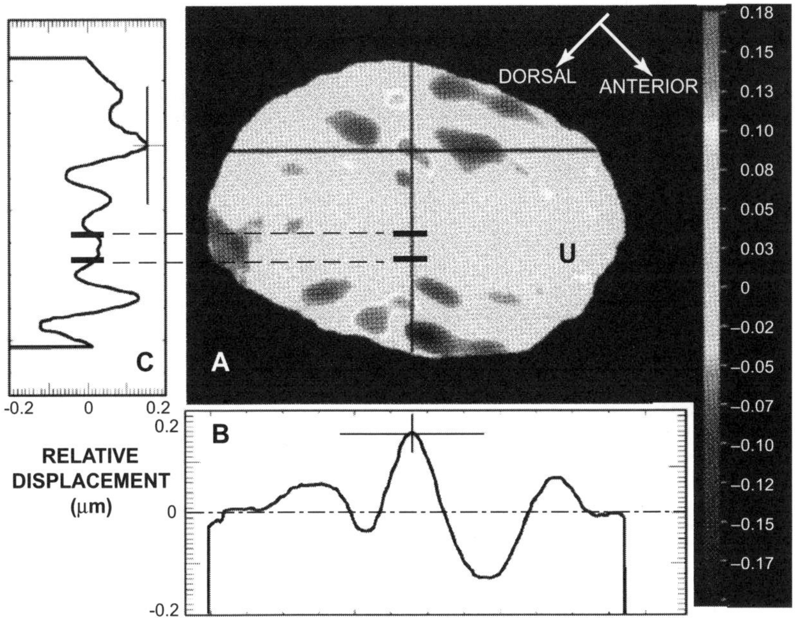

Fig. 2 (A) Stroboscopic hologram in cat at 8,776 Hz. Displacement is coded by shading at right. The short dark bars mark where the vertical line crosses the manubrium; the umbo is marked by "U". (B) and (C) Displacement profiles along the horizontal and vertical lines in (A), respectively.

The difference in cat TM displacement between the two stimulus phases at 8,776 Hz is shown in Fig. 2A. Multiple positive and negative maxima are apparent across the TM – a *complex* displacement pattern. Figs. 2B and 2C show that several points on the TM move in the opposite direction as the manubrium (bars). The peak-to-peak surface displacement is about 0.35 μm. The biphasic spatial variations seen in Figs. 2B and 2C are similar to those reported by others [4,5,6].

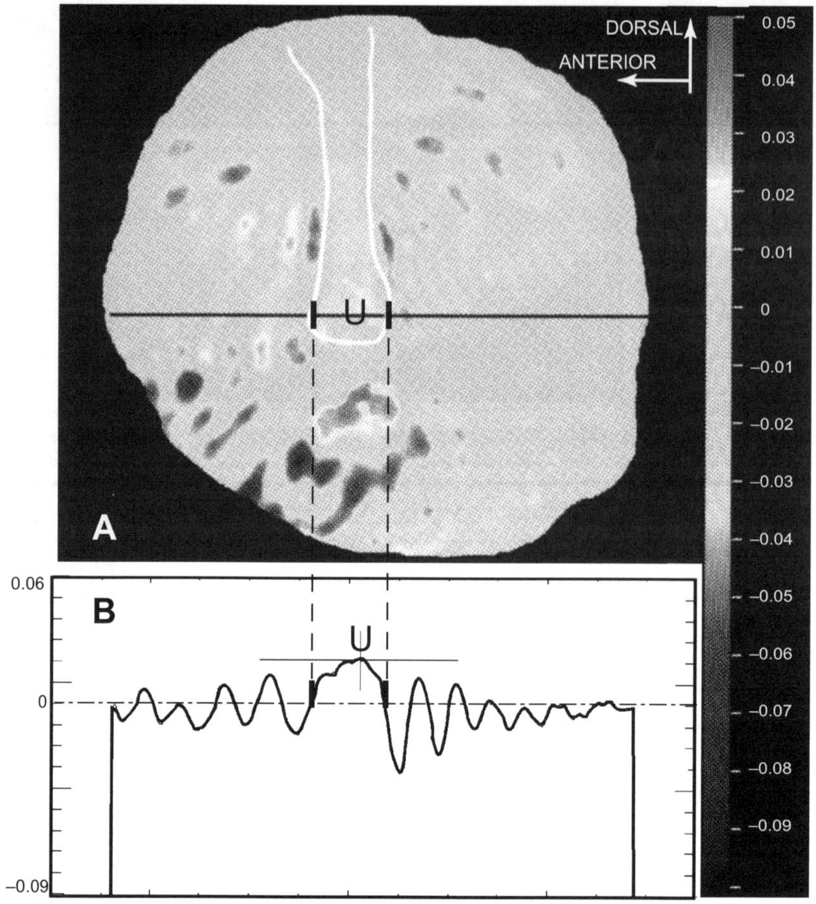

Fig. 3 (A) Stroboscopic hologram in chinchilla at 15,700 Hz. Displacement is coded by shading at right. The short dark bars mark where the horizontal line crosses the manubrium (outlined); the umbo is marked by "U". (B) Displacement profile along the horizontal line in (A).

The difference in chinchilla TM displacement at 15,700 Hz is shown in Fig. 3A – an **ordered** displacement pattern. The circumferential arrangement of displacement maxima rings is clear in this example, while the rays are less clear. The circumferential maxima are arranged such that rings of peak positive displacements alternate with rings of peak negative displacements. The patterns are somewhat blurred ventral to the umbo, where a large positive displacement maximum is surrounded by an arc of negative displacement maxima. Along the horizontal line (8 mm distance) there are >11 cycles of displacement (Fig. 3B). The peak-to-peak surface displacement is 0.05 μm.

4. Discussion

4.1 Comparison of TM displacements in cat and chinchilla

Differences in TM motion were observed between cat and chinchilla, perhaps related to the fact that the TM in chinchilla is larger and rounder than in cat. Chinchilla TM displacement patterns change from simple to complex to ordered at lower frequencies than in cat (Fig. 1). The chinchilla TM and umbo move more than cat for a given sound level, indicating a greater compliance and a greater sensitivity to sound. Umbo displacements computed from cat and chinchilla holograms are consistent with previous single-point measurements [7,8].

4.2 Evidence for standing waves on the TM

The circumferential ring pattern of displacement maxima in Figs. 1C and 3 is consistent with the presence of standing waves on the TM surface. (Any traveling wave-like displacement is averaged out of Fig. 1C.) Standing waves may result from the interaction of surface waves moving inward from the tympanic ring toward the umbo and outward toward the tympanic ring (possibly reflected at the umbo). The wave speed cw can be computed from the stimulus frequency f and the spatial separation of the displacement maxima (the distance between + and – magnitude maxima in the stroboscopic measurements) x:

$$c_w = 2\,x f\,.$$

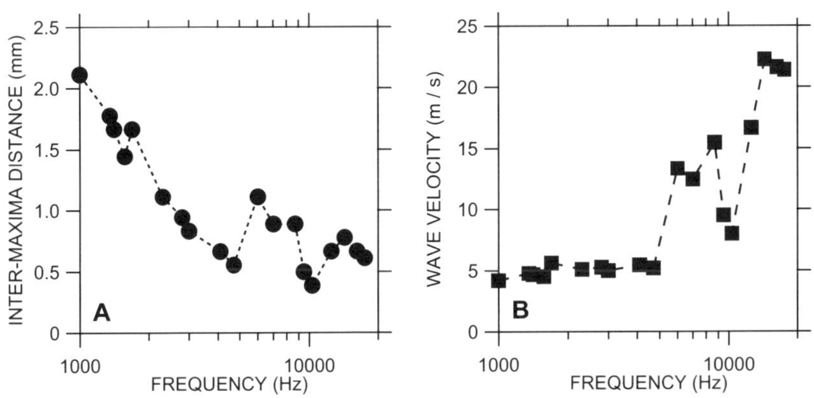

Fig. 4 (A) Separation between displacement maxima in stroboscopic holograms from a chinchilla ear at various frequencies. (B) Wave speed computed from data in (A) by Eq. 4.

Fig. 4A shows displacement maxima separation in a chinchilla ear determined from holograms at various frequencies; Fig. 4B shows the wave velocity computed from Fig. 4A. The computed wave speeds are 5–25 m/s, within the range computed by Fay et al. [6]. The delay associated with the 4mm distance between tympanic ring and umbo varies from 800 μsec at low frequencies to 160 μsec at high frequencies. These delays are 4–20 times larger than the 0.040 msec middle-ear transmission delays observed in gerbil [9,10] or predicted for wave motion along the TM of cat [1].

5. Conclusions

- Opto-Electronic Holography techniques provide rapid measurements of the displacement of the entire TM surface. Stroboscopic holography provides displacement resolution superior to time-averaged holography as well as phase information.
- The time-averaged holographic measurements in cat are similar to previous measurements but are extended to higher frequencies.
- TM displacements progress from SIMPLE to COMPLEX to ORDERED patterns as frequency increases. The difference in TM displacement pattern transition frequencies between cat and chinchilla is consistent with differences in TM mechanical properties.
- The time-averaged and stroboscopic measurements in both cat and chinchilla indicate standing waves on the TM at frequencies above 1–4 kHz.

Acknowledgments

Suppported by the NIDCD and the WPI.

References

1. Puria S. and Allen J.B., Measurements and model of the cat middle ear: Evidence of tympanic membrane acoustic delay. *J. Acoust. Soc. Am.* **104** (1998): 3463–3481
2. Khanna S.M. and Tonndorf J., Tympanic membrane vibrations in cats studied by time-averaged holography. *J. Acoust. Soc. Am.* **51** (1972): 1904–1920
3. Furlong C. and Pryputniewicz R.J., Non-destructive damage evaluation of composite structures by optoelectronic holography methodologies. *Proc. SEM, Dr. C. P. Burger Symposium – Testing and Modeling of Structures* (2003), Charlotte NC.
4. Wada H., Ando M., Takeuchi A., Sugawara H., Koike T., Kobayashi T., Hozawa K., Gemma T. and Nara M., Vibration measurement of the tympanic membrane of

guinea pig temporal bones using time-averaged speckle pattern interferometry. *J. Acoust. Soc. Am.* **111** (2002): 2189–2199

5. Decraemer W.F., Khanna S.M., and Funnell W.R.J.,Vibrations at a fine grid of points on the cat tympanic membrane measured with a heterodyne interferometer. *EOS/SPIE International Symposia on Industrial Lasers and Inspection, Conference on Biomedical Laser and Metrology and Applications* (1999), München.
6. Fay J., Puria S., Decraemer W.F., and Steele C., Three approaches for estimating the elastic modulus of the tympanic membrane. *J Biomech.* **38** (2005): 1807–1815
7. Buunen T.J.F. and Vlaming M.S.M.G., Laser-Doppler velocity meter applied to tympanic membrane vibrations in cat. *J. Acoust. Soc. Am.* **69** (1981): 744–750
8. Ruggero M.A., Rich N.C., Robles L., and Shivapuja B.G.. Middle ear response in the chinchilla and its relationship to mechanics at the base of the cochlea. *J. Acoust. Soc. Am.* **87** (1990): 1612–1629
9. Olson E.S., Observing middle and inner ear mechanics with novel intracochlear pressure sensors. J. Acoust. Soc. Am. **103** (1998): 3445–3463
10. Overstreet E.H. III and Ruggero M.A., Development of wide-band middle-ear transmission in the Mongolian gerbil. *J. Acoust. Soc. Am.* **111** (2002): 261–270

AN ANIMAL MODEL OF SUPERIOR CANAL DEHISCENCE

J.E. Songer[1], M.L. Wood, J.J. Rosowski[2]
Eaton-Peabody Lab, Massachusetts Eye and Ear Infirmary 243 Charles St. Boston, MA, 02114, USA, Email: jocelyns@mit.edu

[1] Speech and Hearing Biosciences and Technology Program, Harvard-Massachusetts Institute of Technology
[2] Department of Otology and Laryngology, Harvard Medical School

Superior canal dehiscence (SCD) syndrome is a non-middle-ear source of conductive hearing loss [3, 5]. The purpose of this study is to develop a better understanding of the physiology and mechanics behind SCD-induced changes in auditory sensitivity to both air-conducted (AC) and bone-conducted (BC) stimuli. To achieve this goal we surgically introduced a hole (dehiscence) into the chinchilla superior canal (SC) and then monitored cochlear potential (CP) in response to both BC and AC stimuli. As a result of SCD, low frequency sensitivity to BC stimuli increased and in response to AC stimuli it decreased, producing an air-bone gap of 12dB. Our results support the hypothesized 'third window' mechanism, which suggests that the SCD introduces a pathological shunt pathway that alters inner-ear fluid motion and results in an air-bone gap.

1. Introduction

Superior canal dehiscence (SCD) syndrome is characterized by a hole in the bone between the membranous SC and the cranial cavity. Patients with SCD often present with vestibular symptoms [2, 4, 6]; however, some present with auditory symptoms [1, 3, 5] including increased AC and decreased BC thresholds at low frequencies. The dB difference between the BC and AC auditory thresholds, called the air-bone gap, is indicative of a conductive hearing loss. SCD patients may present with air-bone gaps of up to 60dB.

A pathological 'third window', has been proposed as the mechanism for the SCD-induced conductive hearing loss [6, 7, 10]. In response to AC stimuli a pathological fluid pathway shunts volume velocity away from the cochlea and through the dehiscent SC resulting in decreased auditory sensitivity. In response to BC stimuli the shunt pathway alters the pressure difference across the basilar membrane resulting in increased sensitivity to BC sound.

We expand on previous work [9–11] by pairing measurements of cochlear potential (CP) in response to both AC and BC stimulation to look at the air-bone gap in each animal. Developing a better understanding of the effect of SCD on both AC and BC hearing may provide insight into the mechanisms of hearing and improve the diagnosis and treatment of patients with SCD syndrome.

2. Methods

Seven anesthetized chinchillas were used following a protocol approved by the Massachusetts Eye and Ear Infirmary. Measurements were made in response to both AC and BC log-chirp stimuli according to procedures described previously [8–11] and summarized here. The stimulus was presented via an earphone in the ear-canal for AC and via a clinical BC vibrator fixed to the skull for BC sound. CP in response to the stimuli was measured at the round window in the intact state. An SCD was then introduced by shaving away the bony roof of the SC within the middle ear. CP measurements were made with the SCD both open and patched with Superglue. Measurements were repeated after removing and after re-applying the Superglue patch. The difference between the patched and the re-patched condition was evaluated to determine the reversibility of the SCD-induced effects. The patch-unpatch-repatch series was evaluated because it exhibited the greatest stability over time and across animals.

3. Results

3.1 SCD and bone conduction

Figure 1 illustrates data from the patched, SC hole open and re-patched states in one ear as well as the effect of smoothing. In this ear introducing a SC hole results in a low-frequency increase in CP in response to BC stimuli for frequencies below 800Hz as well as a decrease in CP for some frequencies above 1kHz. Repatching the SCD returns the CP to close to the value seen in the initial patched condition. Thus, the effects appear to be reversible between the patched and repatched states.

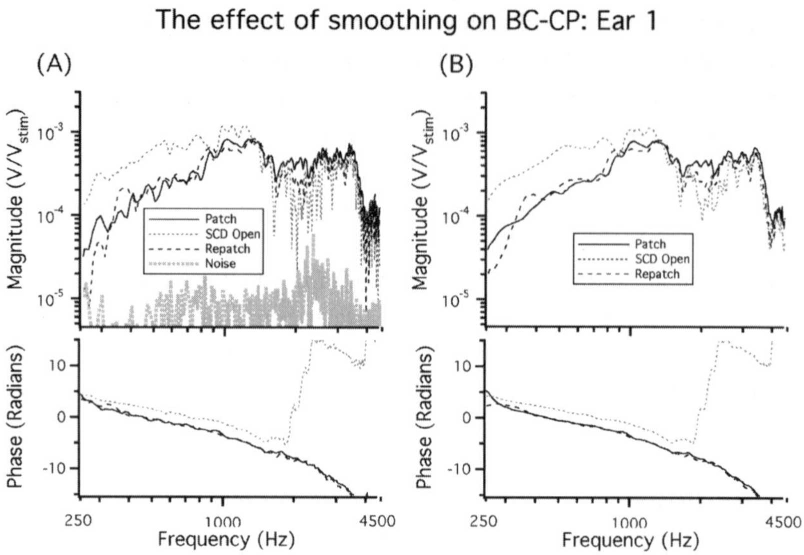

Fig. 1 The CP in response to BC stimuli A) recorded from an ear in the patch-unpatch (SCD Open)-repatch states. B) after the data is smoothed using the loess smoothing algorithm.

To evaluate the reversibility of the effect of SC opening on CP, we calculate the mean dB difference in magnitude ($20 \times log10(\frac{repatched}{patched})$) as well as the difference in phase between the patched and the repatched states in the seven ears. The mean dB difference between the patched and repatched condition (Figure 2A) is not statistically different from zero across the measured frequency range. Therefore the preparation was stable and the effects of SC opening are reversible. There are no statistically significant changes in phase angle between the patch and the repatch states. For frequencies below 500Hz and above 3000Hz the 95% confidence interval includes almost 2 radians; this is a result of an unwrapping artifact due to rapid phase cycling observed in many of the ears.

The difference in CP between the unpatched and patched conditions in response to BC sound in the same ears is presented as a dB difference in magnitude (Figure 2B). There is a mean increase in CP as a result of SC opening for frequencies below 1kHz. The increase is near 10dB at 300Hz and is statistically significant ($p < 0.05$). Additionally, there is a mean phase lead for frequencies between 400Hz and 4000Hz that is significant over a small range of frequencies (1500Hz–1800Hz).

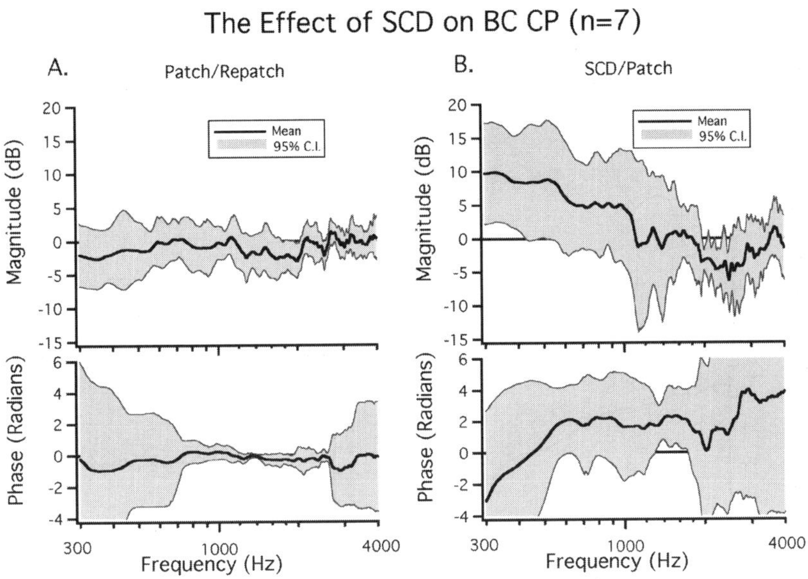

Fig. 2 The mean change in BC CP between A) the patched and repatched conditions and B) the SCD open and patched conditions. The 95% confidence intervals as well as the means are plotted (n=7).

3.2 SCD and air conduction

While the CP produced by BC stimulation was normalized by the stimulus voltage, the CP in response to AC sound stimuli is normalized by P_{TM} [10] because P_{TM} is considered to be the effective stimulus for AC sound.

Figure 3 shows measurements from an ear in which there is a low-frequency decrease in CP in response to AC sound even as there is a low-frequency increase in CP in response to BC sound. The SCD-induced changes in response to both stimuli are reversible.

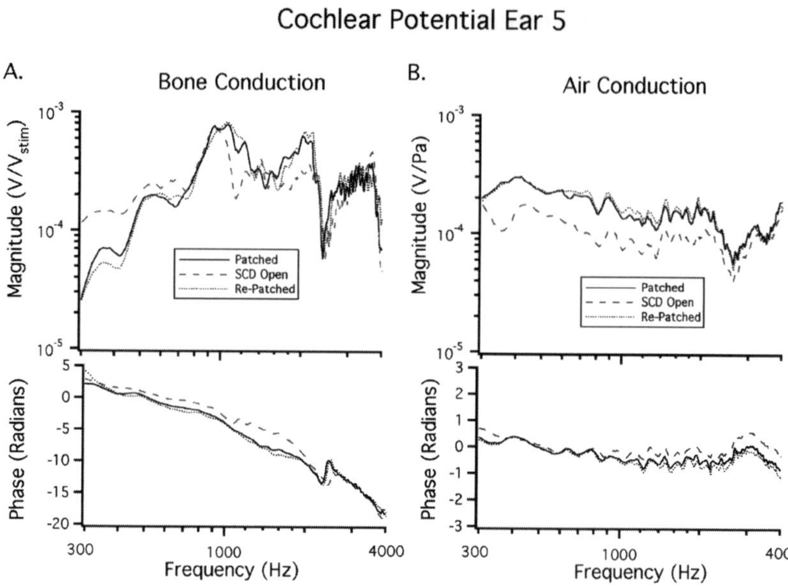

Fig. 3 Changes in CP in response to both AC and BC sound stimuli in an example ear. A) A reversible increase in sensitivity to BC sound. B) A reversible decrease in sensitivity to AC sound.

The mean difference between the patched and repatched state in response to AC stimuli in seven ears (Figure 4A) shows a slight decrease that is fairly constant with frequency but is not statistically different from zero. The mean difference in CP between the SC hole and the patched states (Figure 4B) is a decrease of 2–5dB between 500Hz and 4kHz ($p < 0.05$).

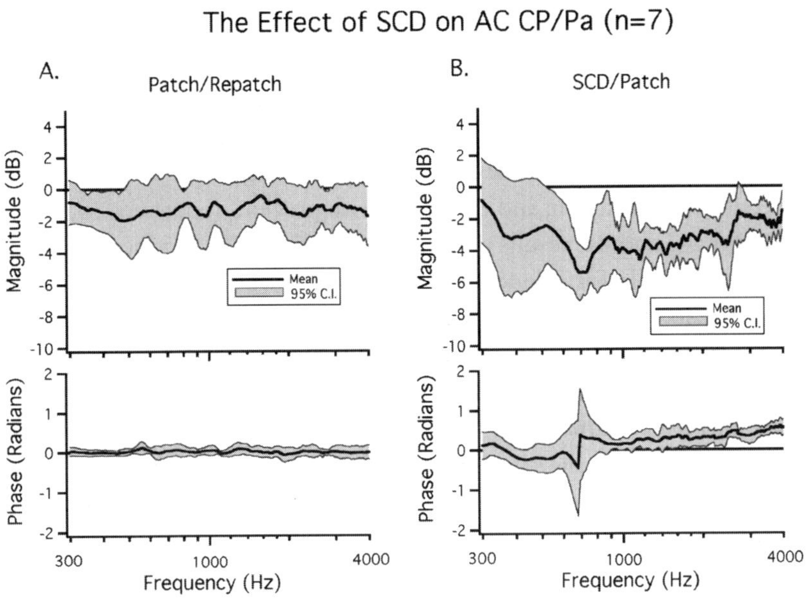

Fig. 4 The mean change in AC CP A) between the patch and repatch state and B) between the SCD open and the patched state along with the 95% confidence intervals (n=7).

3.3 SCD and air-bone gap

We define the SCD induced air-bone gap in chinchilla as the dB difference between the SCD-induced changes in response to BC and AC stimuli. We observe a mean air-bone gap of as much as 12 dB for frequencies below 2kHz (Figure 5). The air-bone gap is significant ($p < 0.05$) for frequencies between 300Hz and 900Hz.

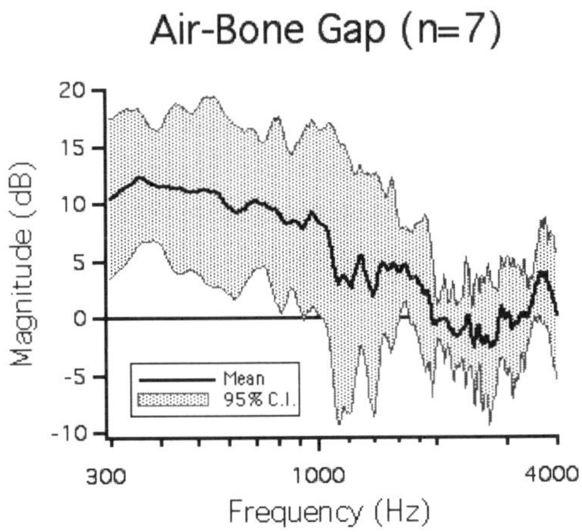

Fig. 5 The mean air-bone gap with 95% confidence intervals (n=7).

4. Discussion

4.1 Summary of results

We observed an increase in CP sensitivity to BC sound after introducing SC holes in seven ears (Figure 2). With AC sound we observed a significant decrease in CP after SCD. These changes in CP are largest for low frequencies, reversible with patching and consistent with previous reports [9, 10].

Our AC and BC results are consistent with an SCD-induced air-bone gap in chinchilla for frequencies below 1kHz. This air-bone gap is largest at the lowest frequencies with a mean near 12dB and is affected by the increased sensitivity to BC stimuli and the decreased sensitivity to AC stimuli. The repeatability and reversibility observed between the patch-unpatch-repatch conditions (n=7) both within and across animals are consistent with hearing changes that are tied to the mechanical effects of opening and closing the SCD and not uncontrolled changes in the sensitivity of the inner ear.

4.2 Comparison to clinical findings

Air-bone gaps of 24 ± 7dB for frequencies between 250 and 4000Hz [5] and a mean air-bone gap of 37dB at 500Hz [3] have been reported in human patients. The air-bone gap we report for chinchilla (12dB) is smaller than that observed clinically. This difference is primarily due to the smaller changes in sensitivity to AC as a result of SCD in chinchillas compared to that observed in patients. Interspecies variation may be one reason for the difference in magnitude of the air-bone gap [10]: 1) the SC hole in chinchilla opens into an air-filled middle-ear air space whereas the SCD in human patients opens into the cranial cavity, and 2) differences in middle-ear dynamics.

For patients with SCD syndrome, important information can be obtained by fully exploring the sensitivity to both AC and BC sound stimuli. Specifically, increased sensitivity to BC stimuli may aid in the differential diagnosis of SCD syndrome and otosclerosis. In both of these conditions patients may present with a conductive hearing loss, however, patients with SCD syndrome and a conductive hearing loss usually exhibit a super-sensitivity to BC stimuli, whereas patients with otosclerosis do not.

5. Conclusions

We have demonstrated an SCD-induced air-bone gap in chinchilla. This air-bone gap is similar in frequency range, though smaller in magnitude, to that observed in patients with SCD syndrome. The reversible physiological changes we observed demonstrate that the hearing loss associated with

SCD syndrome results from changes in inner-ear mechanics and should therefore resolve when the dehiscence is patched.

Acknowledgments

We thank M.E. Ravicz, W.T. Peake, S.N. Merchant and H.H. Nakajima for their input and advice. This work was supported by the NSF and the NID-CD.

References

1. K. Brantberg, J. Bergenius, L. Mendel, H. Witt, A. Tribukait, and J. Ygge., Symptoms, findings and treatment in patients with dehiscence of the superior semicircular canal. *Acta Otolaryngol,* 121: 68–75, 2000
2. P. Cremer, L. Minor, J. Carey, and C. Santina., Eye movements in patients with superior canal dehiscence syndrome align with the abnormal canal. *Neurology,* 55: 1833–1841, 2000
3. A. Mikulec, M. McKenna, M. Ramsey, J. Rosowski, B. Herrmann, S. Rauch, H. Curtin, and S. Merchant., Superior semicircular canal dehiscence presenting as conductive hearing loss without vertigo. *Otol. and Neurotol.,* 25: 121–129, 2004
4. L. Minor., Superior canal dehiscence syndrome. *Amer. J. of Otol.,* 21: 9–19, 2000
5. L. Minor, J. Carey, P. Cremer, L. Lustig, and S. Streubel., Dehiscence of bone overlying the superior canal as a cause of apparent conductive hearing loss. *Otol. and Neurotol.,* 2003
6. L. Minor, D. Solomon, J. Zinreich, and D. Zee., Sound and/or pressure-induced vertigo due to bone dehiscence of the superior semicircular canal. *Arch Otolaryngol Head Neck Surg,* 124: 249–258, 1998
7. J. Rosowski, J. Songer, H. Nakajima, K. Brinsko, and S. Merchant., Investigations of the effect of superior semicircular canal dehiscence on hearing mechanisms. *Otol. and Neurotol.,* 25: 323–332, 2004
8. J. Songer., *Superior Canal Dehiscence: Auditory Mechanisms.* PhD thesis, Massachusetts Institute of Technology, 2006
9. J. Songer, K. Brinsko, and J. Rosowski., Superior semicircular canal dehiscence and bone conduction in chinchilla. In K. Gyo, H. Wada, N. Hato, and T. Koike, editors, *The proceedings of the Third International Symposium on Middle Ear Reasearch and Oto-Surgery,* pages 234–241. World Scientific, 2004
10. J. Songer and J. Rosowski., The effect of superior canal dehiscence on cochlear potential in response to air-conducted stimuli in chinchilla. *Hear. Res.,* 210: 53–62, 2005
11. J. Songer and J. Rosowski., The effect of superior-canal opening on middle-ear input admittance and air-conducted stapes velocity in chinchilla. *J. Acoust. Soc. Amer.,* 120: 258–269, 2006

EPIDEMIOLOGY OF PRESSURE REGULATION. INCIDENCE OF VENTILATION TUBE TREATMENTS AND ITS PRELIMINARY CORRELATION TO SUBSEQUENT EAR SURGERY

Michael Gaihede[1], Kirsten Hald[1], Mette Nørgaard[2], Pia Wogelius[2], Daniel Buck[2], Kjell Tveterås[1]
Department of Otolaryngology, Head and Neck Surgery[1] and
Department of Clinical Epidemiology[2], Aalborg University Hospital, Hobrovej 18–22, DK 9000 Aalborg, Denmark

Michael Gaihede, mlg@rn.dk, Phone +45 9932 2911, Fax +45 9932 2938
Kirsten Hald, kirsten.hald@rn.dk, Phone +45 9932 2911, Fax +45 9932 2938
Kjell Tveterås, kt@rn.dk, Phone +45 9932 2911, Fax +45 9932 2938
Mette Nørgaard, m.noergaard@rn.dk, Phone +45 9932 6903, Fax +45 9932 6914
Pia Wogelius, pia.wogelius@rn.dk, Phone +45 9932 6894, Fax +45 9932 6914
Daniel Buck, DB@DCE.AU.DK, Phone +45 9932 6903, Fax +45 9932 6914

Corresponding author: Michael Gaihede

Keywords: ventilation tubes, incidence, secretory otitis media, otitis media sequelae, otosurgery

Purpose: Treatment with ventilation tubes (VT) in secretory otitis media and related conditions is a very common procedure based on the rationale of equilibrating the middle ear pressure (MEP) with ambient. Repeated VT treatments are also common in more severe cases, which increase the risk of permanent perforation of the tympanic membrane. The purpose of the present study was to describe the current incidence of VT treatments in children (<15 years) during 2000 to 2005 in a Danish County as well as the number of children subsequently admitted to a tertiary hospital setting for subsequent reconstructive ear surgery.

Materials and Methods: Database information was obtained from the County Health Authorities with information on all VT treatments in children in primary otological practices for the period. Cross reference of this information for year 2000 was made with our database on ear surgery for the identification of patients, who subsequently had been referred for surgery to our department.
Results: The incidence of VT insertions was determined for the group of children born in 2000 and followed for a 6-year period. The incidence peaked between the age of 1 to 2 years at 137 per 1,000 children, while the cumulated incidence was 28 %. Repeated insertions were found amounting to 45, 22, and 11 % for 2nd, 3rd, and 4th+ insertions, respectively. A total of 3544 children were treated with one or more VTs in 2000; in the following observation period 40 of these were identified in our department. A total of 45 surgical procedures were performed in these children: 39 myringoplasties (87 %), 5 tympanoplasty type II (11 %), 1 tympanoplasty type III (2 %); cholesteatoma was found in 9 cases (20 %).
Conclusions: The incidence of VT insertions was high amounting to 28 % by the age of 6 years. Reinsertions were also high and likely to be correlated to subsequent referrals of patients for reconstructive otosurgery. During our limited period of follow up only few children (1 %) were submitted for ear surgery, where the majority had simple myringoplasties (87 %), while the remaining cases consisted of more severe cases with structural damage. Future studies including a longer observation period will increase this number and provide measures of the correlation between the incidence of VT insertions and reinsertions and the need for subsequent otosurgery reflecting complications and sequelae of SOM and VT. Such numbers describe a more complete measure of the epidemiological weight of SOM and the necessity of basic research in MEP regulation.

1. Introduction

The most common indication for treatment with ventilation tubes (VT) is chronic secretory otitis media (SOM) based on ventilation and equilibration of negative middle ear pressure. Since SOM is frequent with a cumulated incidence of >80 % by the age of 4 years [1], insertions of VTs are similarly frequent accounting for the largest number of surgical procedures in children. Though short term effects in hearing and behaviour have been documented, long term effects seem absent and due to risks of complications watchful waiting has been suggested for the majority of children [2–4]. Moreover, the international costs related to insertions of VTs in chronic SOM are high amounting to approximately US $ 2 billion in the United States, and hence, the analysis of the clinical outcome is important [5].

In recurrent or chronic SOM repeated VTs are often employed, which is correlated to increased rates of complication. In particular, permanent perforation of the tympanic membrane (TM) can be found in up to 24 % of cases treated with long-term T-tubes [6]. Moreover, patients with repeated VT insertions also represent the cases with more severe courses of SOM related to the development of sequelae like retraction of the tympanic membrane, atelectasis, and cholesteatoma [7]. These patients are likely candidates for proper ear surgery either because of simple perforations of the TM or more extended reconstruction due to more severe courses and related sequelae. Thus, these patients constitute a larger part of the patients later referred to otosurgical centres.

The current study was conducted in order to describe these aspects by determining the rate of VT insertions including repeated VTs and their correlation with the subsequent referral of these patients to our department for otosurgical procedures. These aspects of VT treatment would add to the overall description of indications, benefits and costs of VT treatments [5].

2. Materials and Methods

The study was conducted in North Jutland County, Denmark, during 2000–2005. Since 1968 a 10-digit civil registration number has been assigned to all Danish citizens shortly after birth, and this allows unambiguous linkage between datasets.

2.1 VT database

Information about VT insertions was obtained from the Health Authorities of North Jutland County. This database covers all surgeries by the private ENT-practioners in our county and includes information on civil registration number, date and type of surgery (uni or bilateral). We included children up to the age of 15 years. Based on these data the incidence of VT insertions could be determined as well as the proportion of reinsertions. It should be noted that the vast majority of VT insertions in Denmark (more than 95 %) are performed by private ENT-practioners, whereas these are not engaged in proper otosurgery, which is restricted to hospital settings.

2.2 Ear surgery database

Systematic registration of all ear surgery is taking place in our department covering the otosurgical service of the entire county. This database relates to the same civil registration numbers as the VT database and it contains types of surgery and extent of pathology. Thus, patients treated with VT inserted in 2000 and subsequently referred during 2000 to 2005 could be identified and described.

2.3 Statistics Denmark

From Statistics Denmark we obtained information on the number of residents in North Jutland County born in the year 2000.

3. Results

Among 5769 children born in 2000 a total of 1610 (28 %) had at least one VT inserted during the study period. From this group the incidence of VT insertions according to age was determined (Fig. 1); maximum incidence of 137 VTs per 1,000 children was found at 1-year. The proportion of these children, who had more VTs inserted during the study period, is described in Fig. 2, where the last group (4+) describes 4 or more surgeries. For simplicity, uni and bilateral VTs have been described together (overall ratio = 1:4).

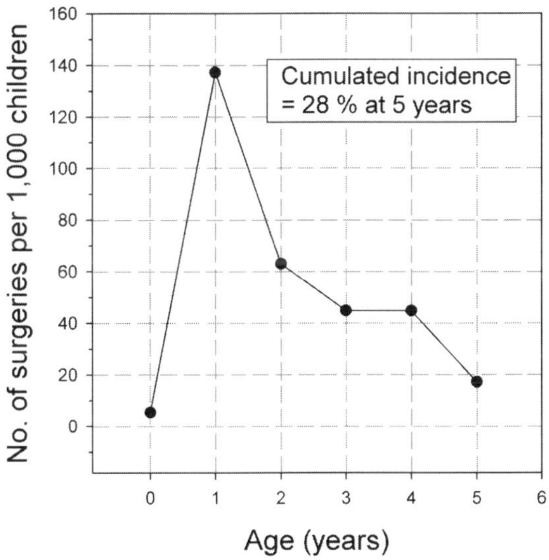

Fig. 1 First time insertions of VT's according to age among 1,610 children born in 2000 (0 → 0 to < 1 years; etc.). The cumulated incidence over time until the end of the 5th year was 28 %.

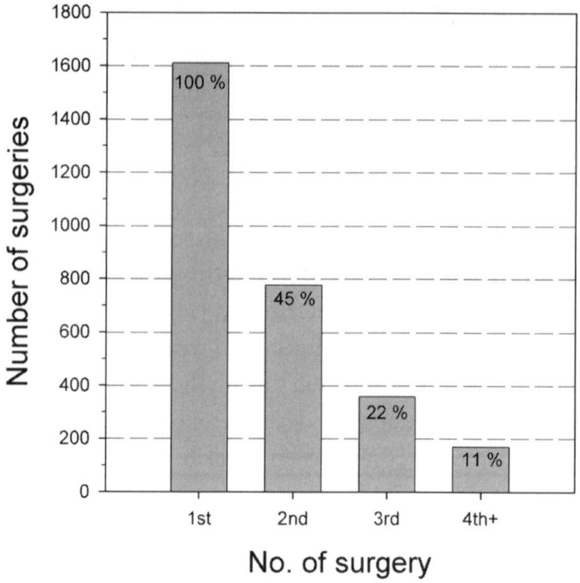

Fig. 2 Proportions of repeated surgeries among 1,610 children born in 2000 and followed until the end of the 5th year (corresponding to a 6-year study period).

In total 3544 children had VTs inserted in 2000. Forty-five of these children were identified in our ear surgery database during 2000–05. Five patients were excluded, since the conditions were unrelated to the VT; in the remaining 40 patients, bilateral surgery was performed in five. In Table 1 these 45 cases have been described according to the distribution of types of surgery.

Table 1 Distribution of oto-surgeries during a 5-year period after previous treatment.

Type of surgery	No. of cases (%)
Tympanoplasty I*	39 (87)
Tympanoplasty II	5 (11)
Tympanoplasty III	1 (2)

* including myringoplasties. In total nine cases of cholesteatoma was found (20 %).

4. Discussion

The current study basically described two groups of children: 1) a group born in 2000 and followed over a 6-year period describing the incidence of VT insertions and reinsertions and 2) a group with VT insertions in 2000 subsequently referred until the end of 2005 for proper otosurgery due to either complications and/or sequelae.

In the group born in 2000 more than a quarter of the children from our County were treated with at least one VT from birth until the age of six years (Fig. 1). This proportion is considered to be representative for Denmark, since the same clinical practice applies in the whole country, and it exceeded previously reported proportions of 20 % in 1987 [8]. Only few data comparing national rates of VT treatments have been reported, but they may vary from 2 to 20 per 1,000 children in the United Kingdom and The Netherlands, respectively [9]. These rates, however, are not directly comparable to the current results, since our proportion only described the incidence of VT insertions, i.e. the number of new cases during the 6-year study period and not the total number of insertions. Hence, repeated VTs were not included, and consequently the total rate of VTs would be even larger.

We have not found similarly high numbers of VT insertions in the literature, but several factors may explain this. In Denmark a relatively high proportion of children are attending day care, since the majority of mothers are working, and hence, the infection load of these children is high as well as parents tolerance may be low [3]. Furthermore, access to ENT-practioners is relatively easy with one practioner per 30,000 to 40,000 inhabitants. Finally, our registration of insertions is almost 100 %, since our health system is predominantly public, and reimbursements of ENT-practioners are based on their registrations and reports of procedures to the County; hence, the enticement for reporting procedures is high.

In the majority of cases with SOM bilateral VT insertions would be performed, since unilateral SOM generally is considered a relatively peaceful condition, and also reinsertions are likely to be performed only in bilateral cases. In approximately 20 % of our material unilateral insertions were registered, and these are largely expected to reflect other indications, i.e. acute otitis media (AOM). We have no records of the actual indications in each case, but in a survey of VT insertions from various Swedish centres 70 % of VTs have been reported to be on the basis of SOM, while only 24 % due to AOM [10]. Hence, in our group of children 70 to 80 % were likely to have VTs due to recurrent or chronic SOM, and consequently, due to disturbances in their ventilation and equilibration of middle ear pressure.

The numbers of reinsertions were also high amounting to 45, 22, and 11 % of the cases having 2, 3, or 4+ VTs, respectively (Fig. 2). These patients were especially likely to be candidates for later referral to hospital based reconstructive otosurgery. However, the exact linkage between the numbers of children with repeated VT insertions and subsequent referrals will await future studies with a longer observation time, since the group referred for otosurgery merely consisted of all children having VTs in 2000. Thus, we had no records of any previous VT insertions in this group, i.e. before 2000, but we were only able to demonstrate the possibility of tracking the connection of VTs and subsequent referrals at this point.

In continuation, among the patients treated with VTs in 2000, we currently only received 45 cases (1 %) for subsequent otosurgery over the 6-year period. The majority of cases were simple myringo or tympanoplasties (87 %), whereas structural damages with ossicular reconstruction constituted 13 % (Table 1: type II and III tympanoplasty). These cases were all related to cholesteatoma, which was found in 20 % of the cases, and hence, in three cases an intact ossicular chain could be maintained (Table 1). Obviously, these numbers reflect that the current referral proportion was small, since referrals of these patients often increase by the age of 7–8 years, where the results of otosurgery also are improved. Thus, our observation period was short and referral rates are likely to increase markedly by extending the study period by only a few years.

A general impression from our clinical work is a decreasing occurrence of extended cholesteatomas. This has previously been related to the benefits of increasing VT treatments without any significant correlation [11]. However, based on our unique linkage of information between primary ENT practices and hospitals due to civil registration numbers, a more detailed linkage could be obtained applying a longer observation period. Hence, the current study demonstrates the future possibility for the description of such relationships and changes in surgical practice over time.

5. Conclusions

The incidence of VT insertions amounted to 28 % of children at the age of 6 years, and repeated insertions were frequent. Future studies employing longer observation time can describe the correlation between the needs for subsequent otosurgery, and hence, provide a wider perspective to cost-effectiveness analysis and health economic decisions [5]. The high incidence reflects the large costs related to VT treatments and development of late sequelae, which in the vast majority of cases can be explained by dysregulation of MEP. These factors emphasize the need for basic research in otitis media and pressure regulation of the middle ear.

References

1. Zielhuis G. A., Rach G. H., van-den-Broek P., The occurrence of otitis media with effusion in Dutch pre-school children. *Clinical Otolaryngol.* **15** (1990) pp. 147–153
2. Issa A., Bellman M. and Wright A., Short-term benefits of grommet insertion in children. *Clin Otolaryngol* **24** (1999) pp. 19–23
3. Rovers M. M., Black N., Browning G. G., Maw R., Zielhuis G. A., Haggard M. P., Grommets in otitis media with effusion: an individual patient meta-analysis. *Arch Dis Child* **90** (2005) pp. 480–485
4. Lous J., Burton M. J., Felding J. U., Ovesen T., Rovers M. M., Williamson I., Grommets (ventilation tubes) for hearing loss associated with otitis media with effusion in children. *Cochrane Database Syst Rev.* **25** (2005) CD001801
5. Hartman M., Rovers M. M., Ingels K., Zielhuis G. A., Severens J. L., van der Wilt G. J., Economic evaluation of ventilation tubes in otitis media with effusion. *Ann Otolaryngol Head Neck Surg* **127** (2001) pp. 1471–1476
6. Strachan D., Hope G., Hussain M., Long-term follow-up of children inserted with V-tubes as a primary procedure for otitis media with effusion. *Clin Otolaryngol* **21** (1996) pp. 537–541
7. Sadé J., Ar A., Middle ear and auditory tube: Middle ear clearance, gas exchange, and pressure regulation. *Otolaryngol Head Neck Surg* **116** (1997) pp. 499–524
8. Secretory otitis media. Consensus report. (The Danish Medical Research Council and Danish Hospital Institute, Copenhagen, Denmark 1987) pp1–24 (In danish)
9. Schilder A. G. M., Lok W. and Rovers M. M., International perspectives on management of acute otitis media: a qualitative review. *Int J Pediatr Otorhinolaryngol* **68** (2004) pp. 29–36
10. Annual Report 2003. National registry for ENT Health Service. https://kvalitet.onh.nu (in swedish)
11. Padgham N., Mills R. and Christmas H., Has the increasing use of grommets influenced the frequency of surgery for cholesteatoma? *J Laryngol Otol* **103** (1989) pp. 1034–1035

MORPHO-FUNCTIONAL PARTITION OF THE MIDDLE EAR CLEFT

B.M.P.J. Ars[1,3] , J.J.J. Dirckx[2], N.M. Ars-Piret[3]
[1] Department NKO, UZA, University of Antwerp
[2] Laboratory of Biomedical Physics, Department of Physics, University of Antwerp
[3] Temporal Bone Foundation, Brussels

Correspondence: Avenue du Polo, 68, B 1150, Brussels, Belgium
Phone: 32 2 771 25 05, Fax: 32 2 762 39 68, Email: ArsBernhard@hotmail.com

1. Introduction

The middle ear cleft and the fibrocartilaginous eustachian tube form an integrated whole. It is a complex system. The middle ear cleft is made up of the mastoid gas cells system and the tympanic cavity, with tympanum and four annexes, epi and hypo-tympanum, retro and pro-tympanum. This latter corresponds to the bony eustachian tube.

Since the year 1997 [1], we are defending and demonstrating the original and personal concept of a specific fitting of the middle ear cleft which consists in a morpho-functional partition that separates the middle ear cleft in two different compartments: antero-inferior and postero-superior [2,3,4,5,6,7]. We will try to share our conviction that this partition is not an idle fancy, but well a concrete reality that expresses itself under numerous aspects, among others, anatomy, organogenesis, histology, histo-pathology, clinic and leads to clinical as well as surgical inferences.

2. Morpho-functional Partition of the Middle Ear Cleft

2.1 Anatomical approach

The tympanic cavity is constricted, in its superior third, by a bony-membranous barrier, perforated by two openings, known as «inter-attico-tympanic diaphragm». This anatomical barrier divides the middle ear cleft in two separate compartments. It forms a diaphragm which is made up of two complementary types of structures: mucosal folds and bony with muscular structures: the head and neck of the malleus, the body and short process of the incus, the tensor tympani muscle, the anterior and lateral mallear as well as the double posterior incudal ligaments.

This barrier is not impenetrable. There are two small permanent openings: the anterior tympanic isthmus which is situated between the tensor tympani tendon and the stapes, and the posterior tympanic isthmus between the double posterior ligament of the incus and the bony posterior tympanic wall. (Fig. 1).

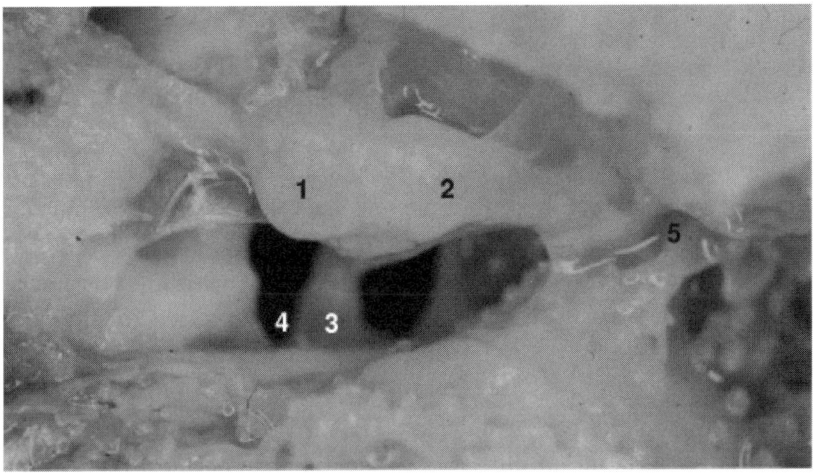

Fig. 1 The inter-attico-tympanic diaphragm. Superior view of a right tympanic cavity in a fresh human temporal bone specimen. The tegmen tympani has been removed. 1.: Malleus head / 2.: Body of the incus / 3.: Stapes / 4.: Anterior tympanic isthmus / 5.: Posterior tympanic isthmus.

In 1946, H.P. Chatellier and J. Lemoine [8] published a histological description of the inter-attico-tympanic diaphragm, in the newborn. They linked their study to clinically important aspects encountered in treating patients with complications of acute otitis media.

In 1971, B. Proctor [9] used the term: "tympanic diaphragm" and demonstrated that this diaphragm and the aditus play a very important role in determining the degree to which middle ear suppurations may progress.

In 1995, T. Palva and L.G. Johnsson [10] used the term "epitympanic diaphragm" and presented a sketch of this diaphragm that was based upon serial sections of temporal bones.

In 1997, B. Ars and N. Ars-Piret resume the term of H.P. Chatellier in the justification of a personal concept of "morpho-functional partition of the middle ear cleft" [1]. They include the notion of inter-attico-tympanic diaphragm in the description of the partition.

2.2 Developmental approach

The development and the progression of the sacci in the middle ear cleft [11] lead to the formation of the inter-attico-tympanic diaphragm and the accompanying folds. They also pave the way for the settlement of two different epithelia with specific functions into the separate antero-inferior and postero-superior compartments of the middle ear cleft.

2.3 Histological approach

The normal middle ear cleft mucosa is an extension of the mucosa of the rhinopharynx.

In the antero-inferior compartment of the middle ear cleft, the epithelial layer is pseudo-stratified; There are numerous mucous and ciliated cells. The connective tissue is thick and relatively dense.

In the postero-superior compartment of the middle ear cleft, the epithelial layer is monocellular. They are only flat cells, no ciliated or mucous cells. The connective tissue is loose.

In order to investigate the extent of the gas exchanges, we measured the distance between the centre of gravity of the blood vessels and the basal membrane of the mucosa, in the different regions of the middle ear cleft.

The mean distance of the antero-inferior part was 70 microns and of the postero-superior part, 40 microns (Fig. 2). These measurements imply that there is a significant difference in the diffusion of the gases between the two separate compartments of the middle ear cleft [12].

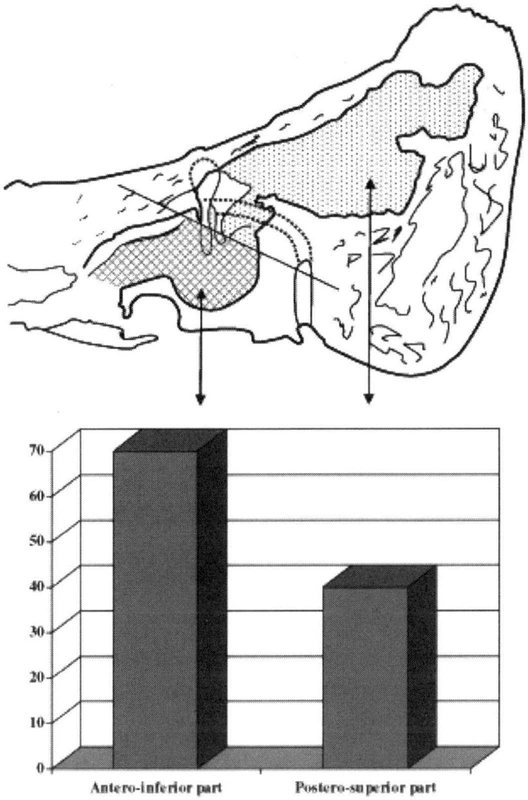

Fig. 2 Distance (μm) between the center of the blood vessels and the basal membrane of the normal mucosa in the antero-inferior and postero-superior compartments of the middle ear cleft.

We also noted that the connective tissue in the postero-superior part was looser than that in the antero-inferior part. All these facts point to the importance of gaseous exchange in the postero-superior compartment of the middle ear cleft.

2.4 Histo-pathological approach

Does an inflammatory process modify the behaviour of the middle ear cleft mucosa?

We conducted similar histo-morphometric studies on mucosal samples of middle ear cleft collected in patients having chronic inflammatory mucosa disease with otorrhea and undergoing surgery for chronic suppurative otitis media.

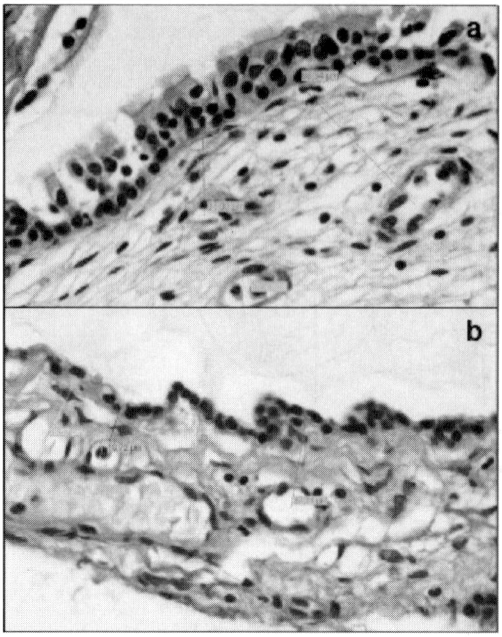

Fig. 3 Epithelium of the mucosa of the middle ear cleft: Two different types of epithelium according to the localization.

a: The antero-inferior compartment of the middle ear cleft appears with a pseudo-stratified epithelial layer, numerous mucous and ciliated cells. The connective tissue is thick and relatively dense.

b: The postero-superior compartment shows a mono-cellular epithelial layer with only flat cells, no ciliated nor mucous cells. The connective tissue is loose.

Examples of the distance measurements: The blood vessel centers are determined as the middle point of the longest axis of the vessels. The measurements were performed on the distance between the blood vessel's center and the basal membrane perpendicular to the long axis of the cross-section vessel.

To objectively estimate the importance of the tissular barrier that separates, under these inflammatory situations, the blood compartment and the gas-containing spaces of the middle ear cleft, we measured the distance between the center of the blood vessels and the basal membrane of the mucosa, in the different regions of the middle ear cleft, of mucosal pathological samples (Fig. 3a & b) [13].

We observed that the inflammatory process respects and reinforces the morpho-functional partition of the middle ear cleft. The mean distance is 45 microns in the antero-inferor compartment, and 22 microns in the postero-superior compartment (Fig. 4).

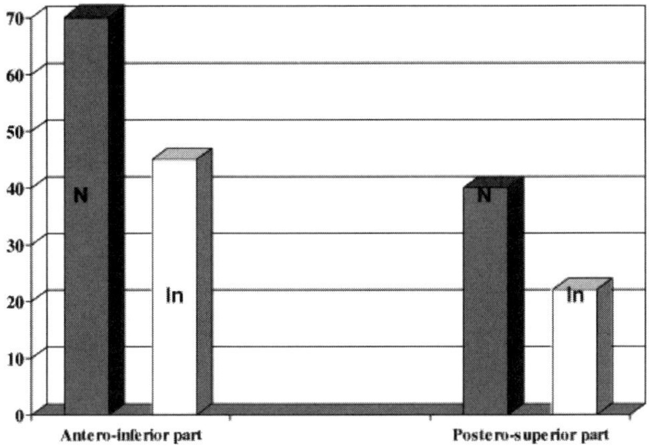

Fig. 4 Distance (μm) between the center of the blood vessels and the basal membrane of the inflamed mucosa in the two different compartments: comparison between healthy (N = normal) and inflamed mucosa (In = inflamed) in the antero-inferior and postero-superior parts of the middle ear cleft.

2.5 Clinical approach

Tympanosclerosis usually occurs in the antero-inferior part of the drum. Tympanic membrane retraction pockets are more often located in the postero-superior part of the tympanic membrane.

3. Clinical and Surgical Inferences

3.1 Clinical inferences

The antero-inferior compartment of the middle ear cleft, situated under the diaphragm, includes the pro, meso and hypo-tympanum. It is covered by secretory or non secretory, ciliated cells, usually with a muco-ciliary clearance function. It consists of a less rigid chamber because of the presence of the drum. Thanks to the fibrocartilaginous eustachian tube, it opens in an intermittently ventilated gas pocket. It communicates with the postero-superior compartment by both the anterior and posterior tympanic isthmus. It is probably the site of predilection of secondary bacterial infections from the rhinopharynx.

An inflammatory process involving the mucosa of the antero-inferior middle ear cleft compartment leads to muco-ciliary clearance problems, and to the accumulation of mucus, which could generate, among other things, serous or sero-mucous otitis.

Additional infection is possible. A rare consequence could be tympanosclerosis.

The postero-superior compartment of the middle ear cleft, situated above the diaphragm, includes the epi and retro-tympanum, aditus ad antrum, antrum and mastoid gas cell system. It is covered by a richly vascularized cuboidal epithelium, mainly devoted to gas exchange. It consists of a rigid chamber, and an open, non ventilated gas-pocket which communicates with the antero-inferior compartment by way of both openings. It is probably the site of predilection of viral haematogenous infections.

An inflammatory process involving the mucosa of the postero-superior middle ear cleft compartment, causes problems in the exchange of gas, leading to the development of a "gas deficit" in the middle ear cleft and, later on, to the development of a tympanic membrane retraction pocket, which could eventually deteriorate into cholesteatoma.

3.2 Surgical inferences

Simple mastoidectomy is not sufficient. An antro-attico-mastoidectomy, taking care to preserve the scutum and the posterior bony canal wall, and, if necessary, completed with the posterior tympanotomy, must be performed with the aim of restoring the function of gas exchange to the postero-superior part of the middle ear cleft.

References

1. Ars B., Ars-Piret N., Morphofunctional partition of the middle ear cleft. *Acta Oto-Rhino-Laryngologica Belgica,* **51** (1997) pp. 181–184
2. Ars B., Middle Ear Cleft: Three structural sets, two functional sets. *Otorhinolaryngol. Nova,* **8** (1998) pp. 273–276
3. Ars B., Ars-Piret N., L' oreille moyenne: trois ensembles structurels; deux ensembles fonctionnels. *Revue officielle de la Société française d'O.R.L.* **52**(6) (1998) pp. 27–32

4. Ars B., Ars-Piret N., Compartimentation morpho-fonctionnelle de l'oreille moyenne. *Journal français d' Oto-Rhino-Laryngologie.* (Lyon) **47**(2) (1998) pp. 82–88
5. Ars B., Pathogenesis of Acquired Cholesteatoma, In: *Pathogenesis in Cholesteatoma,* edited by B. Ars, Kugler Pub., The Hague, The Netherlands (1999) pp. 1–18
6. Ars B., Middle Ear Cleft Atelectasis. In: *Cholesteatoma & Ear Surgery,* edited by J. Magnan, A. Chays, Label Production Pub. (2001) pp. 279–293
7. Ars B., Balance of Pressure Variation in the Middle Ear Cleft. In: *Fibrocartilaginous eustachian tube – Middle ear cleft.,* edited by B. Ars, Kugler Pub., The Hague, The Netherlands (2003) pp. 57–66

8. Chatellier H. P., Lemoine J., Le diaphragme inter-attico-tympanique du nouveau-né. *Ann. Otolaryngol. Chir. Cervico-Fac.* (Paris) **13** (1946) pp. 534–566
9. Proctor B., Attic-Aditus block and the tympanic diaphragm. *Annals of Otology, Rhinology and Laryngology* **80** (1971) pp. 371–376
10. Palva T., Johnsson L. G., The epitympanic compartments, surgical considerations. *Ann. J. Otol.* **16** (1995) pp. 505–513
11. Proctor B., The development of the middle ear spaces and their surgical significance. *J. Laryngol. Otol.* **78**(7) (1964) pp. 630–649
12. Ars B., Wuyts F., van de Heyning P., Miled J., Bogers J., Van Marck E., Histomorphometric study of the normal middle ear mucosa. *Acta Otolaryngol. (Stockh)* **117** (1997) pp. 704–707
13. Matanda R., Van de Heyning P., Bogers J., Ars B., Behaviour of middle ear cleft mucosa during inflammation: Histomorphometric study. *Acta Oto-Laryngol.* **126** (2006) pp. 905–909

LASER DOPPLER VIBROMETRY DATA OF THE CLIP PISTON MVP

A. Arnold, Ch. Stieger, R. Häusler
Dept. of Otorhinolaryngology, Inselspital, Universität Bern, 3010 Bern, Switzerland
Email: Christof.Stieger@dkf.unibe.ch

Keywords: malleus grip stapedectomy, malleo-vestibulopexy, prosthesis, laser Doppler vibrometry

Introduction: A new malleus handle prosthesis for malleo-vestibulopexy and revision stapedotomy has been used successfully for the last two years. A CliP®-mechanism facilitates attachment to the malleus handle and a ball joint provides easy position adjustment intra-operatively. The present study was devised to determine if the ball joint of the CliP Piston MVP specially developed by Haeusler causes a loss of sound transfer from the malleus grip to the vestibulum.

Methods: A middle ear model was set up, consisting of a vibrator normally used in an active implantable hearing device with a metal arm in the shape and size of an actual malleus handle, where the CliP Piston MVP was attached with the ball joint bent to an angle of about 120°. The piston was dipped into the hole of a plastic container filled with water, simulating a piston hole in the footplate. A second hole served as the round window. The excitation level was more than 110 dB SPL for frequencies between 100 Hz –10000 Hz. The movements were picked up at different spots above and below the ball joint with a laser Doppler vibrometer. Vaseline simulated slight fibrosis around the piston in a second measurement.

Results: The overall characteristics of sound transfer were virtually identical above and below the ball joint (difference < 3dB). Additionally, biphasic resonance peaks (5-10 dB) were observed around 1000 Hz.

Discussion: Our results show very stable transfer properties over the frequency band. The resonance peaks of 5–10 dB are very probably below a level of significance in clinical pure tone audiometry. This is in accordance with our clinical practice experience.

Conclusion: The ball joint of the CliP Piston MVP has good transfer characteristics with virtually no loss.

1. Introduction

Malleo-vestibulopexy or malleus grip stapedotomy is employed for patients with otosclerosis, either as a primary procedure or as a revision stapes surgery.

The technique of malleus grip stapedotomy is complicated by the varying angle and distance of the malleus handle and the distance from the oval window. This is in contrast to a standard incus stapedotomy, where the incus prosthesis is clamped onto the long process of the incus and oriented vertically to the oval window.

The new malleus handle prosthesis for malleo-vestibulopexy and revision stapedotomy has been developed in our department and used successfully during the last two years. The piston prosthesis features a ball joint for easy and accurate positioning of the piston on the oval window intra-operatively. The CliP®-mechanism, modified from the àWengen Clip [1], facilitates attachment to the malleus handle.

The study was devised to determine if the specially developed ball joint of the CliP Piston MVP causes a loss of sound transfer from the malleus grip to the vestibulum.

2. Material and Methods

2.1 MVP cliP prosthesis

The MVP CliP Piston by Häusler is a new malleus grip prosthesis and is characterized by the following features: 1) a clip which obviates the need for the usual crimping and can easily accommodate the malleus handle; the rear of the clip bears a convenient tab for easy grasping with forceps and sliding for secure attachments; 2) a ball joint connection bendable for adjustment of the angle; 3) rounded piston edges to minimize connective tissue adhesion and trauma to surrounding tissues; and 4) titanium construction (ASTM F67 medical grade), diameters of 0.4 mm and 0.6 mm and length from 5.25 to 6.25 mm (0,25mm-increments). The prosthesis is grasped by the tab on the rear end of the clip and carefully slid onto the malleus handle. Once the attachment is secure, the angle is adjusted by stabilizing the upper component and pushing the piston medially towards the oval window. In this experiment a piston of 0.4 mm in diameter and 5.25 mm in length was used.

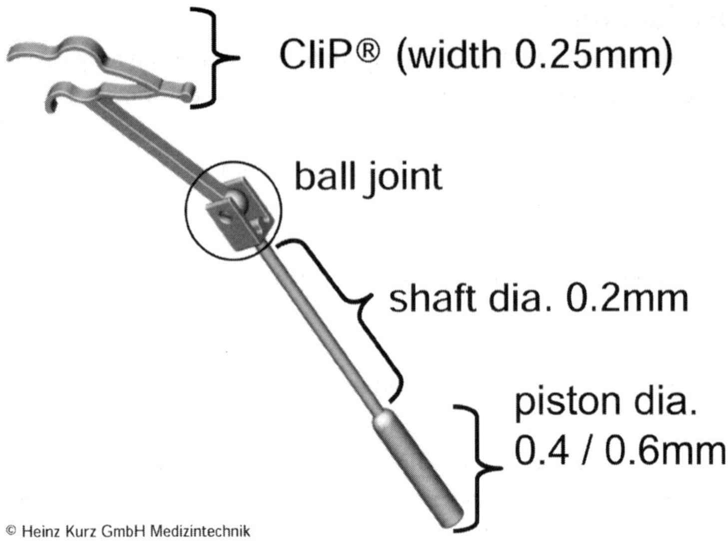

Fig. 1 CliP Piston MVP by Haeusler.

2.2 Model

A middle ear model was set up. It consists of the vibrator of an active implantable hearing device [2]. A hermetically sealed electro-mechanical system drives a tiny rod which features a metal arm in the shape and dimension of an actual malleus handle. The CliP Piston MVP was attached on this artificial malleus handle with the ball joint bent to an angle of approximately 120°. The piston was dipped into a hole which has a size comparable to that of a stapedotomy piston hole. A plastic container filled with water represented the inner ear fluid, thus the piston was directly coupled to fluid, representing qualitative simulation of the cochlear impedance. A second hole served as the round window (Fig. 2).

In order to simulate the higher impedance of a slight fibrosis around the stapedotomy site in a second set of measurements, the piston was sealed with Vaseline at the piston hole.

2.3 Laser Doppler Vibrometer (LDV) measurements

To investigate the performance of the ball joint the Clip piston MVP was mechanically excited and the vibrations above and below the ball joint were measured. The excitation level was more than 110 dB SPL for frequencies between 100 Hz–10000 Hz. Displacements above and below the ball joint were measured with a Laser Doppler Vibrometer (Polytec, HLV). Measurements were averaged fifty times. The results were confirmed with repetition of the experiment for each setup (without and with Vaseline). Noise floor was measured at the end of the experiments.

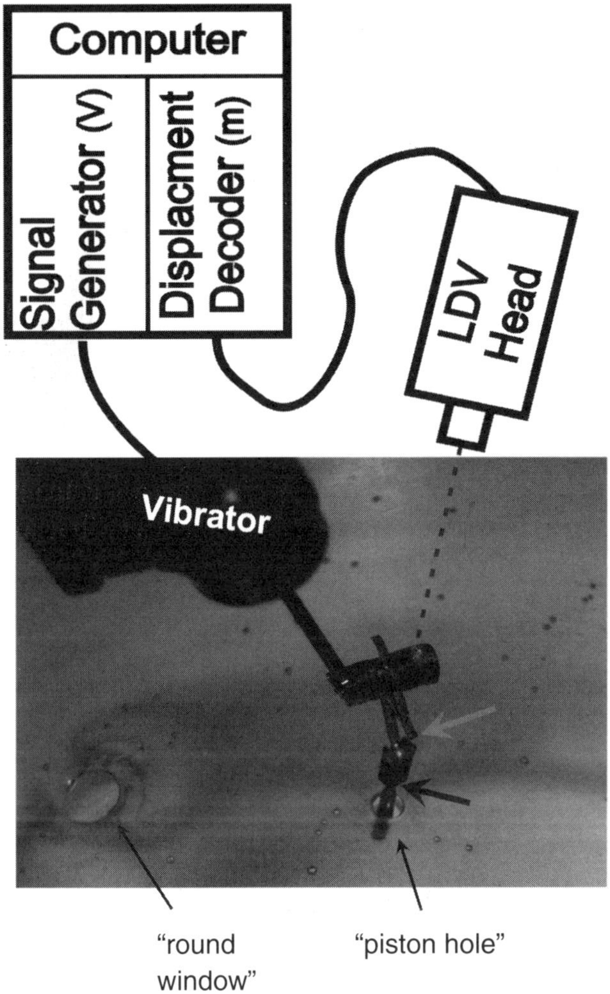

Fig. 2 Setup of the Laser Doppler Vibrometer measurements.

3. Results

Figure 3 and 4 show the displacement amplitude above and below the ball joint, with repeated tests for each site measured. In figure 3, the MVP piston Clip was not sealed with Vaseline at the point in which it was sealed in figure 4. In both cases, the measurements above and below the ball joint were virtually the same (mean deviation < 3dB for frequencies above 300 Hz). A resonance peak was observed at 1500 Hz. An additional biphasic resonance peak (5–10 dB) was observed around 1000 Hz when the CliP piston MVP was not sealed with Vaseline. The dotted line denotes the idealized stapes displacement for an excitation of 100 dB SPL. All MVP measurements were above the noise.

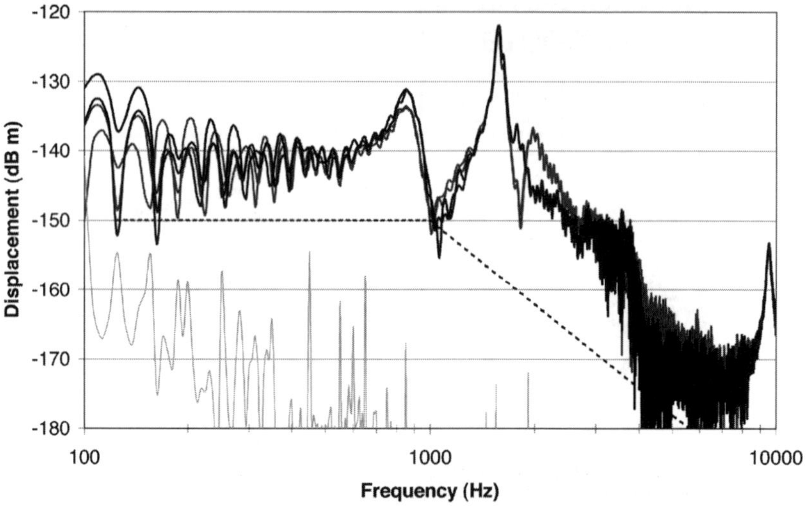

Fig. 3 Displacement above (bold grey lines) and below (black lines) the ball joint of the CliP Piston MVP and idealized middle ear function at 100 dB SPL (dotted line). Single test repetition is shown by two lines for each site measured. Noise floor is depicted by the lowest line.

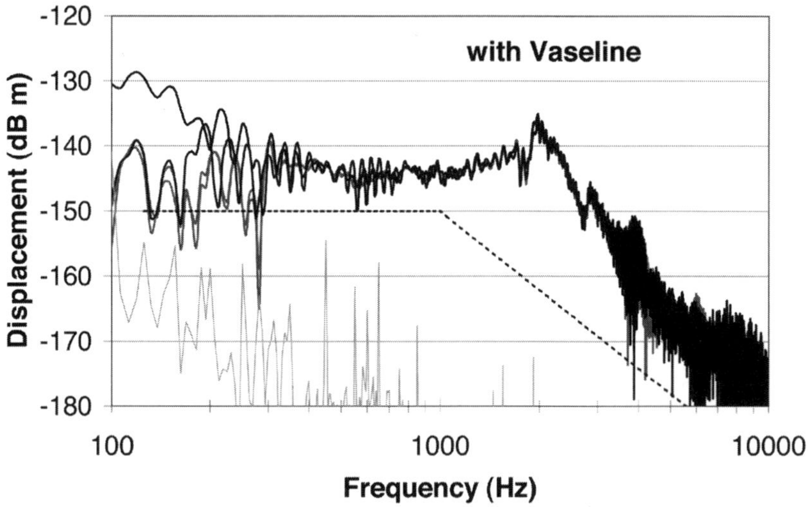

Fig. 4 Displacement above (bold grey lines) and below (black lines) the ball joint of the CliP Piston MVP with Vaseline applied around the piston and idealized middle ear function at 100 dB SPL (dotted line). Single test repetition is shown by two lines for each site measured. Noise floor is depicted by the lowest line.

4. Discussion

Our results show no evident loss of ball joint sound transfer of the CliP piston MVP by Haeusler over the entire frequency band. The resonance peak at 1500 Hz is in accordance with the resonance peak of the vibrator. The biphasic resonance peak at 1000 Hz is probably caused by the flexural mode of the CliP piston MVP. However fibrosis (scarring) at the oval window, which was simulated using Vaseline around the piston, seems to dampen resonance peaks and to reduce the loss in the ball joint.

The additionally noticed resonance peaks of 5–10 dB are very probably below levels of significance in clinical pure tone audiometry. This is in accordance with our clinical practice experience.

5. Conclusion

The ball joint of the CliP Piston MVP has good transfer characteristics with virtually no loss.

References

1. Grolman W., Tange R.A., First experience with a new stapes clip piston in stapedotomy. *Otol Neurotol.* Jul; 26(4) (2005) 595–8
2. Stieger C., Bernhard H., Haller M., Kompis M., Häusler R., A novel implantable hearing system with direct acoustical cochlear stimulation (DACS). In: EMBEC; 2005; Prague: *IFMBE Proceedings*, Vol. 11; 2005
3. Voss S.E., Rosowski J.J., Merchant S.N., Peake W.T., Acoustic responses of the human middle ear. *Hear Res.* 150(1–2) (2000) 43–69